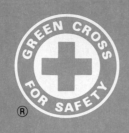

National Safety Council

First Aid and CPR

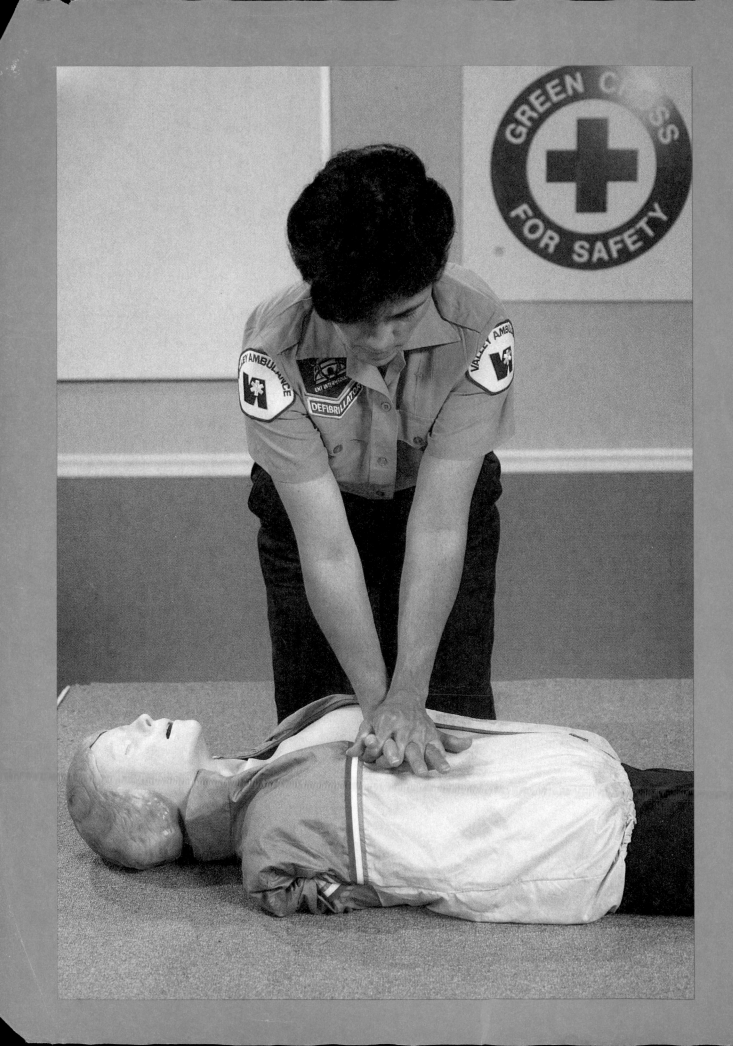

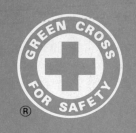

National Safety Council

First Aid and CPR

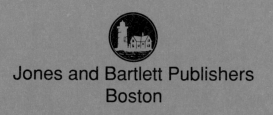

Jones and Bartlett Publishers
Boston

Eight records of fact reprinted with permission of the publisher, Guinness Publishing Ltd (copyright © 1989 Guinness Publishing Ltd), appear on pages 37,119,120,147,159,160, 220, and 243.

The first aid and CPR procedures in this book are based on the most current recommendations of responsible medical sources. The National Safety Council and the publisher, however, make no guarantee as to, and assume no responsibility for, the correctness, sufficiency or completeness of such information or recommendations. Other or additional safety measures may be required under particular circumstances.

Library of Congress Cataloging-in-Publication Data

First aid and CPR: / National Safety Council.
       p. cm.
   Includes index.
   ISBN 0-86720-193-2
   1. First aid in illness and injury. 2. CPR (First aid)
I. National Safety Council.
   [DNLM: 1. Emergencies. 2. First aid. 3. Resuscitation. WA 292
F5266]
RC86.7.F5575 1991
DNLM/DLC   91-6996
for Library of Congress   CIP

Vice-President and Publisher ■ Clayton E. Jones

Copy Editor ■ Anne Benaquist
Design and Production ■ PC&F, Inc.
Cover Design ■ Hannus Design Associates
Anatomical Art: Appendix A ■ Vincent Perez
Principal Photographer ■ Rick Nye
Illustrations ■ Chris Young, artist
Greg Kyle, Larry Hall, Matt Hall, illustrators

Other full-color illustrations ■
   Bruce Argyle, M.D.
   H.B. Bectal, M.D.
   Michael D. Ellis
   Murray P. Hamlet, D.V.M.
   Axel W. Hoke, M.D.
   Sherman A. Minton, M.D.
   Eugene Robertson, M.D.
   Richard C. Ruffalo, D.M.D.
   Jeffrey Saffle, M.D.
   Clifford C. Snyder, M.D.

ISBN: 0-86720-193-2

Jones and Bartlett Publishers
20 Park Plaza
Boston, MA 02116
617-482-3900

Printed in the United States of America
10 9 8 7 6 5 4 3 2 1

Brief
Table of Contents

Expanded Table of Contents

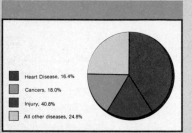

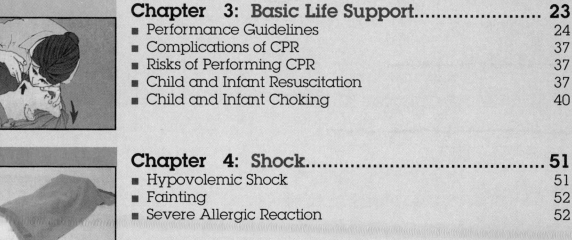

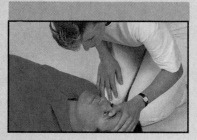

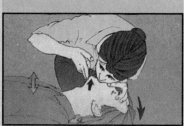

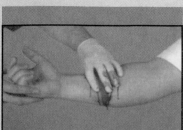

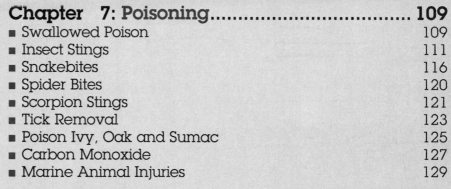

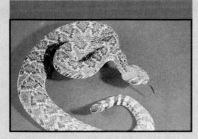

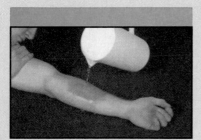

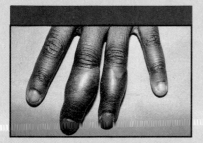

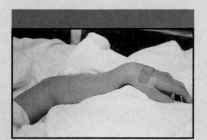

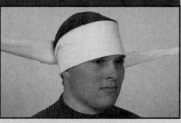

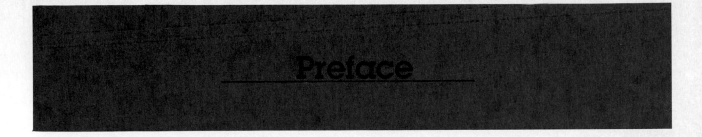

Preface

The National Safety Council is pleased to present **FIRST AID AND CPR** as successor to the best-selling text, **FIRST AID AND EMERGENCY CARE WORKBOOK** (1987). **FIRST AID AND CPR** provides accurate, comprehensive, and up-to-date information and procedures on first aid and CPR. Extensively reviewed by over 30 national organizations, **FIRST AID AND CPR** meets the needs of all first aid and CPR courses.

Background

When we first published the National Safety Council **FIRST AID AND EMERGENCY CARE WORKBOOK**, educators called it the finest text ever published in first aid. For the first time, a nationally recognized first aid text was authoritative, challenging, and written specifically for the academic setting. No longer would students and instructors have to struggle and improvise with out-dated and inappropriate materials.

World Authority

The National Safety Council, the world's leading authority on saftey/injury education, has trained tens of millions of students for nearly eight decades. Its sole focus is upon education and is not distracted by other pursuits. Founded in 1913, the National Safety Council is a nongovernmental, not-for-profit public service organization dedicated to the reduction of accidental deaths, injuries, and preventable illnesses.

A New Standard

The National Safety Council's previous text set a new standard for first aid instruction. Over 150,000 students at nearly 1,000 institutions have learned first aid and CPR the innovative National Safety Council way. Now, listening to your needs and feedback, we are proud to present a new and improved program featuring the new student text, **FIRST AID AND CPR**.

Special Features of First Aid and CPR

Nationally Recognized Certification: All students successfully completing a course utilizing **FIRST AID AND CPR** are eligible to receive FREE National Safety Council certification cards in both first aid and/or CPR.

American Heart Association BLS: Includes complete American Heart Association Basic Life Support techniques and procedures, reprinted with their permission from the Heartsaver Manual.

Authoriatative: In addition to the American Heart Association, **FIRST AID AND CPR** incorporates the latest information, reviews, and techniques from over 30 national organizations.

Full-Color Design: Dramatic full-cover photographs and illustrations, combined with a functional full-color design, provide an attractive text which is easy to learn from.

Class Tested: All materials have been successfully class-tested and refined in thousands of classrooms over the past four years.

Skill Scan Pages: Over 20 skill scan pages present key first aid skills in a format that enhances student comprehension.

Flowcharts: Over 35 full-page, full-color flowcharts depict decision making and appropriate first aid procedures.

Learning Activities: End-of-chapter self-tests and case studies can be used to evaluate student mastery of the subject. Perforated learning activity pages allow students to hand in completed materials to the instructor.

Informational Tables: Numerous tables throughout the text present key data and information to stimulate student interest and thought.

Anecdotal Boxes: Many anecdotal boxes provide interesting, humorous, and unique first aid information.

Award-Winning Anatomical Art: A special appendix containing beautiful anatomical art serves as an excellent reference for students.

Glossary of Key Medical Terms: Hundreds of key first aid terms with their meanings are presented in an appendix.

Quick Emergency Index: Conveniently placed opposite the back-inside cover, this index allows the student to rapidly find important information.

To the Instructor

"Training of individuals in first aid in the United States is carried out through a variety of mechanisms...The National Safety Council, through Jones and Bartlett Publishers, provides educational materials to train individuals in basic first aid knowledge and skills."

Occupational Safety and Health Administration (OSHA)
Guidelines for First Aid Training Programs

As stated in the OSHA first aid guidelines, the National Safety Council is the recognized source for first aid training in the educational marketplace. With the publication of this new text, **FIRST AID AND CPR**, the National Safety Council will continue to set the standard for first aid instruction in classrooms across the country.

Nationally Recognized Certification Program

Finally, a nationally recognized first aid/CPR certification program that academic departments can administor. No longer will your first aid program be subject to the hassles and expense associated with off-campus certifying organizations.

Academic departments become eligible for this program by having a department head complete a simple, one-page application. Once approved, your department qualifies as an official Educational Training Agency of the National Safety Council.

All students successfully completing a course using **FIRST AID AND CPR** qualify to receive FREE National Safety Council certifications in both first aid and CPR. The first aid certification is valid for three years and the CPR is valid for one year. The certification cards are recognized nationally and like other similar cards, signify successful course completion.

Free Instructor Supplements

To assist the instructor in teaching this course, we have assembled an **Instructor's Teaching Package for FIRST AID AND CPR** containing the following seven components:

- **First Aid Video** (VHS, Color, 60 minutes) This authoritative, full-feature video is designed for all first aid training classes. It combines dramatic first aid emergencies with an instructional classroom format to effectively teach your students how to handle emergency situations. This video is designed in a modular/topical format that corresponds with the material in the text.

- **CPR Video** (VHS, Color, 22 Minutes) This video applies to all CPR training classes and follows the latest American Heart Association standards as published in the JAMA Supplement. It combines dramatic, real-life emergencies with an instructional classroom format to effectively teach your students basic life support.

- **Instructor's Resource Manual** This manual includes lesson plans, teaching strategies, proficiency tests, supplemental information and answers to all learning activities in the text. This manual clearly explains how best to utilize the slides, transparencies and videos.

- **Instructor's Transparency Set** A set of 33 full-color acetate transparencies depicting the most important flowcharts in the text. An essential teaching tool to explain proper sequence of procedures and to review important techniques.

- **Instructor's Slide Set** A set of 80, 35mm color slides depicting key first aid topics and actual injuries. The topical slides outline the most important information in the text while the injury slides prepare your students to handle a real-life emergency.

- **Instructor's Test Bank** A manual containing over 1,000 test questions. An excellent reference source for exam construction.

- **Instructor's Computerized Test Bank** A computerized version of the above test manual. Available in IBM/Apple formats.

All of the above supplements are conveniently packaged in an **Instructor's Teaching Package for FIRST AID AND CPR**. All academic departments qualifying as official Educational Training Agencies of the National Safety Council are eligible to receive this package free.

For additional information on any aspect of this program, please contact Jones and Bartlett Publishers Marketing Department at 1-800-832-0034 or (617) 482-3900.

1

Introduction

■ **Size of the Injury Problem** ■ **Need for First Aid Training** ■
■ **Legal Aspects of First Aid** ■

Size of the Injury Problem

Injuries are one of the most serious public health problems. Injuries are the leading cause of death and disability in children and young adults. They destroy the health, lives, and livelihoods of millions of people.

- Each year, more than 140,000 Americans die from injuries (this includes accidents, suicides, and homicides), and one person in three suffers a nonfatal injury.
- Preceded by heart disease, cancer, and stroke, injury is the fourth leading cause of death among all Americans.
- One of every eight hospital beds is occupied by an injured patient.

Percentages of years of potential life lost to injury, cancer, heart disease, and other diseases before age 65. Modified from Centers for Disease Control.

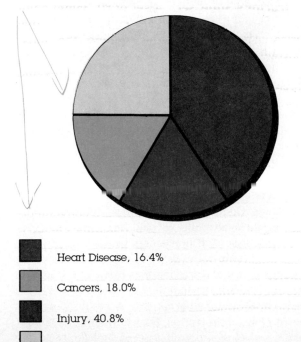

■ Heart Disease, 16.4%

■ Cancers, 18.0%

■ Injury, 40.8%

■ All other diseases, 24.8%

- Every year, more than 80,000 Americans suffer unnecessary but permanently disabling injuries of the brain or spinal cord.
- Injury is the leading reason for physician contacts. And more than 25 percent of hospital emergency room visits are for the treatment of injuries.

Need for First Aid Training

Because of the size and magnitude of the injury problem, everyone must expect sooner or later to be present when an injury or sudden illness strikes. The outcome of such misfortune frequently depends not only on the severity of the injury or illness, but on the first aid rendered. Therefore, every person should be trained in first aid.

First aid is the immediate care given to the injured or suddenly ill person. First aid does *not* take the place of proper medical treatment. It consists only of furnishing temporary assistance until competent medical care, *if needed*, is obtained, or until the chance for recovery without medical care is assured. *Most injuries and illnesses require only first aid care.*

Properly applied, first aid may mean the difference between life and death, rapid recovery and long hospitalization, or temporary disability and permanent injury.

Legal Aspects of First Aid

Duty to Act

No one is required to render aid when no legal duty to do so exists. For example, even a physician could ignore a stranger suffering a heart attack or a fractured bone. Moral obligations exist, but they may not be the same as a legal obligation to give aid.

Duty to act may occur in the following situations:

1. *When employment requires it.* If your employment has designated you to render first aid and you are called to an accident scene, then you have a duty to act. Examples include law enforcement officers, park rangers, lifeguards, and teachers

1

who have a job description usually designating the giving of first aid.

2. When a preexisting responsibility exists. You may have a preexisting relationship with another person which demands being responsible for them (e.g., parent-child, driver-passenger) although it is not spelled out in your job description. You must give first aid should they need it.

3. After beginning first aid. Once you start first aid, you cannot stop. Duty to give first aid is usually questioned only when a person fails to act.

Standards of Care

Standards of care ensure quality care and protection for injured or suddenly sick victims. The elements making up a standard of care include:

1. The type of rescuer. A first aider should provide the level and type of care expected of a reasonable person with the same amount of training and in similar circumstances.

2. Published recommendations. Emergency care-related organizations and societies publish recommended first aid procedures. For example, the American Heart Association publishes procedures for giving CPR.

Obtain Consent to Help

You should obtain the victim's approval or permission before starting first aid. This permission is known as **consent.**

- When a victim gives permission to a first aider to help, this is known as **actual consent.** Oral or written permission is valid.
- Consent should be obtained from every conscious, mentally competent adult.
- Permission is implied for giving care for an unconscious victim and is known as **implied consent.** A first aider should not hesitate to treat an unconscious victim.
- Consent should be obtained from the parent or guardian of a victim who is a child, or of one who is an adult but is mentally incompetent. If a parent or guardian is not available, emergency first aid to maintain life may be given without consent. Do *not* withhold first aid from a minor just to obtain parental or guardian permission.
- Psychological emergencies present difficult problems of consent. Under most conditions, a police officer is the only person with the authority to restrain and transport a person against the person's will. However, if the victim is not violent, the situation is similar to that for minors.

Abandonment

Abandonment refers to the behavior of a first aider who begins giving care and then leaves the victim before another person arrives to take over. After starting first aid, you must remain with the victim until he or she is under the care of another person with equal or more training, or until the victim refuses treatment or transportation.

The Right to Refuse Care

A difficult problem involves the conscious, rational, adult victim who is suffering from an actual or potential life-threatening injury or illness but who refuses treatment or transportation. In such situations, make every reasonable effort to convince the victim, or anyone who can influence the victim, to accept first aid and/or transportation. When such a victim refuses to consent, do *not* give first aid or transportation. In such cases, document everything on paper, and if possible, have witnesses.

Parent Refusing Permission to Help a Child

Very rarely will a first aider encounter a parent who refuses permission—usually on moral, ethical, or religious grounds—to care for a seriously injured or ill child. If refusal does occur, make every effort to convince the parent about the seriousness of the problem and the necessity of first aid. If you do not succeed, call the police, document everything, and, if possible, have witnesses.

The Intoxicated or Belligerent Victim

If an intoxicated or belligerent victim refuses first aid, make every effort to persuade him or her of the need for such care. If refused, document everything in writing; if possible, have witnesses.

If the intoxicated person consents to first aid, take the greatest possible care. Alcohol and drugs may hide signs and symptoms. Because first aiders may be repulsed by the appearance and/or attitude of the intoxicated person, they may overlook injuries. It's important to focus on helping the victim.

Good Samaritan Laws

First aiders are covered by a Good Samaritan law in some states. Good Samaritan laws protect only those acting in good faith and without gross negligence or willful misconduct. If first aiders provide care within the scope of their training, lawsuits are rare. However, if a minor injury is worsened by a first aider, litigation is possible even if the first aider or medical person is covered by a Good Samaritan law. Actually, these laws provide no legal protection. Protection for a first aider consists of being properly trained and applying appropriate procedures and skills.

The table below shows estimates of injuries, deaths, and participants associated with various sports. Methods and coverage of reporting may vary among sources and can affect comparisons among sports. Because this list is not complete and the number of participants varies greatly, no inference should be made concerning the relative hazard of these sports or rank with respect to risk of injury.

Sport	Participants	Injuries	Fatalities
Archery	5,500,000	4,490	(a)
Baseball	13,400,000	327,620	1[b]
Basketball	23,100,000	460,420	7[b]
Bicycle riding	53,800,000	525,026	(a)
Boating	32,500,000	3,635[c]	896[c]
Bowling	37,900,000	17,382	(a)
Boxing	(a)	4,439	(a)
Fishing	45,700,000	66,605	(a)
Football	12,400,000	323,112	6[d]
Golf	22,700,000	19,836	(a)
Gymnastics	(a)	37,671	1[b]
Handball	(a)	2,857	(a)
Hang gliding	30,000[c]	(a)	6[e]
Ice hockey	1,800,000	18,910	0[b]
Ice skating	7,000,000	23,010	(a)
Parachuting	115,000[f]	(a)	36[f]
Racquetball	9,300,000	16,190	(a)
Roller skating	20,500,000	72,109	(a)
Scuba diving	2,500,000[g]	(a)	66[g]
Skateboarding	7,400,000	80,242	(a)
Snow skiing	18,200,000	(a)	1[b]
Soccer	8,700,000	94,569	0[b]
Softball	20,600,000	(a)	(a)
Swimming	71,100,000	99,161	1,700[h]
Tennis	17,300,000	21,201	1[b]
Volleyball	22,000,000	88,617	(a)
Water skiing	12,800,000	21,828	21[c]
Wrestling	(a)	37,122	0[b]

Source: Participants—National Sporting Goods Association (1988), except where noted; figures include those who participate more than one time per year except for bicycle riding and swimming, which include only those who participate more than six times per year. *Injuries—*Consumer Product Safety Commission (1988), except where noted; figures include only hospital emergency room treated injuries. Fatalities—[b]National Collegiate Athletic Association (NCAA) (1987–1988 school year); figures are for school or college sponsored sports only. [c]U.S. Coast Guard (1989), [d]NCAA (calendar year 1988), [e]U.S. Hang Gliding Association (1989), [f]U.S. Parachute Association (1989), [g]National Underwater Accident Data Center (1988), [h]National Safety Council (1989). [a]Estimate not available.

most dang - men

most region N.Y. EAstern north & Calf.
dangerous

age group - 4-5 - teenagers
biggest suicide next 40d50
acc. death in motor vechicles - 2lane deaths
- Weekends, Holidays

The following list of items found in and around the home was selected from the U.S. Consumer Product Safety Commission's National Electronic Injury Surveillance System (NEISS) for 1988. The NEISS estimates are calculated from a sample of statistically representative hospitals in the U.S. Injury totals represent estimates of the number of hospital emergency room-treated cases nationwide associated with various products. However, product involvement may or may not be the cause of the accident.

Estimated Injuries Related to Selected Consumer Products, 1988

Product	Injuries[a]
Home Maintenance:	
Noncaustic cleaning equip., detergents	19,338
Cleaning agents (except soaps)	36,344
Miscellaneous household chemicals	14,348
Paints, solvents, lubricants	21,928
Home Workshop Equipment:	
Batteries, all types	12,080
Hoists, lifts, jacks, etc.	15,165
Miscellaneous workshop equipment	33,726
Power home tools, except saws	24,208
Power home workshop saws, all	64,232
Welding, soldering, cutting tools	13,940
Wires, cords, not specified	14,298
Workshop manual tools	99,016
Packaging & Containers, Household:	
Cans, other containers	183,023
Glass bottles, jars	67,439
Paper, cardboard, plastic products	34,174
Housewares:	
Cookware, pots, pans	29,226
Cutlery, knives, unpowered	337,464
Drinking glasses	114,923
Miscellaneous housewares	51,383
Scissors	19,566
Small kitchen appliances	35,484
Tableware and accessories	114,628
Home Furnishings, Fixtures and Accessories:	
Bathtub, shower structures	121,600
Beds, mattresses, pillows	299,222
Carpets, rugs	82,235
Chairs, sofas, sofa beds	291,446
Desks, cabinets, shelves, racks	166,661
Electric fixtures, lamps, equipment	40,517
Ladders, stools	128,818
Mirrors, mirror glass	23,013
Miscellaneous household covers, fabrics	14,545
Other misc. furniture, accessories	39,417
Sinks, toilets	42,016
Tables, all types	269,255
Home Structures and Construction Materials:	
Cabinets or door hardware	17,209
Ceilings, walls, panels (inside)	186,328
Counters, counter tops	23,088
Fences	113,331
Glass doors, windows, panels	176,393
Handrails, railings, banisters	35,899
Miscellaneous construction materials	59,829
Nails, carpet tacks, etc.	220,640
Nonglass doors, panels	281,649
Porches, open side floors, etc.	92,508
Stairs, ramps, landings, floors	1,477,887
Window, door sills, frames	41,457

Product	Injuries[a]
General Household Appliances:	
Cooking ranges, ovens, etc.	41,442
Irons, clothes steamers (not toys)	18,805
Miscellaneous household appliances	22,124
Refrigerators, freezers	26,615
Washers, dryers	19,075
Heating, Cooling, and Ventilating Equipment:	
Air conditioners	10,476
Chimneys, fireplaces	14,682
Fans (except stove exhaust fans)	19,384
Heating stoves, space heaters	30,992
Pipes, heating and plumbing	24,188
Radiators, all	17,976
Home Communication, Entertainment and Hobby Equipment:	
Miscellaneous hobby equipment	11,868
Pet supplies, equipment	13,576
Sound recording, reproducing equipment	37,440
Television sets, stands	31,754
Personal Use Items:	
Cigarettes, lighters, fuel	20,878
Clothing, all	115,058
Grooming devices	25,680
Holders for personal items	14,895
Jewelry	43,087
Paper money, coins	29,418
Pencils, pens, other desk supplies	42,130
Razors, shavers, razor blades	36,122
Sewing equipment	29,996
Yard and Garden Equipment:	
Chain saws	36,145
Hand garden tools	35,427
Hatchets, axes	16,458
Lawn, garden care equipment	39,421
Lawn mowers, all types	53,830
Other power lawn equipment	15,300
Sports & Recreation Equipment:	
All-terrain vehicles, mopeds, minibikes	112,571
Barbecue grills, stoves, equipment	13,239
Bicycles, accessories	525,027
Exercise equipment	65,029
Nonpowder guns, BBs, pellets	22,240
Playground equipment	204,726
Skateboards	80,242
Toboggans, sleds, snow disks, etc.	28,818
Trampolines	13,944
Miscellaneous Products:	
Dollies, carts	32,604
Elevators, other lifts	11,539
Fireworks, flares	10,330
Gasoline and diesel fuels	15,964
Nursery equipment	84,193
Toys	141,755

Source: Consumer Product Safety Commission, National Electronic Injury Surveillance System.
[a]Estimated number of product-related injuries in the U.S. and territories which were treated in hospital emergency departments in 1988. Not all product categories are shown.

2

Victim Assessment

■ Primary Survey ■ Secondary Survey ■

Do *not* move the injured or suddenly ill person until you have a clear idea of the injury or illness and have applied first aid. The exception occurs when the victim is exposed to further danger at the accident scene. If the injury is serious, if it occurred in an area where the victim can remain safely, and if emergency medical service (EMS) attention is readily available, it is sometimes best not to attempt to move the person, but to use first aid at the injury scene until the EMS system responds.

When making a victim assessment, a first aider will consider what witnesses to the accident can tell about the accident, what is observed about the victim, and what the victim can tell.

The first aider must not assume that the obvious injuries are the only ones present because less noticeable injuries may also have occurred. Look for the causes of the injury which may provide a clue as to the extent of physical damage.

In all actions taken during the initial survey the first aider should be especially careful not to move the victim any more than necessary to support life. Any unnecessary movement or rough handling should be avoided because it might aggravate undetected fractures or spinal injuries.

In order to provide good first aid, a person should be able to identify a victim's injury or sudden illness and its seriousness. To find out what is wrong and how extensive it is, the first aider should follow a systematic approach known as a victim assessment.

A victim assessment attempts to:

- Get the victim's consent
- Gain the victim's confidence
- Identify the victim's problem(s) and determine which of them requires immediate first aid
- Get information about the victim that may prove useful later to the EMS responders and attending medical personnel

A victim assessment of either an injured victim or a medically ill victim is divided into two steps:

- Primary survey
- Secondary survey

Primary Survey

The primary survey covers these areas:

- A—Airway open?
- B—Breathing?
- C—Circulation at carotid pulse?
- H—Hemorrhage—severe bleeding?

The primary survey is the first step in assessing a victim and always takes precedence over all other aspects of the victim assessment. Its purpose is to find and correct life-threatening conditions. Many times the primary survey will be quickly completed (e.g., in the case of an alert victim with a sudden illness). At other times, however, close examination will be needed (e.g., with a victim who is unconscious or suffering a severe injury).

If the primary survey uncovers any problems, such as an obstructed airway or massive bleeding, you must attend to them immediately before proceeding with the victim assessment.

Airway. Ask: Does the victim have an open airway? If the person is talking or is conscious, the airway is open. Refer to page 24 for the correct and detailed procedures for opening an airway.

Breathing. Ask: Is the victim breathing? Conscious victims are breathing. However, note any breathing difficulties or unusual breathing sounds. If the victim is unconscious, keep the airway open and *look* for the chest to rise and fall, *listen* for breathing, and *feel* for air coming out of the victim's nose and mouth. See page 25 for the correct and detailed procedures.

Circulation. Ask: Is the victim's heart beating? Determine this by feeling for a pulse at the side of the neck (carotid pulse). Refer to page 26 for the correct and detailed procedures.

Hemorrhage. Ask: Is the victim severely bleeding? Check for severe bleeding by looking, if necessary, over the victim's entire body for blood-soaked clothing as a sign of severe bleeding. See page 63 for the correct and detailed procedures.

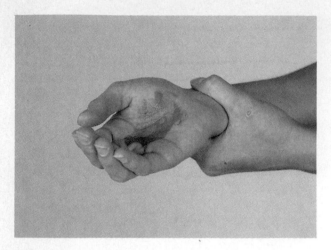

Blood represents a sign.

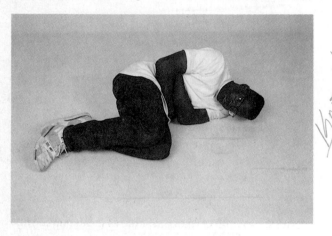

Abdominal pain represents a symptom.

Secondary Survey

Having completed the primary survey and attended to any life-threatening problems it uncovers, take a closer look at the victim and make a systematic assessment called the secondary survey.

Look for important signs and symptoms of injury. A **sign** is something the first aider sees, hears, or feels (e.g., pale face, no respiration, cool skin). A **symptom** is something the victim tells the first aider about (e.g., nausea, back pain, no sensation in the extremities).

The secondary survey is done to discover problems that do not pose an immediate threat to life but may do so if they remain uncorrected. The secondary survey has three parts:

- Interview
- Vital signs
- Head-to-Toe Exam

Interview

If the victim is conscious, identify yourself and get his or her consent for you to give first aid. See page 2 for more information on consent and its legal implications.

The interview usually involves only the victim. Start by introducing yourself and asking for the victim's name (use it during the assessment). Get the victim's consent before giving first aid. In some cases the victim's family and any bystanders may be involved. Ask the victim about his or her chief complaint. Often it is obvious (e.g., bleeding). Most chief complaints are characterized by pain or an abnormal function.

For an unconscious victim, monitor breathing and pulse, and if needed, render rescue breathing or CPR.

After finding out about the chief complaint and if time permits, two mnemonic devices might help you identify a victim's problem: taking a S-A-M-P-L-E history and, since pain is one of the most common chief complaints, using P-A-I-N as a way of describing the victim's pain:

Symptoms (chief complaint)
Allergies (may give a clue as to the problem and helps prevent the giving of wrong medication)
Medications (may give a clue as to the problem and helps prevent the giving of wrong medication)
Preexisting illnesses (relating to the problem)
Last food (in case of needed surgery, or in case of food poisoning)
Events prior to the injury

Period of pain (How long? What started it?)
Area (Where?)
Intensity (How strong?)
Nullify (What stops it? such as rest, certain position)

Vital Signs

First aiders involve themselves with the following vital signs: pulse, respirations, and, if indicated, skin condition. Check these every five or so minutes while wait-

TABLE 2–1 Normal Pulse Rates	
60–70	Men
70–80	Women
80–90	Children over seven years
80–120	Children from one to seven years
110–130	Infants
Pulse Classified in Adults	
60 and below	Slow or subnormal
60–80	Normal (men, women)
80–100	Moderate increase
100–120	Quick
120–140	Rapid
140 and above	Running (hard to count)

Source: U.S. Public Health Service, The Ship's Medicine Chest and Medical Aid at Sea.

TABLE 2-2 What Body Temperatures Mean

	Fahrenheit (F)		Centigrade (C)
	108°	Usually fatal	42.2°
	107 ⎤		41.7 ⎤
	106 ⎬	Critical condition	41.1 ⎬
	105 ⎦		40.6 ⎦
	104 ⎤		40.0 ⎤
	103 ⎬	High fever	39.4 ⎬
	102 ⎦		38.9 ⎦
	101 ⎤		38.3 ⎤
	100 ⎬	Moderate fever	37.8 ⎬
	99 ⎦		37.2 ⎦
	98.6	Healthy (normal) temperature in mouth	37.0
	98 ⎤		36.7 ⎤
	97 ⎬	Subnormal	36.1 ⎬
	96 ⎬	temperature	35.6 ⎬
	95 ⎦		35.0 ⎦

Source: U.S. Public Health Service. The Ship's Medicine Chest and Medical Aid at Sea.

ing for the EMS to respond or while transporting the victim to a medical facility.

Pulse. Place two fingertips (do *not* use a thumb since it has its own pulse) over either the radial pulse point (on thumb side of inside wrist) or the carotid pulse point (in the groove beside the Adam's apple on the neck). Generally, use the radial pulse of a conscious victim and the carotid pulse of an unconscious victim. Do *not* feel both carotid arteries at the same time. Do *not* put too much pressure on or massage the carotid artery area because either will disturb the heart's rhythm.

Count the beats for 30 seconds and multiply by two. Normal pulse at rest for adults is from 60 to 80 beats per minute. A physically fit person may have a lower resting pulse rate. For children, it is 80 to 100; and for babies, it is 100 to 140 beats per minute.

Respiration. During the primary survey, the concern focuses upon whether or not the victim is breathing. However, in the secondary survey, the respiration rate is determined.

Count the number of breaths for one minute. Between 12 and 20 breaths per minute is normal for resting adults and older children. Up to 30 breaths per minute is normal for children, and 40 is normal for babies. Do *not* let victims know you are counting their respirations since the knowledge may alter their breathing.

As you determine the respiration rate, listen for sounds, for example:

- A whistle or wheeze—constricted airway
- A crowing sound—constricted airway
- A gurgling sound—fluid in airway

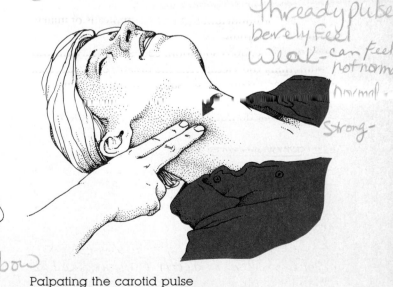

Palpating the radial pulse   Palpating the carotid pulse

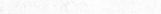

9

Skin Condition. Skin condition refers to three things:

- **Temperature.** It is important to record body temperature in cases of heat stroke or high fever. When a person cannot receive medical care for some time, as in a rural area when snow or high water prevents the immediate transfer of a sick or injured person to a medical facility, body temperature should be monitored. If a person is very sick, take the temperature at least four times each day and write it down. Body temperature is best taken with a thermometer that is held for a short time under the tongue, inside the rectum, or in the armpit (referred to respectively as oral, rectal, and axillary). A standard glass thermometer should *not* be used when there is a chance that the victim will bite through it. The temperature at the axilla is usually one degree lower than that measured under the tongue, and rectal temperature is generally a degree higher. Although 98.6°F is considered normal, the body temperature of healthy individuals may vary from 97°F to 99°F.

  Devices for taking temperatures include the well-known mercury thermometer, the electronic thermometer, and a color-changing temperature device which attaches to the forehead. If a thermometer is not available, you can get a rough idea of the temperature by putting the back of one hand on the victim's forehead and the other on your own or that of another healthy person. If the victim has a fever, you should feel the difference. Fingertips and palms may be insensitive because of calluses.
- **Color.** Skin color, especially in light-skinned people, reflects the circulation under the skin as well as oxygen status. In darkly pigmented people, these changes may not be apparent in the skin, but may be assessed by examining the mucous membranes (inside mouth, inner eyelids, and nailbeds). If the skin's blood vessels constrict or pulse slows, the skin becomes pale, mottled, or cyanotic (bluish discoloration). If the skin's blood vessels dilate or blood flow increases, the skin becomes warm and pink.
- **Moisture.** Notice if the skin appears (a) wet or dry and (b) hot or cold. This gives four possible variations: hot and dry, hot and moist, cold and dry, or cold and moist.

Head-to-Toe Exam

The victim assessment's final step involves a head-to-toe exam. It consists of looking for other injuries. Tell the victim what is being done and why. Do *not* aggravate injuries or contaminate wounds. Do *not* move the victim in case of neck and spinal injuries. Removing of clothing from the victim during this exam is *not* usually necessary except in the injured area.

Head and Neck. Use both hands to check the scalp for bleeding or deformity ("goose egg" or depression). Do *not* move the head during this procedure. Check the ears and nose for a clear fluid or bloody discharge. Look in the mouth for blood or foreign materials.

Eyes. Notice whether *pupils are constricted or dilated.* Use a flashlight to determine if the pupils are reactive. If there is no flashlight, cover an eye with your hand and notice the pupil reaction when the eye is uncovered. Normally, the pupil contracts (gets smaller) within 1 second. No pupil reaction to light could mean death, coma, cataracts (in older persons), or an artificial eye. Pupil dilation happens within 30 to 60 seconds of cardiac arrest.

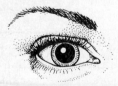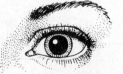   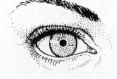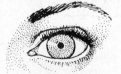

Dilated pupils   Constricted pupils

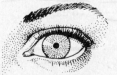

Unequal pupils

Changes in pupil size can have medical significance.

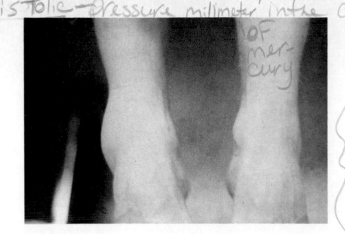
OF
mer-
cury

Sprained ankle (Compare one with the other.)

Look for *unequal pupils*. A difference in the size of the two pupils is almost always a sign of a medical emergency, such as a stroke or a brain injury. However, the unequal condition occurs normally in 2 to 4 percent of the population. An artificial eye may give the appearance of unequal pupils. Look at the inner eyelid surface—pink is normal in all healthy people regardless of skin pigmentation. A pale color may indicate anemia or blood loss.

Chest. Check the chest for cuts, bruises, penetrations, and impaled objects. Warn the victim that you are going to apply pressure to the sides of the chest. Pain from squeezing or compressing the sides may indicate a rib fracture.

Abdomen. Anything protruding from the abdomen will be obvious, but check for penetrating objects. If a chief complaint is abdominal pain, ask the victim to point to where it hurts. Then, beginning on the opposite side from the spot, press gently on different parts of the abdomen to see where it hurts the most. Feel for abnormal lumps and hardened areas. Do *not* push too deeply. The victim may "guard" an area if it is tender by tightening abdominal muscles or protecting that area with his or her hands. Feel the four abdominal quadrants. (Divide the abdomen into four parts by two imaginary lines intersecting at right angles at the navel.)

Extremity Assessment. Check the arms and legs for injury, deformity and tenderness. Compare the two sides of the body with each other. Blood circulation can be checked by feeling the pulse, the warmth of the part, and capillary refill in a nailbed. To assess capillary refill, gently press on the nailbed's surface to whiten the underlying tissue. Then, release the pressure and observe the rate at which the nailbed becomes pink again. Instant refilling indicates good circulation. Refill time greater than two seconds is definitely abnormal. Check the radial pulse (in the wrist) and the foot pulse (on the inside of the ankle or the top of the foot) for blood circulation.

In examining injured victims, the first aider should look for abnormal positioning of the legs. For example, a leg that is externally rotated suggests a hip fracture.

Spine and Back Assessment. If you suspect spinal injury or stroke, check sensation and strength in all extremities by having the victim press each foot against your hand and use each hand to squeeze your hand. The spinal injured victim may show paraplegia (paralysis of both legs) or quadriplegia (paralysis of all four extremities); the stroke victim is likely to have hemiplegia (paralysis of an arm or leg on the same side of the body).

Putting It All Together

The victim assessment will be influenced by whether the victim is suffering from a medical problem or an injury, whether the victim is conscious or unconscious, and whether life-threatening conditions are present. Remember to first conduct a primary survey and correct any problems it uncovers before going on to the secondary survey.

Medical Alert Tag

A medical alert emblem tag worn as a necklace or as a bracelet attracts attention in an emergency situation. These tags contain the wearer's medical problem and a 24-hour telephone number to call in case of an emergency that offers access to your medical history plus names of doctors and close relatives.. Do *not* remove a medical alert tag from an injured or sick person. Necklaces and bracelets are durable, instantly recognizable, and less likely than cards to be separated from the victim in an emergency.

Calling the Emergency Medical Services (EMS) System for Help*

In many communities, to receive emergency assistance of every kind you just phone 9-1-1. Check to see if this is true in your community. An emergency number should be listed on the inside cover of your telephone directory

*Adapted from Consumer's Union, Consumer Reports.

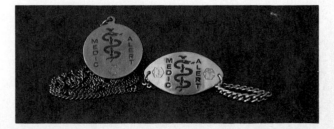

Medical alert tag

TABLE 2-3 Diagnostic Signs

Observation	Examples
Pulse	
Rapid, strong	fright, apprehension, heat stroke
Rapid, weak	shock, bleeding, diabetic coma, heat exhaustion
Slow, strong	stroke, skull fracture
None	cardiac arrest, death
Respirations	
Shallow	shock, bleeding, heat exhaustion, insulin shock
Deep, gasping, labored	airway obstruction, chest injury, diabetic coma, heart disease
None	respiratory arrest due to any number of illnesses/injuries
Bright, frothy blood coughed up	lung damage possible due to fractured ribs or penetrating objects
Skin temperature	
Cool, moist	shock, bleeding, heat exhaustion
Cool, dry	exposure to cold
Hot, dry	heat stroke, high fever
Face color	
Red	high blood pressure, heat stroke, diabetic coma
Pale/white/ashen	shock, bleeding, heat exhaustion, insulin shock
Blue	heart failure, airway obstruction, some poisonings

Note: Blue results from poor oxygenation of circulating blood. For people with dark skin pigmentation, blue may be noted around the fingernails, palms of hands and mouth.

Pupils of eyes	
Dilated	shock, bleeding, heat stroke, cardiac arrest
Constricted	opiate addiction
Unequal	head injury, stroke
State of consciousness	
Confusion	most any illness/injury, fright, apprehension, alcohol, drugs
Coma	stroke, head injury, severe poisoning, diabetic coma
Inability to move upon command (an indicator of paralysis)	
One side of the body	stroke, head injury
Arms and legs	damage to spinal cord in neck
Legs	damage to spinal cord below neck
Reaction to physical stimulation (an indicator of paralysis)	
No sensation in arms and/or legs	damage to spinal cord as indicated above
Numbness in arms and/or legs	damage to spinal cord as indicated above

Note: No sensation or indication of pain when there is an obvious injury can also be due to hysteria, violent shock, or excessive alcohol or drug use.

Source: *National Highway Traffic Safety Administration, Emergency Medical Services: First Responder Training Course (Washington, D.C.: U.S. Superintendent of Documents).*

To receive the best emergency medical help fast, you should keep a list of phone numbers for important services near your telephone.

1. *The rescue squad.* Often part of the local fire department, these specially trained paramedics are likely to respond swiftly and competently.

2. *The police.* They may or may not be able to respond with medically trained personnel; however, they can get someone to the hospital quickly.

3. *Ambulance service.* Some services have trained paramedics; others do not.

4. *Your doctor.* Your own doctor may not be available, but he or she should be alerted if an emergency has occurred.

5. *Poison control center.* In some communities, this service will give information to doctors only. Call before an emergency occurs to find out.

TABLE 2-4 Victim Assessment

Primary Survey	Performed?	
	Yes	No
A = Airway open? B = Breathing? C = Circulation at carotid? H = Hemorrhage—severe?		

Secondary Survey	Performed?	
	Yes	No
Interview S = Symptom (chief complaint)? A = Allergies? M = Medications? P = Preexisting illnesses? L = Last food? E = Events prior to emergency? P = Period of pain (how long?) A = Area (where?) I = Intensity? N = Nullify (what stops it?)		
	Yes	No
Vital Signs Pulse rate? Respiration rate? Skin temperature? Skin color?		
	Yes	No

Head-to-Toe Examination
Head: Bleeding?
            Deformity?
            CSF?
            Cyanosis?
 	
Eyes: Pupils equal?
            Pupils react?
            Eyelid color?
 	
Chest: Pain?
            Wounds?
 	
Abdomen: Pain?
            Wounds?
 	
Extremities: Deformity?
            Pulses?
            Sensation?
            Capillary refill?
 	
Spine, Back: Finger/toe wiggle?
            Finger/toe touch?
            Hand squeeze/foot push?
 	
Medical alert tags?		

Give the following information over the phone:

1. *The victim's location.* Give city or town, street number, and street name. Give names of intersecting streets or roads and other landmarks if possible. Describe the building. The victim's location may be the single most important information you can provide.

2. *Your phone number.* This information is required not only to help prevent false calls but, more importantly, to allow the center to call back for additional information.

3. *What has happened.* Tell the nature of the emergency (traffic accident, heart attack, dog bite, and so on).

4. *Number of persons needing help and any special conditions.* Tell the number of people involved. Tell about any special problems, such as

What To Expect When You Dial 9-1-1

Modern emergency services provide a wide variety of assistance to those who call for help today. It is estimated that on the average, every individual in the U.S. will require some kind of emergency assistance at least twice during their lifetime. The emergency number that we are now most familiar with in seeking this help is "9-1-1."

But how do you know when to call, how to call, and what to expect when calling in the event of an emergency?

9-1-1 began in the 1970s, as a method by which citizens could get assistance more easily, without having to look up a long 7-digit number and possibly misdial, causing unnecessary delays in the response times of available emergency services. As this program has matured nationally over the years, more and more municipalities have chosen to implement a 9-1-1 service, and many now have enhanced computerized systems showing instantly the address and telephone number from where the call originated.

When To Call For Help:

There is a natural tendency in all of us to be independent and self-reliant; this sometimes causes delays in calling for assistance in the event of an emergency while the potential caller decides whether or not it is appropriate to dial 9-1-1. It is estimated that an average two minute lapse of time passes before the actual decision to call for help is made—often two *deadly* minutes.

Whenever you are faced with a situation or crisis in which you have no personal control or ability to provide adequate assistance yourself, call someone for help—dial 9-1-1. Thanks to modern technology, police, fire, or emergency medical assistance is within a finger's reach at any time, day or night, to help you in your time of need.

As a general rule, if you are *ever* faced with the dilemma of whether or not to call, *make the call.* If you are in doubt, you probably do need some extra assistance, and it certainly cannot hurt to ask.

How To Call 9-1-1:

In cities with 9-1-1 in place, getting help quickly is as easy as picking up a phone and dialing "9-1-1." An important hint to remember is never to tell your children to dial "Nine-Eleven," simply because there is not an "eleven" on the telephone dial and this may cause some confusion if an emergency does arise. *Always* think "Nine-One-One."

If your town does not have a 9-1-1 system in place yet, or if you are not sure, *call your local department of public safety* to find out more information and to learn what emergency numbers to call in your area. You should post emergency numbers near each phone in your house. Many cities produce stickers with these numbers already printed on them for quick reference. Discuss with your children when and how to call so that they can get help if they are ever in need.

When your call for help is answered you will be speaking to a trained professional dispatcher and telecommunicator with experience and specialized training in dealing with crises over the phone. They may ask you to explain briefly what your exact situation is so they will know whether to alert police, fire, or medical assistance and know what level of response to send you. Many dispatchers today are also trained in pre-arrival instructions, so they may be able to assist you with certain life-saving techniques, such as CPR or the Heimlich Maneu-

several flights of stairs and no elevators, or the presence of a guard dog.

5. **Condition of the victim(s).** Tell about such things as no breathing or pulse, severe bleeding, unconsciousness.

6. **What is being done for the victim(s).** Tell about CPR, how the bleeding is being controlled, and so on.

Always be the last to hang up the phone. The EMS system dispatcher may need to ask more questions about how to find you. They may also tell you what to do until help arrives.

Speak slowly and clearly. Shouting is difficult to understand.

More than 50 percent of the United States population has access to 9-1-1 telephone service from their homes. Most large cities have 9-1-1 service. Record your local community emergency telephone numbers and other information on this book's back cover.

What To Expect When You Dial 9-1-1 (continued)

ver before professional help can arrive. They will continue to talk with you or immediately connect you with a dispatcher in one of their specialty areas. In either case, be confident that *help is on the way.*

What happens next:

The dispatcher will ask you for your phone number and address, and will then ask certain *key questions* that enable them to send the proper response. Public safety agencies have multiple skilled teams at their disposal, often including helicopters, fireboats, police, SWAT teams, search and rescue teams, firefighters, advanced life support paramedics and emergency medical technicians to name a few. The dispatcher *must* ask you specific questions to ensure that you get the kind of help you need. If a previous caller, for example, failed to answer these questions correctly, the dispatcher might send advanced paramedics to a call requiring only a basic technician. The result could be that a special unit is unavailable to respond as quickly to your call or someone else's with a more severe or complicated emergency. *The point is that while it may seem as though you are answering a lot of questions, this is not to establish need, but to determine the level of need required.*

What To Know When Calling:

The most important thing to remember when calling 9-1-1 for help is to LISTEN and do what the dispatcher(s) asks you to do. After the necessary key information has been exchanged (usually in less than 30 seconds), they may ask you to stay on the line and assist in handling the emergency situation. You may be asked to get near the victim(s) and then told ways you can help them. Remember, *trained dispatchers never ask questions that are unnecessary.* Hundreds of lives have been saved by callers, with the help of a trained dispatcher, during the five to seven critical minutes it usually takes before first responders or advanced life support paramedics can arrive. You may be asked to do nothing, or to get out of an unsafe environment; in any case, do what the dispatcher suggests. They have the *experience and training* to help you.

Four Key Questions:

Appropriate response of emergency medical technicians or paramedics *depends on you* to relay the following minimal information through your dispatcher:

- Patient problem or type of incident
- Approximate age
- Conscious: yes/no (or alert)?
- Breathing: yes/no (or difficulty)?

Unless you can answer these key, critical questions, it is difficult for the dispatchers to put their knowledge and experience to work quickly and effectively.

9-1-1 is here for you whenever you need it. If you are faced with what you think is an emergency and you have no way of adequately helping yourself, there is something you can do; dial 9-1-1 and alert emergency medical services. *They are there for you when you need them most.*

Reproduced by permission, © 1989
Medical Priority Consultants, Inc.

■ PRIMARY SURVEY ■

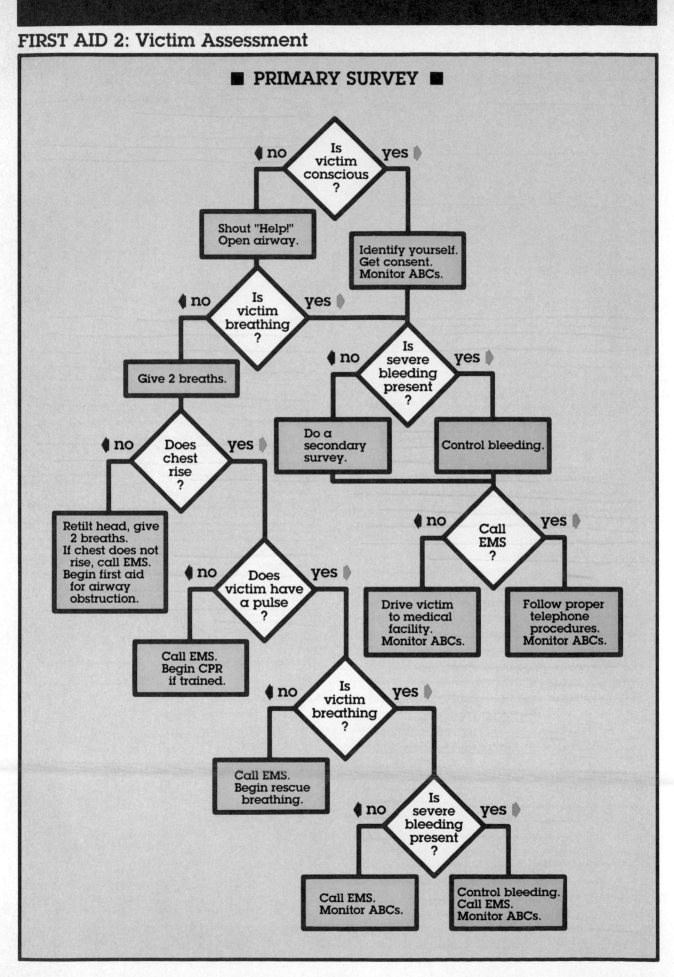

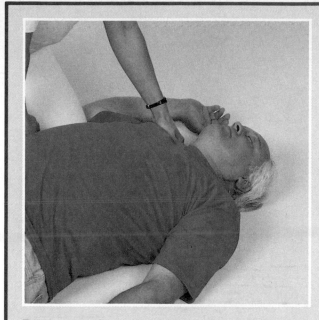

Responsive?

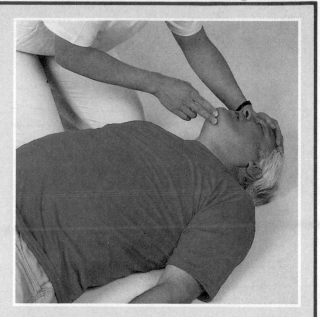

A = Airway open?

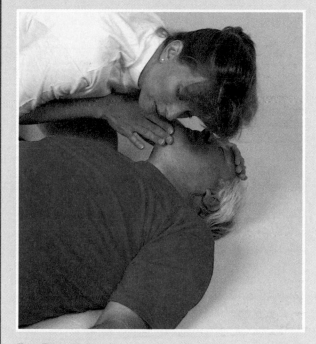

B = Breathing?

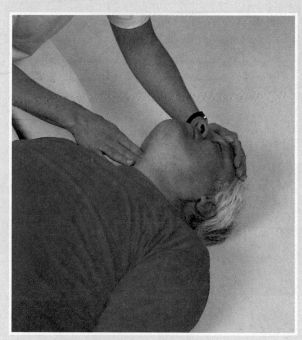

C = Circulation at carotid pulse?

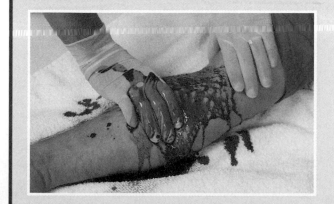

H = Hemorrhage—severe bleeding?

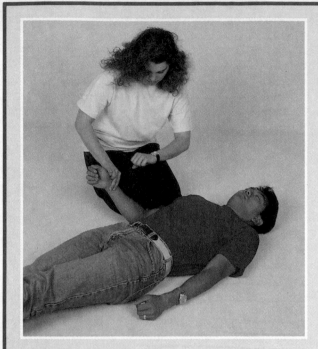

Pulse rate: Radial

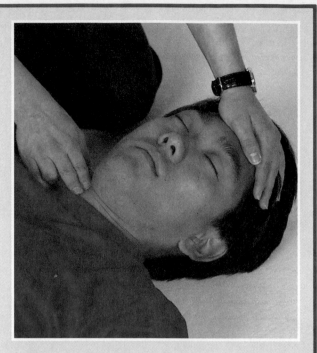

Pulse rate: Carotid

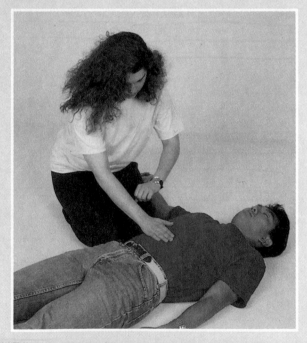

Respiration rate

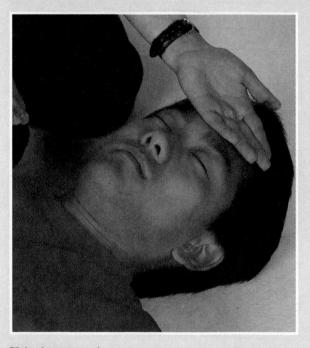

Skin temperature

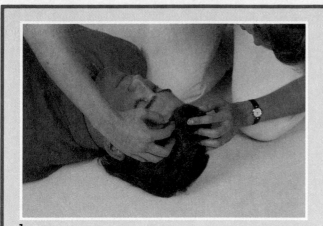

1.

1. Check scalp and head for bleeding or deformity. Do not move head.

2. Check ears and nose for clear fluid or blood.

3. Check mouth for blood or foreign materials.

4. Check pupils for size, equality, and reaction.

5. Check inner eyelid color.

6. Check chest for wounds.

7. Squeeze sides of chest for tenderness.

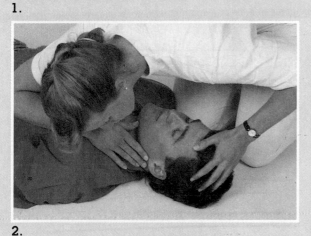

2.

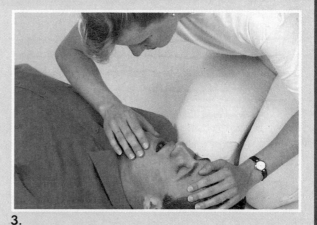

3.

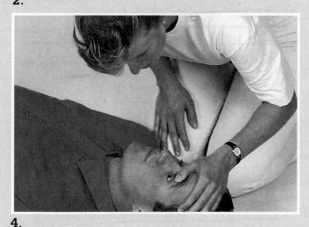

4.

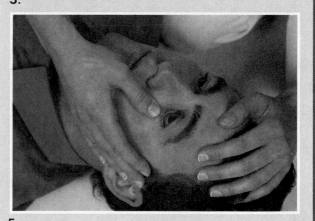

5.

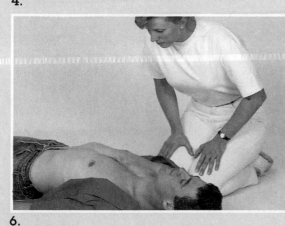

6.

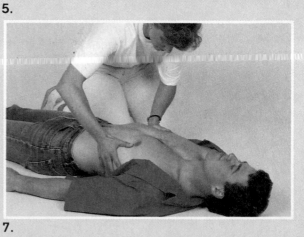

7.

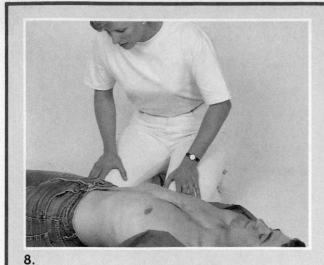

8.

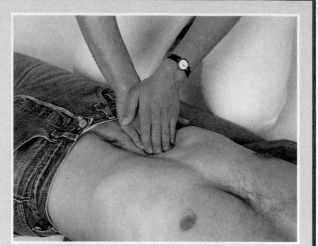

9.

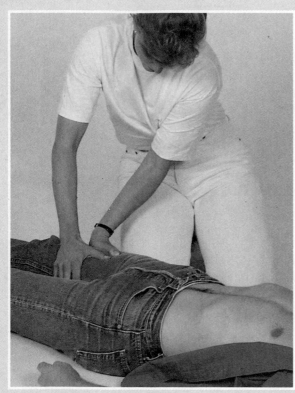

10.

8. Check abdomen for wounds.

9. Gently press abdomen for tenderness.

10. Check arms and legs for deformity and tenderness. Compare two sides with each other.

11. Pinch fingernail or toenail (capillary refill test).

12a. and b. Check pulses.

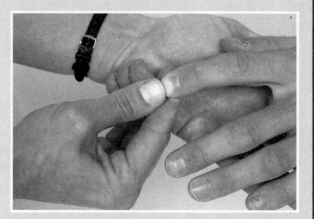

11.

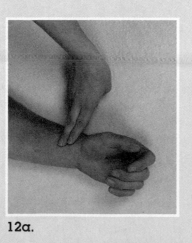

12a.

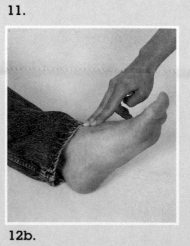

12b.

3

Basic Life Support*

■ **Performance Guidelines** ■ **Complications of CPR** ■ **Risks of Performing CPR** ■
■ **Child and Infant Resuscitation** ■ **Child and Infant Choking** ■

Sudden death from heart disease accounts for the most prominent medical emergency today. Prompt action providing early cardiopulmonary resuscitation (CPR) and entry into the emergency medical services (EMS) system can prevent a large number of deaths.

Successful resuscitation offers the only survival chance for many persons experiencing cardiac arrest. Early bystander CPR remains a critical element in the prevention of sudden death. When coupled with an efficient emergency medical services (EMS) system and advanced cardiac life support capability, the chances for survival increase to more than 40%. Larger numbers of trained lay people and a rapid response system of well-trained paramedical personnel could save an estimated 100,000 to 200,000 lives each year in the United States. In addition, prompt and proper application of CPR could save a number of victims who die of drowning, electrocution, suffocation, and drug intoxication.

The first two hours after the onset of symptoms represent the greatest risk of death from heart attack. Lay people, both those recognized to be at high risk and their immediate family and friends, must first be educated to recognize the unusual manifestations of heart attack. They then must know how to gain access to the emergency medical services (EMS) system. The use of a universal emergency telephone number, such as 9-1-1, is the fastest way for an emergency medical team to respond.

Young adults who are not often exposed to high-risk individuals compose the majority of lay people taking CPR courses. An emphasis, however, must be placed on the need to train families, neighbors, and coworkers of high-risk individuals.

Most CPR training stresses one-rescuer CPR by the lay individual. Two-rescuer CPR is seldom, if ever, used by lay rescuers, because when help is summoned it most often comes in the form of EMS personnel, who then relieve the lay rescuer. Learning the skills of two-rescuer CPR adds complexity, likely leading to decreased retention of the main techniques of one-rescuer CPR.

*Source: American Heart Association; reprinted with permission.

Common CPR Mistakes

- Pivoting at knees instead of hips
- Bending elbows
- Shoulders not above sternum (arms not vertical)
- Fingers touching chest
- Heel of bottom hand not in line with sternum
- Hands not remaining on chest between compressions
- Compression rate incorrect
- Compressions given in jerks rather than smoothly

—American Heart Association

When Not To Start CPR

First aiders should initiate CPR to the best of their knowledge and capability when they recognize pulselessness. However, if positive signs of death are present, CPR should *not* be started. Positive signs of death include:

- Decapitation
- Rigor mortis
- Evidence of tissue decomposition
- Lividity (purple-redish color showing on parts of body closest to the ground).

Effective CPR

The rescuer must periodically check to determine if the CPR being provided is effective. Check by:

- Having another person feel for a carotid pulse while you are giving chest compressions. A pulse should be felt each time a compression is made.
- Looking to see if the victim's color improves or if normal color is retained. This is especially noticeable around the nailbeds and lips.

The resuscitation procedures for adults are reprinted with permission from the American Heart Association's *Heartsaver Manual*. These procedures are based upon the Standards and Guidelines for Cardiopulmonary Resuscitation (CPR) and Emergency Cardiac Care (*JAMA*, June 6, 1986, American Heart Association).

Performance Guidelines One-Rescuer CPR: Adult

	Objectives	Critical Performance	Reason
	Airway Assessment: Determine unresponsiveness. Get help if possible.	Tap or gently shake shoulder. Shout "Are you OK?" Call out "Help!"	One concern about teaching people CPR is the risk of possible damage from unnecessarily resuscitating sleepers, fainters, etc. Call for help will summon nearby bystanders.
	Position the victim (4–10 seconds).	Turn on back as a unit, if necessary, supporting head and neck.	Frequently the victim will be facedown. Effective CPR can be provided only with the victim flat on back. The head cannot be above the level of the heart or CPR is ineffective.
	Open the airway (head-tilt/chin-lift).	Kneel beside victim's shoulder; lift the chin up gently with one hand while pushing down on the forehead with the other to tilt the head back. The chin should be lifted so that the teeth are brought almost together. Avoid completely closing the mouth.	Airway must be opened to establish breathlessness. Many victims may be making efforts at breathing that are ineffective because of obstruction by the tongue.

Performance Guidelines One-Rescuer CPR: Adult (continued)

Objectives	Critical Performance	Reason
Breathing Assessment: Determine breathlessness (3–5 seconds).	Maintain open airway. Turn your head toward victim's chest with your ear directly over and close to victim's mouth. Look at the chest for movement. Listen for the sounds of breathing. Feel for breath on your cheek.	Hearing and feeling are the only true ways of determining the presence of breathing. If there is chest movement but you cannot feel or hear air, the airway is still obstructed. Accurate diagnosis is important; rescue breathing should not be performed on someone who is breathing.
Give 2 full breaths (1 to 1½ seconds per breath.)	Pinch off nostrils with thumb and forefinger of upper hand while maintaining pressure on victim's forehead to keep the head tilted. Open your mouth wide, take a deep breath, and make a tight seal. Breathe into victim's mouth 2 times with complete refilling of your lungs after each breath. Watch for victim's chest to rise. Rescue breaths are given at the rate of 1 to 1½ seconds each, allowing the lungs to deflate between breaths. (If you cannot give rescue breaths to a victim, start the obstructed airway sequence (see Step 7, p. 42.))	When you are beginning rescue breathing, it is important to get as much oxygen as possible to the victim. If your rescue breathing is effective, you will: . feel air going in as you blow . feel the resistance of the victim's lungs . feel your own lungs emptying . see the rise and fall of the victim's chest and belly.

Performance Guidelines One-Rescuer CPR: Adult (continued)

Objectives	Critical Performance	Reason
Circulation Assessment: Determine pulse-lessness (5–10 seconds)	Place 2–3 fingers on the Adam's apple (voice box) just below chin. Slide fingers into the groove between Adam's apple and muscle, on the side nearest you. Maintain head-tilt with the other hand. Feel for the carotid pulse.	This activity should take 5 to 10 seconds because it takes time to find the right place, and the pulse itself may be slow or very weak and rapid. The victim's condition must be properly assessed.
Activate the EMS system.	Know your local EMS or rescue unit telephone number. Send second rescuer to call.	Notification of the EMS system at this time allows the caller to give complete information about the victim's condition.
Begin first cycle of rescue breathing with chest compressions:	To begin first cycle: Move your hands to the victim's chest. Run the index and middle fingers up the lower margin of the rib cage and locate the sternal notch with your middle finger. With index finger on sternum, place heel of the hand closest to the head on the sternum next to, but not covering the index finger. Place second hand on top of first.	Precise hand placement is essential to avoid serious injury.

Performance Guidelines One-Rescuer CPR: Adult (continued)

Objectives	Critical Performance	Reason
	Position body. Compress with weight transmitted vertically downward, elbows straight and locked, and shoulders over hands.	
	Between compressions, the pressure must be released and the chest allowed to return to its normal position, but the hands should not be lifted off the chest. Say mnemonic at proper rate and ratio. (Count aloud to establish rhythm: "one-and-two-and-three-and-four-and . . .")	50% of compression/relaxation is downward to empty the heart; 50% of compression/relaxation is upward to fill the heart. With each compression, you want to squeeze the heart or increase pressure within the chest so that blood moves to the vital organs.
	Compress smoothly and evenly, keeping fingers off victim's ribs. The rescuer must apply enough force to depress the sternum 1½–2 inches (4–5 cm), at a rate of 80–100 compressions per minute.	

Performance Guidelines One-Rescuer CPR: Adult (continued)

Objectives	Critical Performance	Reason
15 compressions (9 to 11 seconds) and 2 ventilations	Ventilate properly: After every 15 compressions, deliver 2 rescue breaths.	Adequate oxygenation must be maintained.
At the end of 4 cycles (52–73 seconds), check for return of pulse for 5 seconds.	Check pulse. If no pulse, resume CPR. If there is a pulse but no breathing, give 1 rescue breath every 5 seconds (12 per minute).	To establish whether there is a spontaneous return of pulse or breathing.

Entrance of a 2nd Rescuer to Replace the 1st Rescuer

1st rescuer ends cycle with 2 breaths.

Second rescuer appears and identifies him or herself:
1) "I know CPR; can I help?"
2) checks pulse for 5 seconds.

If no pulse, second rescuer starts one-rescuer CPR with two breaths.

1st rescuer assesses the adequacy of 2nd rescuer by

- watching for chest to rise during rescue breaths
- checking the pulse during chest compressions.

Performance Guidelines Obstructed Airway: Conscious Adult

Objectives	Critical Performance	Reason
Rescuer must identify complete airway obstruction by determining if victim is able to speak or cough. Victim may be using the "Universal Distress Signal" of choking: clutching the neck between thumb and index finger.	Rescuer asks, "Are you choking?"	In the conscious victim it is essential to recognize the signs of an airway obstruction and take action immediately. If the victim is able to speak or cough effectively, do not interfere with his or her attempts to expel the foreign body. Continually check for success.
Perform the Heimlich maneuver (subdiaphragmatic abdominal thrusts) until the foreign body is expelled or the victim becomes unconscious.	SUBDIAPHRAGMATIC ABDOMINAL THRUSTS (the Heimlich maneuver): Stand behind victim and wrap your arms around victim's waist. Grasp one fist with your other hand and place thumb side of your fist in the midline slightly above the navel. Press fist into abdomen with quick inward and upward thrusts. Each abdominal thrust should be delivered decisively, with the intent of relieving the obstruction.	Such thrusts can force air upward into the airway from the lungs with enough pressure to expel the foreign body.
For victims in late pregnancy or who are obese:	CHEST THRUSTS: Stand behind victim and place your arms under victim's armpits to encircle the chest. Grasp one fist with other hand and place thumb side on the middle of the breastbone. Press with quick backward thrusts.	Chest thrusts are more easily done than abdominal thrusts when the abdominal girth is large, as in gross obesity or in advanced pregnancy.

Abdominal Thrust

Chest Thrust

Performance Guidelines Obstructed Airway: Conscious Adult Who Becomes Unconscious

Objectives	Critical Performance	Reason
Position the victim and get help. Activate the EMS system.	Turn victim on back as a unit, if necessary, supporting head and neck. Call out "Help!" Activate EMS; or if someone responds to call for help, send them.	The victim must be properly positioned on his or her back in case CPR becomes necessary. It is vitally important to gain access to advanced life support.

Performance Guidelines Obstructed Airway: Conscious Adult Who Becomes Unconscious
(continued)

Objectives	Critical Performance	Reason
Foreign body check.	Perform tongue-jaw lift. Sweep deeply into mouth to remove foreign body.	This can be done only in the unconscious victim.
Open airway and give rescue breaths.	Use head-tilt/chin-lift. Attempt rescue breathing.	Complete airway obstruction by a foreign body is assumed present, but at this point an attempt must be made to get some air into the lungs just in case the victim's fall has dislodged the foreign body.

Performance Guidelines Obstructed Airway: Conscious Adult Who Becomes Unconscious
(continued)

Objectives	Critical Performance	Reason
Airway remains obstructed? Give 6–10 abdominal thrusts.	SUBDIAPHRAGMATIC ABDOMINAL THRUSTS (the Heimlich maneuver): Straddle the victim's thighs. Place heel of one hand on the abdomen in the midline slightly above the navel and well below the tip of xiphoid. Place the second hand directly on top of the first hand. Press into the abdomen with quick upward thrusts. Perform 6–10 thrusts.	Such thrusts can force air upward into the airway from the lungs with enough pressure to expel the foreign body.
	Continually check for success. Each abdominal thrust should be delivered with the intent of relieving the obstruction.	
	(CHEST THRUSTS: Same hand position as that of for applying external chest compression. Exert quick downward thrust.)	Chest thrusts are preferred in the presence of large abdominal girth (advanced pregnancy or obesity). Downward thrusts generate effective airway pressure.
Check for foreign body using finger sweep.	Turn head up, open mouth with tongue-jaw lift technique and sweep deeply into mouth along cheek with hooked finger.	A dislodged foreign body may now be manually accessible if it has not been expelled. Dentures may need to be removed to improve finger sweep.

Performance Guidelines Obstructed Airway: Conscious Adult Who Becomes Unconscious
(continued)

Objectives	Critical Performance	Reason
Open airway and give rescue breaths.	Open airway by the head-tilt/chin-lift maneuver, and attempt rescue breathing.	By this time another attempt must be made to get some air into the lungs.
Repeat sequence until successful.	Alternate the above maneuvers in rapid sequence: • Abdominal thrusts • Finger sweep • Attempt rescue breathing	Persistent attempts are rapidly made in sequence in order to relieve the obstruction. As the victim becomes more deprived of oxygen, the muscles will relax and maneuvers that were previously ineffective may become effective.

Performance Guidelines Obstructed Airway: Unconscious Adult

Objectives	Critical Performance	Reason
Establish unresponsiveness, call for help, and position victim. Allow 4–10 seconds if turning is required.	Tap, gently shake shoulder, shout "Are you OK?" Call out "Help!" Turn on back as a unit, if necessary, supporting head and neck.	This initial call for help is to alert bystanders.

Performance Guidelines Obstructed Airway: Unconscious Adult (continued)

Objectives	Critical Performance	Reason
Open airway. Establish breathlessness.	Kneel properly. Head-tilt with one hand and chin-lift with other hand. Ear over mouth, observe chest: look, listen, and feel for breaths.	
Give rescue breaths.	Attempt rescue breathing.	Complete airway obstruction by a foreign body is assumed present, but at this point an attempt must be made to get some air into the lungs.
Airway remains obstructed? Open airway and give rescue breaths.	Reposition head; attempt again to give rescue breaths.	Improper head-tilt is the most common cause of airway obstruction.

Performance Guidelines Obstructed Airway: Unconscious Adult (continued)

Objectives	Critical Performance	Reason
Activate the EMS system.	If unsuccessful, and a second person is available, he or she should activate EMS system. Know your local EMS or rescue unit number.	Advanced life support capability may be required.
Give 6–10 subdiaphragmatic abdominal thrusts.	SUBDIAPHRAGMATIC ABDOMINAL THRUSTS (the Heimlich maneuver): Straddle the victim's thighs. Place heel of one hand on the abdomen midline slightly above the navel and well below the tip of the xiphoid. Place the second hand directly on top of the first hand. Press into the abdomen with quick upward thrusts. (CHEST THRUSTS: Same hand position as that for applying chest compression. Exert quick downward thrusts.)	Such thrusts can force air upward into the airway from the lungs with enough pressure to expel the foreign body. Chest thrusts are preferred in the presence of large abdominal girth (advanced pregnancy or obesity). Downward thrusts generate effective airway pressure.

Performance Guidelines Obstructed Airway: Unconscious Adult (continued)

Objectives	Critical Performance	Reason
Remove foreign body.	Turn head up, open mouth with tongue-jaw lift technique, and sweep deeply into mouth along cheek with hooked finger.	A dislodged foreign body may now be manually accessible if it has not been expelled. Dentures may need to be removed to improve finger sweep.
Open airway and give rescue breaths.	Reposition head using head-tilt/chin-lift. Attempt to give rescue breaths.	By this time another attempt must be made to get some air into the lungs.
Repeat sequence until successful.	If the airway remains obstructed, alternate the above maneuvers in rapid sequence: ■ Abdominal thrusts ■ Finger sweep ■ Attempt to ventilate	Persistent attempts are rapidly made in sequence in order to relieve the obstruction. As the victim becomes more deprived of oxygen, the muscles will relax and maneuvers that were previously ineffective may become effective.

- Looking at the eyes' pupils for their reaction to light. They will constrict (get smaller) if the brain is receiving oxygenated blood.

Remember to stop after the first minute and every few minutes thereafter to check the carotid pulse for the starting of a heartbeat. Be aware that this usually does not happen without advanced life support procedures. Your CPR effort serves as a holding action until advanced life support arrives.

When To Stop CPR

First aiders should continue resuscitation efforts until one of the following occurs:

1. Victim recovers (regains breathing and pulse).

2. Resuscitation efforts have been transferred to another responsible person, who continues efforts to resuscitate.

3. A physician or a physician-directed person or team assumes responsibility.

4. The victim is transferred to properly trained personnel charged with responsibilities for emergency medical services (EMS).

5. The rescuer is exhausted and unable to continue resuscitation.

Complications of CPR

Vomiting

Vomiting frequently happens while giving CPR. If vomiting occurs, turn the victim's head and body on the side to allow the vomitus to flow out of the mouth, wipe the victim's mouth, and then continue CPR.

Air in the Stomach

When the stomach is filled with large amounts of air, it bulges and appears bloated. This condition is known as stomach or gastric distention and happens more often in children than in adults. This condition can develop in three ways:

- Rescue breaths are given too fast.
- Rescue breaths are given too forcefully.
- The airway is partially or completely blocked so that the rescuer gives larger breaths to fill the victim's lungs, and air goes not only into the lungs, but also into the stomach.

The bloated stomach pushes up on the diaphragm and prevents the lungs from being fully inflated.

Large amounts of air in the stomach can cause vomiting. The vomited stomach contents could go into the lungs and lead to death.

Avoid breathing air into the stomach by: (1) not breathing too hard (use the rise and fall of the chest as a gauge); (2) not giving breaths too fast (pause between them so you can take another breath); and (3) properly tilting the head.

Do *not* relieve a bloated stomach by pressing the victim's abdomen, since he or she is certain to vomit—especially if the stomach is full. If vomiting does occur, follow the recommendations given in the previous section.

If severe gastric distention makes it difficult for a rescuer's breaths to enter the victim, turn the victim's head and body on the side and press the victim's abdomen. Expect vomiting to occur. If it does, follow the instructions given in the previous section.

Chest Compression-Related Injuries

Even properly performed chest compressions can injure a pulseless victim. The most common chest compression-related injuries include broken ribs and sternum, heart and lung contusions, and lacerations of the lung, liver and spleen. Prevent injuries by properly performing CPR. Despite the possibility of injury, do *not* stop or deviate from properly giving CPR, since the alternative would mean death for a victim.

Risks of Performing CPR

No instance is known in which a lay person who has performed CPR reasonably has been successfully sued.

To date, no evidence exists that AIDS is transmitted by casual personal contact, by indirect contact with inanimate surfaces, or by the airborne route. The risk of transmission of any infectious disease by manikin practice appears to be low. No documented case of transmission of bacterial, fungal, or viral disease by a CPR training manikin exists.

Child and Infant Resuscitation

Events necessitating resuscitation in children include: (1) injuries, (2) suffocation caused by foreign objects, (3) smoke inhalation, (4) sudden infant death syndrome, (5) infections of the respiratory tract, and (6) drownings.

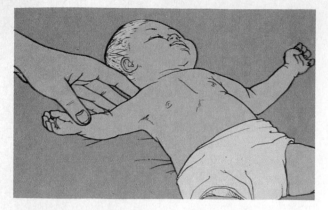

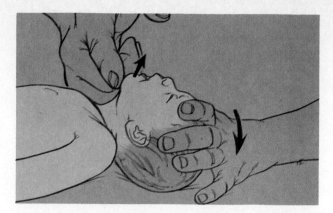

1. **Check for unresponsiveness.** Check a child's or an infant's unconsciousness by gently shaking.

2. **Shout for help.** If the first aider is alone and the child is not breathing, perform CPR for one minute before calling for help.

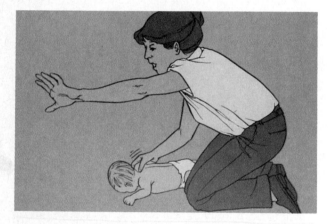

3. **Position the victim.** Carefully position the child on his or her back on a firm, flat surface. If a head or neck injury is suspected, carefully place the child on his or her back. Turn the entire body as one unit, with the head and neck firmly supported. Don't let the head roll, twist, or tilt backward or forward, especially if you think the head or neck is injured.

4. **Open the airway.** Open the child's airway so air can get to his or her lungs. How you do this depends on whether you think the child's neck may be injured:

- **If there is any sign of neck injury.** The safest way to open the airway is to move the lower jaw forward without tilting the head. Rest your elbows on the surface the child is lying on. Place two or three fingers under each side of the child's jaw, just beneath the ears, and lift the jaw upward.
- **If you are sure the neck is not injured:** Place one hand on the child's forehead and hook the fingers, not the thumb, of the other hand under the bony tip of the child's chin. Lift the chin gently while pressing down on the

forehead. Tilt the head gently back, taking care not to close the mouth.

5. **Check for breathlessness.** If you are unsure whether the child is breathing, place your ear close to his mouth and nose. Listen and feel for exhaled air. At the same time, look at the chest and stomach for movement.

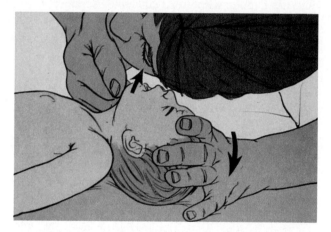

6. **Give two breaths.** If the child is breathing, keep the airway open. If she is not breathing, you must breathe for her.

- **For an infant:** Cover the mouth and nose with your mouth. Be sure your lips make a tight seal. Also be sure to support the tip of the baby's chin with your finger. Without this support, you won't be able to get air into the

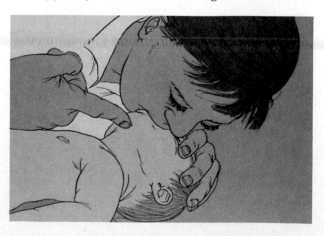

baby's lungs. Gently blow a little air into the infant's mouth and nose—just enough to make the baby's chest rise. If you breathe too hard, you may hurt the infant's lungs. Breathe slowly to give enough air at the lowest possible pressure. Give two slow breaths to the child, between 1 and 1½ seconds per breath— then pause to give yourself time to take another breath. Repeat.

- **For an older child:** Pinch the nose tightly with the fingers of the hand resting on the forehead. Take a breath and seal the child's mouth with yours. Give two slow breaths to the child—between 1 and 1½ seconds per breath—and pause to give yourself time to take another breath. Repeat.

7. *Check for a pulse.*

- **For an infant:** Infants younger than one year of age have short, chubby necks, making the carotid pulse difficult to locate. Therefore, use the pulse in the upper arm (brachial pulse) instead. Its location can be found on the inside of the upper arm between the elbow and the shoulder. Place your thumb on the outside of the arm and press gently with your index and middle fingers on the inside of the arm to feel the pulse. Do this for 5 to 10 seconds.

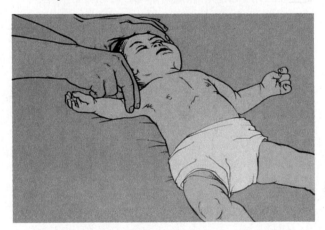

- **For an older child:** Check the carotid pulse the way you would for an adult. Locate the Adam's apple with the index and middle fingers of one hand while keeping the head tilted back with a hand on the forehead. Then slide your fingers toward you into the groove next to the windpipe at the side of the neck. Gently press to feel for a pulse. Do this for 5 to 10 seconds.

8. *Phone the EMS system.*

If a person arrives to help, have him or her call the local emergency telephone number. If this person is trained, he or she could relieve you while you call for help. If unable to telephone for help, the only option is to continue CPR.

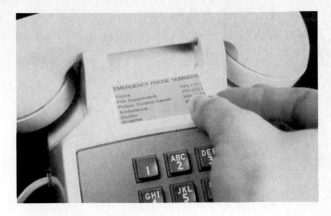

9. *Compress the chest.*

- **For an infant.** If there is no pulse, place two fingers on his or her breastbone, one finger-width below the nipple line, and give five chest compressions for every breath. Compressions should be a half to one inch deep. All five should be given in the three-second interval between each breath (100 times per minute, or 5 in 3 seconds). The count will go quickly— one, two, three, four, five, PUFF.

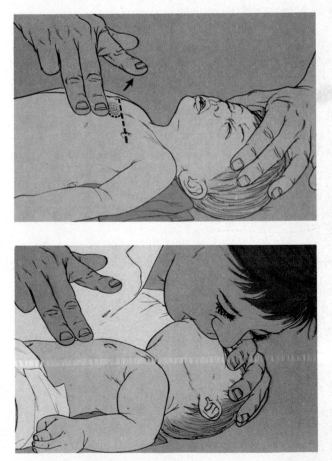

- **For a child.** Locate the lower edges of the rib cage to the "notch" where the ribs meet the breastbone in the center of the lower part of the chest. Place the middle finger on the notch, then the index finger next to it.

TABLE 3-1 Variations in CPR Techniques for the Infant, Child, and Adult

Age	Infant 0–1 yr	Child 1–8 yr.	Adult < 8 yr.
Shake and shout	Shake only	Yes	Yes
Call for help	Yes	Yes	Yes
Position victim	Yes	Yes	Yes
Open airway	Yes	Yes	Yes
Look, listen, feel for breath	Yes	Yes	Yes
Two breaths	Yes	Yes	Yes
Check pulse	Brachial	Carotid	Carotid
Activate EMS	Yes	Yes	Yes
Locate hand position	Lower sternum	Lower sternum	Lower sternum
Compress with	2–3 fingers	Heel of one hand	Heel of two hands
Compression depth	½–1 inch	1–1½ inches	1½–2 inches
Compressions per minute	At least 100	80–100	80–100
Compression:ventilation ratio	5:1	5:1	15:2 or 5:1*

*Rates for one-rescuer (15:2) and two-rescuer (5:1) adult CPR.

Source: American Heart Association; used with permission.

Place the heel of your other hand on the breastbone next to the index finger you used to find the "notch." Keep fingers off the chest. The chest is compressed with one hand to the depth of 1 to 1½ inches at a rate of 80 to 100 times per minute (5 per 3–4 seconds). Give one breath every five compressions. If the child is large or older than about eight years, the method described for adults should be used. Compressions should be smooth, not jerky.

Child and Infant Choking

For a child over one year:

1. *Victim standing or sitting (conscious).* Stand behind the victim and wrap your arms around the victim's waist. Make a fist with one hand. Place the fist's thumb side against the victim's abdomen, slightly above the navel and well below the tip of the breastbone. Grasp your fist with the other hand. Press the fist into the victim's abdomen with a quick, upward thrust.

2. *Victim lying (conscious or unconscious).* Place the victim on his or her back with the face up. Straddle the victim's thighs. Place the heel of one hand against the victim's abdomen, slightly above the navel and well below the tip of the breastbone. Place the other hand directly on top of the first hand. Press into the abdomen with a quick, upward thrust.

For a child less than one year old:

1. Place the baby on your forearm, face down and with his/her head down low. Rest your forearm on your thigh for support.

2. Using the heel of your hand, hit the baby four times on the back, high between the shoulder blades.

Food Choking in Children

Foods causing choking in children, ages 9 and under, ranked in descending order:

> Hot dogs
> Candy
> Peanuts
> Grapes

> —*Journal of the American Medical Association*

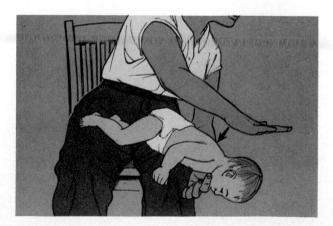

3. If he/she is not yet breathing, support the head and neck and place him/her on the thigh with the head lower than the trunk and give four chest thrusts. These chest thrusts are performed in the same location as external chest compressions but at a slower rate.

Repeat this sequence of back blows and chest compressions until the airway opens or medical help arrives.

Avoid blind finger sweeps in infants and children since the foreign object may be pushed back into the airway, causing further blockage. Remove a foreign object from the mouth *only if it can be seen*.

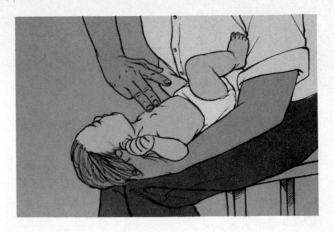

Choking—Causes and Precautions

Obstruction of the airway by choking usually occurs during eating. The National Safety Council reports that choking accounts for about 3,500 deaths yearly.

In adults, meat is the most common cause of choking. Common factors associated with choking on food include: (1) large, poorly chewed pieces of food, (2) alcohol consumption, and (3) dentures. Choking, when it occurs in restaurants, has been mistaken for a heart attack, giving rise to the name "cafe coronary."

The following precautions may prevent choking:

1. Cutting food into small pieces and chewing slowly and thoroughly, especially if wearing dentures.

2. Avoiding laughing and talking during chewing and swallowing.

3. Avoiding excessive intake of alcohol before and during meals.

4. Preventing children from walking, running, or playing with food or foreign objects in their mouths.

5. Keeping foreign objects (e.g., marbles, beads, thumbtacks) away from infants and small children.

—*American Heart Association*

	Objectives	Actions		
		Adult (over 8 yrs.)	**Child** (1 to 8 yrs.)	**Infant** (under 1 yr.)
A. Airway	1. Assessment: Determine unresponsiveness	Tap or gently shake shoulder.		
		Say, "Are you okay?"		Observe
	2. Get help	Call out, "Help!"		
	3. Position the victim.	Turn on back as a unit, supporting head and neck if necessary. (4–10 seconds)		
	4. Open the airway.	Head-tilt/chin-lift		
B. Breathing	5. Assessment: Determine breathlessness.	Maintain open airway. Place ear over mouth, observing chest. Look, listen, feel for breathing. (3–5 seconds)		
	6. Give 2 rescue breaths.	Maintain open airway.		
		Seal mouth to mouth		mouth to nose/mouth
		Give 2 rescue breaths, 1 to 1½ seconds each. Observe chest rise. Allow lung deflation between breaths.		
	7. Option for obstructed airway	**a.** Reposition victim's head. Try again to give rescue breaths.		
		b. Activate the EMS system.		
		c. Give 6–10 subdiaphragmatic abdominal thrusts (the Heimlich maneuver).		Give 4 back blows.
				Give 4 chest thrusts.
		d. Tongue-jaw lift and finger sweep	Tongue-jaw lift, but finger sweep only if you see a foreign object.	
		If unsuccessful, repeat a, c, and d until successful.		
C. Circulation	8. Assessment: Determine pulselessness.	Feel for carotid pulse with one hand; maintain head-tilt with the other. (5–10 seconds)		Feel for brachial pulse; keep head-tilt.
	9. Activate EMS system.	If someone responded to call for help, send them to activate the EMS system.		
	Begin chest compressions: 10. Landmark check	Run middle finger along bottom edge of rib cage to notch at center (tip of sternum).		Imagine a line drawn between the nipples.
	11. Hand position	Place index finger next to finger on notch:		Place 2–3 fingers on sternum, 1 finger's width below line. Depress ½–1 in.
		Two hands next to index finger. Depress 1½–2 in.	Heel of one hand next to index finger. Depress 1–1½ in.	
	12. Compression rate	80–100 per minute		At least 100 per minute
CPR Cycles	13. Compressions to breaths.	2 breaths to every 15 compressions.	1 breath to every 5 compressions.	
	14. Number of cycles.	4 (52–73 seconds)	10 (60–87 seconds)	10 (45 seconds or less)
	15. Reassessment.	Feel for carotid pulse. (5 seconds)		Feel for brachial pulse.
		If no pulse, resume CPR, starting with 2 breaths.	If no pulse, resume CPR, starting with 1 breath.	
Option for pulse return	If no breathing, give rescue breaths.	1 breath every 5 seconds	1 breath every 4 seconds	1 breath every 3 seconds

Foreign Body Airway Obstruction Management

	Objectives	Actions		
		Adult (over 8 yrs.)	**Child** (1 to 8 yrs.)	**Infant** (under 1 yr.)
Conscious Victim	1. Assessment: Determine airway obstruction.	Ask, "Are you choking?" Determine if victim can cough or speak.		Observe breathing difficulty.
	2. Act to relieve obstruction.	Perform subdiaphragmatic abdominal thrusts (Heimlich maneuver).		Give 4 back blows.
				Give 4 chest thrusts.
	Be persistent.	Repeat Step 2 until obstruction is relieved or victim becomes unconscious.		
Victim Who Becomes Unconscious	3. Position the victim; call for help.	Turn on back as a unit, supporting head and neck, face up, arms by sides. Call out, "Help!" If others come, activate EMS.		
	4. Check for foreign body.	Perform tongue-jaw lift and finger sweep.	Perform tongue-jaw lift. Remove foreign object only if you actually see it.	
	5. Give rescue breaths.	Open the airway with head-tilt/chin-lift. Try to give rescue breaths.		
	6. Act to relieve obstruction.	Perform subdiaphragmatic abdominal thrusts (Heimlich maneuver).		Give 4 back blows.
				Give 4 chest thrusts.
	7. Check for foreign body.	Perform tongue-jaw lift and finger sweep.	Perform tongue-jaw lift. Remove foreign object only if you actually see it.	
	8. Try again to give rescue breaths.	Open the airway with head-tilt/chin-lift. Try to give rescue breaths.		
	9. Be persistent.	Repeat Steps 6–8 until obstruction is relieved.		
Unconscious Victim	1. Assessment: Determine unresponsiveness.	Tap or gently shake shoulder. Shout, "Are you okay?"		Tap or gently shake shoulder.
	2. Call for help; position the victim.	Turn on back as a unit, supporting head and neck, face up, arms by sides. Call out, "Help!" If others come, activate EMS.		
	3. Open the airway.	Head-tilt/chin-lift		Head-tilt/chin-lift, but do not tilt too far.
	4. Assessment: Determine breathlessness	Maintain an open airway. Ear over mouth; observe chest. Look, listen, feel for breathing. (3–5 seconds)		
	5. Give rescue breaths.	Make mouth-to-mouth seal.		Make mouth-to-nose-and-mouth seal.
		Try to give rescue breaths.		
	6. Try again to give rescue breaths.	Reposition head. Try rescue breaths again.		
	7. Activate the EMS system.	If someone responded to the call for help, that person should activate the EMS system.		
	8. Act to relieve obstruction.	Perform subdiaphragmatic abdominal thrusts (Heimlich maneuver).		Give 4 back blows.
				Give 4 chest thrusts.
	9. Check for foreign body.	Perform tongue-jaw lift and finger sweep.	Perform tongue-jaw lift. Remove foreign object only if you actually see it.	
	10. Rescue breaths.	Open the airway with head-tilt/chin-lift. Try again to give rescue breaths.		
	11. Be persistent.	Repeat Steps 8–10 until obstruction is relieved.		

CPR and ECC Performance Sheet One-Rescuer CPR: Adult

Step	Activity	Critical Performance	S	U
1. Airway	Assessment: Determine unresponsiveness	Tap or gently shake shoulder		
		Shout, "Are you OK?"		
	Call for help	Call out, "Help!"		
	Position the victim.	Turn on back as unit, if necessary, supporting head and neck (4–10 sec).		
	Open the airway.	Use head-tilt/chin-lift maneuver.		
2. Breathing	Assessment: Determine breathlessness.	Maintain open airway.		
		Ear over mouth, observe chest: look, listen, feel for breathing (3–5 sec.)		
	Ventilate twice.	Maintain open airway.		
		Seal mouth and nose properly.		
		Ventilate 2 times at 1–1.5 sec/inspiration.		
		Observe chest rise (adequate ventilation volume).		
		Allow deflation between breaths.		
3. Circulation	Assessment: Determine pulselessness.	Feel for carotid pulse on near side of victim (5–10 sec).		
		Maintain head-tilt with other hand.		
	Activate EMS system.	If someone responded to call for help, send him/her to activate EMS system.		
		Total time, Step 1—Activate EMS system: 15–35 sec.		
	Begin chest compressions.	Rescuer kneels by victim's shoulders.		
		Landmark check prior to hand placement.		
		Proper hand position throughout.		
		Rescuer's shoulders over victim's sternum.		
		Equal compression—relaxation.		
		Compress 1½ to 2 inches.		
		Keep hands on sternum during upstroke.		
		Complete chest relaxation on upstroke.		
		Say any helpful mnemonic.		
		Compression rate: 100/min (15 per 9–11 sec).		
4. Compression/Ventilation Cycles	Do 4 cycles of 15 compressions and 2 ventilations.	Proper compression/ventilation ratio: 15 compressions to 2 ventilations per cycle.		
		Observe chest rise: 1–1.5 sec/inspiration; 4 cycles/52–73 sec.		
5. Reassessment*	Determine pulselessness. (If no pulse: Step 6.)†	Feel for carotid pulse (5 sec).		
6. Continue CPR	Ventilate twice.	Ventilate 2 times.		
		Observe chest rise; 1–1.5 sec/inspiration.		
	Resume compression/ventilation cycles.	Feel for carotid pulse every few minutes.		

* 2nd rescuer arrives to replace 1st rescuer: (a) 2nd rescuer identifies self by saying, "I know CPR. Can I help?" (b) 2nd rescuer then does pulse check in Step 5 and continues with Step 6. (During practice and testing only one rescuer actually ventilates the manikin. The 2nd rescuer simulates ventilation.) (c) 1st rescuer assesses the adequacy of 2nd rescuer's CPR by observing chest rise during ventilations and by checking the pulse during chest compressions.

† If pulse is present, open airway and check for spontaneous breathing: (a) If breathing is present, maintain open airway and monitor pulse and breathing. (b) If breathing is absent, perform rescue breathing at 12 times/min and monitor pulse.

Instructor _____ Check: Satisfactory _____ Unsatisfactory _____

BLS Performance Sheet Child One-Rescuer CPR*

Step	Objective	Critical Performance	S	U
1. Airway	Assessment: Determine unresponsiveness.	Tap or gently shake shoulder.		
		Shout, ''Are you OK?''		
	Call for help.	Call out, ''Help!''		
	Position the victim.	Turn on back as unit, if necessary, supporting head and neck (4–10 sec).		
	Open the airway.	Use head-tilt/chin-lift maneuver.		
2. Breathing	Assessment: Determine breathlessness.	Maintain open airway.		
		Ear over mouth, observe chest: look, listen, feel for breathing (3–5 sec).		
	Ventilate twice.	Maintain open airway.		
		Seal mouth and nose properly.		
		Ventilate 2 times at 1–1.5 sec/inspiration.		
		Observe chest rise.		
		Allow deflation between breaths.		
3. Circulation	Assessment: Determine pulselessness.	Feel for carotid pulse on near side of victim (5–10 sec).		
		Maintain head-tilt with other hand.		
	Activate EMS system.	If someone responded to call for help, send him/her to activate EMS system.		
		Total time, Step 1—Activate EMS system: 15–35 sec.		
	Begin chest compressions.	Rescuer kneels by victim's shoulders.		
		Landmark check prior to initial hand placement.§		
		Proper hand position throughout.		
		Rescuer's shoulders over victim's sternum.		
		Equal compression—relaxation.		
		Compress 1 to 1½ inches.		
		Keep hand on sternum during upstroke.		
		Complete chest relaxation on upstroke.		
		Say any helpful mnemonic.		
		Compression rate: 80–100/min (5 per 3–4 sec).		
4. Compression/Ventilation Cycles	Do 10 cycles of 5 compressions and 1 ventilation.	Proper compression/ventilation ratio: 5 compressions to 1 slow ventilation per cycle.		
		Observe chest rise: 1–1.5 sec/inspiration (10 cycles/60–87 sec.)		
5. Reassessment†	Determine pulselessness.	Feel for carotid pulse (5 sec).‡ If there is no pulse, go to Step 6.		
6. Continue CPR	Ventilate once.	Ventilate 1 time.		
		Observe chest rise: 1–1.5 sec/inspiration.		
	Resume compression/ventilation cycles.	Feel for carotid pulse every few minutes.		

* If child is above age of approximately 8 years, the method for adults should be used.

† 2nd rescuer arrives to replace 1st rescuer: (a) 2nd rescuer identifies self by saying, ''I know CPR. Can I help?'' (b) 2nd rescuer then does pulse check in Step 5 and continues with Step 6. (During practice and testing only one rescuer actually ventilates the manikin. The 2nd rescuer simulates ventilation.) (c) 1st rescuer assesses the adequacy of 2nd rescuer's CPR by observing chest rise during ventilations and by checking the pulse during chest compressions.

‡ If pulse is present, open airway and check for spontaneous breathing. (a) If breathing is present, maintain open airway and monitor breathing and pulse. (b) If breathing is absent, perform rescue breathing at 15 times/min and monitor pulse.

§ Thereafter, check hand position visually.

Instructor _____ Check: Satisfactory _____ Unsatisfactory _____

CPR and ECC Performance Sheet One-Rescuer CPR: Infant

Step	Activity	Critical Performance	S	U
1. Airway	Assessment: Determine unresponsiveness.	Tap or gently shake shoulder.		
	Call for help.	Call out, ''Help!''		
	Position the infant.	Turn on back as unit, supporting head and neck.		
		Place on firm, hard surface.		
	Open the airway.	Use head-tilt/chin-lift maneuver to sniffing or neutral position.		
		Do not overextend the head.		
2. Breathing	Assessment: Determine breathlessness.	Maintain open airway.		
		Ear over mouth, observe chest: look, listen, feel for breathing (3–5 sec).		
	Ventilate twice.	Maintain open airway.		
		Make tight seal on infant's mouth and nose with rescuer's mouth.		
		Ventilate 2 times, 1–1.5 sec/inspiration.		
		Observe chest rise.		
		Allow deflation between breaths.		
3. Circulation	Assessment: Determine pulselessness.	Feel for carotid pulse (5–10 sec).		
		Maintain head-tilt with other hand.		
	Activate EMS system.	If someone responded to call for help, send him/her to activate EMS system.		
		Total time, Step 1—Activate EMS system: 15–35 sec.		
	Begin chest compressions.	Draw imaginary line between nipples.		
		Place 2–3 fingers on sternum, 1 finger's width below imaginary line.		
		Equal compression-relaxation.		
		Compress vertically, ½ to 1 inches.		
		Keep fingers on sternum during upstroke.		
		Complete chest relaxation on upstroke.		
		Say any helpful mnemonic.		
		Compression rate: at least 100/min (5 in 3 sec or less).		
4. Compression/Ventilation Cycles	Do 10 cycles of 5 compressions and 1 slow ventilation.	Proper compression/ventilation ratio: 5 compressions to 1 slow ventilation per cycle.		
		Pause for ventilation.		
		Observe chest rise: 1–1.5 sec/inspiration; 10 cycles/45 sec or less.		
5. Reassessment	Determine pulselessness. (If no pulse: Step 6.)*	Feel for brachial pulse (5 sec.)		
6. Continue CPR	Ventilate once.	Ventilate 1 time.		
		Observe chest rise; 1–1.5 sec/inspiration.		
	Resume compression/ventilation cycles.	Feel for brachial pulse every few minutes.		

* If pulse is present, open airway and check for spontaneous breathing. (a) If breathing is present, maintain open airway and monitor breathing and pulse (b) If breathing is absent, perform rescue breathing at 20 times/min and monitor pulse.

Instructor _____ Check: Satisfactory _____ Unsatisfactory _____

Name __Rebecca Henf__ Course __First Aid/CPR__ Date __9-13-91__

■ ACTIVITY 1 ■ Adult Resuscitation

Choose the best answer.

1. __B__ Are chest compressions likely to work if the victim is on a soft surface?
    A. Yes, a soft surface is okay.
    B. No, the surface should be hard.

2. __B__ When you tip the head with the chin lift, where do you place your fingertips?
    A. Under the soft part of the throat near the chin
    B. Under the bony part of the jaw near the chin

3. __A__ Which is the safer way to open the airway of a person who may have neck or back injuries?
    A. Push the jaw forward from the corners.
    B. Tip the head very gently, part way back.

4. __A__ How should you check for stopped breathing?
    A. Look at the chest; listen and feel for air coming out of the mouth.
    B. Look at the pupils of the eyes.
    C. Check the pulse.

5. __A__ When you give breaths to an adult, the breaths should be:
    A. Large and full
    B. Fast and full

6. __B__ Before deciding whether to give CPR, check the victim's pulse for:
    A. 1–3 seconds   B. 3–5 seconds
    C. 5–10 seconds   D. 1–20 seconds

7. __B__ To find where to push on the chest for chest compressions, you should measure up:
    A. Two hand-widths from the navel.
    B. One finger-width from the middle finger on the sternal notch.

8. __B__ Give chest compressions:
    A. With a quick jerk
    B. Smoothly and regularly

9. __B__ Push on a victim's chest:
    A. At an angle
    B. Straight down

10. __B__ Compress an adult's chest at least:
    A. ½ to 1 inch
    B. 1½ to 2 inches

11. ____ In one-rescuer CPR, give chest compressions to an adult at the rate, per minute, of:
    A. 100
    B. 80
    C. 60
    D. 40

12. __A__ What is the pattern of compressions and breaths in one-rescuer CPR for an adult victim?
    A. 15 compressions, 2 breaths
    B. 15 compressions, 1 breath
    C. 5 compressions, 2 breaths
    D. 5 compressions, 1 breath

■ ACTIVITY 2 ■ Adult Choking

Choose the best answer.

1. __B__ An adult victim is coughing forcefully. Should you give back blows and thrusts?
    A. Yes
    B. No

2. __A__ A person is coughing weakly and making wheezing noises. You should:
    A. Give abdominal thrusts.
    B. Let the person alone and watch closely.

3. __B__ A victim who seems to be choking *can* speak. Should you give abdominal thrusts?
    A. Yes
    B. No

4. __A__ A conscious person is coughing forcefully, trying to dislodge an object. Then the person stops coughing and cannot speak. You should:
    A. Give abdominal thrusts.
    B. Let the person alone and watch closely.

5. __C__ When you give abdominal thrusts to a conscious victim, what part of your fist do you place against the victim?
   A. The palm side
   B. The little finger side
   C. The thumb side

6. __A__ Give abdominal thrusts quickly:
   A. Inward and upward
   B. Straight back

7. __B__ Where do you place your fist to give abdominal thrusts?
   A. Over the breastbone
   B. Slightly above the navel
   C. Below the navel

8. __A__ To give abdominal thrusts to a victim who is lying down, place the heel of one hand:
   A. Slightly above the navel
   B. On the edge of the breastbone
   C. Below the navel

9. __B__ For a victim who is obese or in advanced pregnancy, it is better to give:
   A. Abdominal thrusts
   B. Chest thrusts

■ ACTIVITY 3 ■ Child and Infant Resuscitation

Choose the best answer.

1. __A__ How should you check for stopped breathing?
   A. Look at the chest; listen and feel for air coming out of the mouth.
   B. Look at the pupils of the eyes.
   C. Check the pulse.

2. __B__ If your amount of breath is enough:
   A. The stomach will form a pouch.
   B. The chest will rise.
   C. Your air backs up against incoming air.

3. __A__ Check a baby's pulse at the:
   A. Middle of the upper arm
   B. Wrist
   C. Neck

4. __A__ To give a baby chest compressions use:
   A. 2 or 3 fingers
   B. The heel of one hand

5. __B__ Push on the chest of a child or baby one finger-width:
   A. Above nipple line
   B. Below nipple line
   C. Above xiphoid notch

6. __B__ How far should you compress a baby's chest?
   A. 1½ to 2 inches
   B. ½ to 1 inch

7. __A__ Give a baby chest compressions at the rate per minute, of:
   A. 100
   B. 80
   C. 60

8. __D__ Give babies and children:
   A. 15 compressions, 2 breaths
   B. 5 compressions, 2 breaths
   C. 15 compressions, 1 breath
   D. 5 compressions, 1 breath

9. __A__ When giving chest compressions to a child, use:
   A. 2 or 3 fingers or heel of one hand
   B. The heel of one hand and the other hand on top

■ ACTIVITY 4 ■ Child and Infant Choking

Choose the best answer.

1. __D__ You believe a baby has an object caught in its airway; it cannot cough or cry. What do you do first?
   A. Let it alone and watch closely.
   B. Give abdominal thrusts.
   C. Give chest thrusts.
   D. Give back blows.

2. __B__ Use your finger to remove an object from an unconscious baby or child's mouth:
   A. Whenever back blows and chest thrusts fail
   B. Only if you see the object

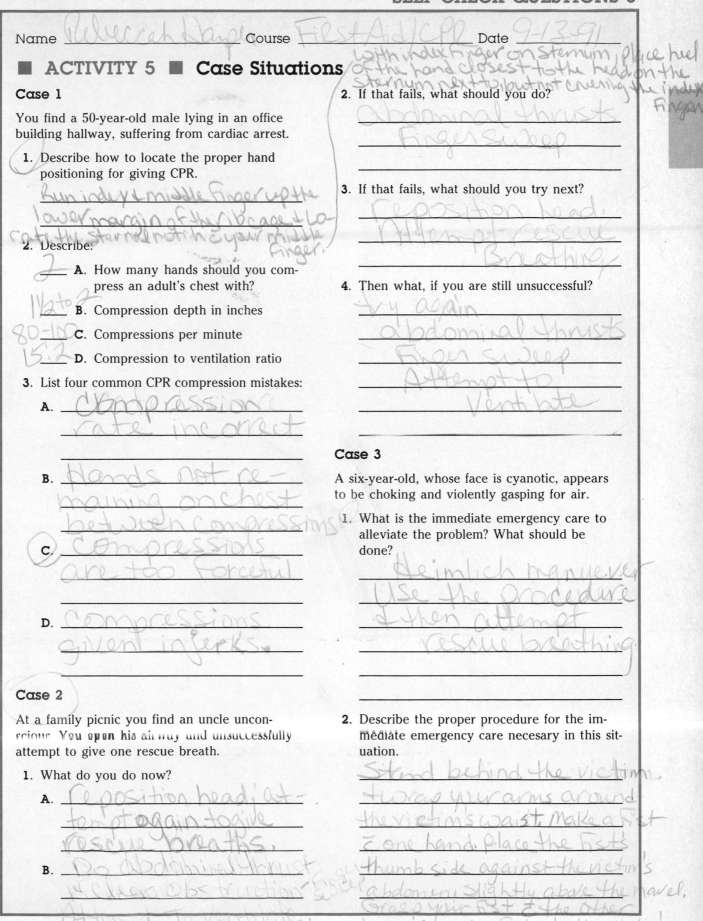

Name *Rebecca Day*   Course *First Aid/CPR*   Date *9-13-91*

■ ACTIVITY 5 ■ Case Situations

Case 1

You find a 50-year-old male lying in an office building hallway, suffering from cardiac arrest.

1. Describe how to locate the proper hand positioning for giving CPR.

   Run index & middle finger up the lower margin of the rib cage & to locate the sternal notch w/ your middle finger.

2. Describe:

   2   A. How many hands should you compress an adult's chest with?

   1½ to 2   B. Compression depth in inches

   80-100   C. Compressions per minute

   15:2   D. Compression to ventilation ratio

3. List four common CPR compression mistakes:

   A. *Compression rate incorrect*

   B. *Hands not remaining on chest between compressions*

   C. *Compressions are too forceful*

   D. *Compressions given in jerks.*

Case 2

At a family picnic you find an uncle unconscious. You open his airway and unsuccessfully attempt to give one rescue breath.

1. What do you do now?

   A. *reposition head, attempt again to give rescue breaths.*

   B. *Do abdominal thrust & clean obstruction, Finger sweep, Attempt to ventilate.*

2. If that fails, what should you do?

   Abdominal thrusts Finger sweep

   With index finger on sternum, place heel of the hand closest to the head on the sternum next to but not covering the index finger

3. If that fails, what should you try next?

   reposition head, Attempt rescue breathing,

4. Then what, if you are still unsuccessful?

   try again abdominal thrusts Finger sweep Attempt to ventilate

Case 3

A six-year-old, whose face is cyanotic, appears to be choking and violently gasping for air.

1. What is the immediate emergency care to alleviate the problem? What should be done?

   Heimlich maneuver Use the procedure & then attempt rescue breathing.

2. Describe the proper procedure for the immediate emergency care necesary in this situation.

   Stand behind the victim, wrap your arms around the victim's waist. Make a fist c̄ one hand. Place the fist's thumb side against the victim's abdomen, slightly above the navel. Grasp your fist & the other hand. Press the fist into the victim's abdomen with a quick, upward thrust.

49

SELF-CHECK QUESTIONS 3

Case 4

A frantic mother calls to report that her infant suddenly has stopped breathing. Within minutes, you cross the street to her house and find the mother giving mouth-to-mouth breathing. A check of the infant's pulse reveals no pulse.

1. What is the immediate emergency care in this situation?

   To get the ~~st~~ a pulse. Keep doing CPR. Check for Any blockage, reposition head (in case your air isn't going thru) Check other signs of death.

2. For an infant, how many cardiac compressions per minute should you complete?

   ____ A. 60–80

   ____ B. 80–100

   ✓ C. 100–120

3. For a small infant, how many inches down should you compress the chest wall?

   ____ A. ¼

   ____ B. ¼ to ½

   ✓ C. ½ to 1

   ____ D. 1 to 1½

4. When taking an infant's pulse, the best location to use is the:

   ____ A. carotid artery

   ____ B. left nipple

   ✓ C. brachial artery

   ____ D. femoral artery

Hypovolemic Shock

Shock refers to circulatory system failure, which occurs when oxygenated blood and nutrients are not provided in sufficient amounts for every body part. Every injury affects the circulatory system to some degree. Therefore, first aiders should automatically treat injured victims for shock. The damage produced by shock depends on which body part is deprived of oxygen and how long it is deprived. For example, without oxygen the brain will be irreparably damaged in 4 to 6 minutes, the abdominal organs in 45 to 90 minutes, and the skin and muscle cells in three to six hours.

To understand shock and its causes, think of the circulatory system as having three components: a working pump (the heart), a network of pipes (the blood vessels), and an adequate amount of fluid (the blood) pumped through the pipes. Damage to any of these components can impair circulation of blood within the tissues and produce the condition known as shock.

The types of shock can be classified according to which component has failed.

1. **Pump failure. Cardiogenic shock** results from a failure of the heart to pump sufficient blood. For example, a major heart attack can cause severe damage to the heart muscle so that the heart cannot squeeze and thereby cannot push the blood through the blood vessels (pipes).

2. **Fluid loss. Hypovolemic shock** happens with the loss of a significant amount of fluid from the system. If the lost fluid is blood, this type of shock is best known as **hemorrhagic shock.** People experiencing dehydration due to vomiting, diarrhea, diabetes, insufficient fluid intake, or misuse of diuretics can lose large amounts of fluid. Profuse sweating can also result in a sizable amount of fluid loss.

3. **Pipe failure.** Blood vessels may enlarge and the blood supply may be insufficient to fill them when the nervous system is damaged, as when a spinal cord is damaged or when the victim takes an overdose of certain drugs. This is known as **neurogenic shock.**

Septic shock develops in some victims with bacterial infection when damaged blood vessels lose their ability to contract. First aiders seldom see this type of shock since victims are usually already hospitalized for a serious illness, injury, or operation.

Hypovolemic Shock results from blood or fluid loss. It is the most common form and its first aid procedures apply to the other forms of shock except anaphylactic shock (severe allergic reaction) and psychogenic shock.

Signs and Symptoms

- Rapid breathing and pulse
- Pale or bluish skin, nailbed, and lips
- Slow capillary filling time
- Cool and wet (clammy) skin
- Heavy sweating
- Dilated (enlarged) pupils
- Dull, sunken look to the eyes
- Thirst
- Nausea and vomiting
- Loss of consciousness in severe shock

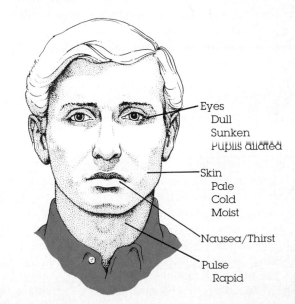

Eyes
Dull
Sunken
Pupils dilated

Skin
Pale
Cold
Moist

Nausea/Thirst

Pulse
Rapid

Signs and symptoms of shock

First Aid

Even if signs and symptoms have not appeared in a severely injured victim, treat for shock. **First aiders can prevent shock; they cannot reverse it.**

- Care for life-threatening injuries and other severe injuries.
- Elevate the legs 8–12 inches unless the injury makes this impossible or unless it is not advised because of chest injuries, unconsciousness, etc. Elevating the legs allows the blood to drain from the legs back to the heart more readily. Do *not* raise the legs more than 12 inches since it affects the victim's breathing by having the abdominal organs push up against the diaphragm. Do *not* lift the foot of a bed or stretcher because breathing will be affected and the blood flow from the brain may be retarded and lead to brain swelling.
- Keep the victim on his or her back. Exceptions are:

  1. Those with head injuries or stroke victims who should have their heads slightly raised if no spine injury is suspected.

  2. Those with breathing difficulties, chest injuries, or a heart attack should be in a semi-sitting position. This helps breathing.

  3. An unconscious, semiconscious, or vomiting victim should lie on his or her side.

- Prevent body heat loss by putting blankets under and over the victim. Do *not* attempt to warm the victim unless he or she is hypothermic.
- Do *not* give the victim anything to eat or drink. It could induce nausea and vomiting, which could be inhaled. This may cause later complications if surgery is needed. If a long distance from a medical facility, allow the victim to suck on a clean cloth soaked in water to relieve a dry mouth.
- Handle the victim very gently.

Fainting

Psychogenic shock (fainting) involves a sudden, temporary loss of consciousness. Fainting is the least serious type of shock. It occurs when the brain's blood flow is interrupted. Numerous causes account for this interruption, the most common being a jolting psychological disturbance, such as seeing blood or hearing unpleasant news. The nervous system dilates blood vessels three to four times their normal size and allows blood to pool. Another type of fainting occurs as the result of spending a long time in an upright position with little movement; for instance, soldiers sometimes faint after standing at attention for a considerable period of time. In such cases blood accumulates in the legs and

does not circulate properly. Other causes of fainting include epilepsy, heart disorder, and cerebrovascular disease.

Signs and Symptoms

Fainting may occur suddenly or may be preceded by warning signs including any or all of the following:

- Dizziness
- Seeing spots
- Nausea
- Paleness
- Sweating

First Aid

When a person appears on the verge of fainting:

- Prevent the person from falling.
- Have the person lie down and elevate the legs 8–12 inches.

If fainting has occurred or if fainting is anticipated:

- Lay the victim down and elevate the legs 8–12 inches.
- If vomiting begins, turn the person on the side to keep the airway open and clear.
- Loosen tight clothing.
- If the victim has fallen, look for injuries.
- Wet a cloth with cool water and wipe the person's forehead and face.
- Do *not* splash or pour water on the victim's face.
- Do *not* use smelling salts or ammonia as inhalants.
- Do *not* slap the victim's face as an attempt to revive him or her.
- Do *not* give the victim anything to drink until fully recovered.

Most fainting cases are not serious and the victim regains consciousness quickly. However, seek medical attention if the victim:

- Is over 40 years old
- Has had repeated attacks of unconsciousness
- Does not waken within four or five minutes
- Loses consciousness while sitting or lying down
- Faints for no apparent reason

Severe Allergic Reaction (Anaphylactic Shock)

Allergies are usually thought of as causing rashes, itching, or some other short-term discomfort that disappears when the offending agent is removed from contact with the allergic person. There is, however, a more powerful reaction to substances ordinarily eaten or injected called anaphylactic shock, which can occur within minutes or even seconds. Such a reaction can cause death if not treated immediately.

Eating of certain foods, such as nuts or shellfish, or using some medications or drugs, such as oral penicillin, can cause severe reactions in sensitive persons.

The sting of a honeybee, wasp, yellow jacket, or hornet can cause very severe, immediate reactions in those allergic to the injected toxin. About one percent of the population is severely sensitive to insect stings.

The injection of a drug such as penicillin or a tetanus antitoxin may cause an immediate severe reaction.

The severe allergic response (anaphylactic shock) is triggered by contact with a substance that the individual has previously encountered and the body has identified as an enemy, causing the development of antibodies called IgE. The antibodies, or body defenders, later come in contact with the offending substance and release chemicals (e.g., histamine) that attack the lungs, blood vessels, intestines, and skin.

It is a life-threatening situation! About 60–80% of anaphylactic deaths are caused by an inability to breathe because swollen airway passages obstruct airflow to the lungs. The second most common cause of anaphylactic deaths—about 24%—is shock, brought on by insufficient blood circulating through the body.

Signs and Symptoms

One or all of these signs and symptoms may appear:

- Coughing, sneezing, or wheezing
- Difficult breathing
- Tightness and swelling in the throat
- Tightness in the chest
- Severe itching, burning, rash, or hives on the skin
- Swollen face, tongue, mouth

- Nausea and vomiting
- Dizziness
- Abdominal cramps
- Blueness (cyanosis) around the lips and mouth
- Unconsciousness

First Aid

The main treatment for anaphylaxis involves injecting epinephrine. The drug, although fast-acting, is rapidly dissipated in the blood. The injection may require repeating as the signs and symptoms recur or worsen.

Often victims may know of their allergies and sensitivity and carry a kit containing epinephrine preloaded in an injecting device. One type contains a notched syringe to ensure the correct dose is given. Other kits contain a syringe-loaded injector that automatically injects a predetermined dose of the drug when it is pressed against the thigh.

In some cases, cardiopulmonary resuscitation (CPR) and intensive medical care are required. It is essential that the offending substance be identified because each anaphylactic response may be more severe than the previous one.

Keep checking the victim after the injection since a second or even a third injection may be needed.

This is a true emergency! Seek immediate medical attention for the victim.

Some other types of emergency conditions are labeled as shock but they are not the type of shock that affects the circulatory system. These include electric shock which may cause cardiac arrest and also produce severe burns; and insulin shock, which occurs in a diabetic who has taken too much insulin.

■ HYPOVOLEMIC SHOCK ■

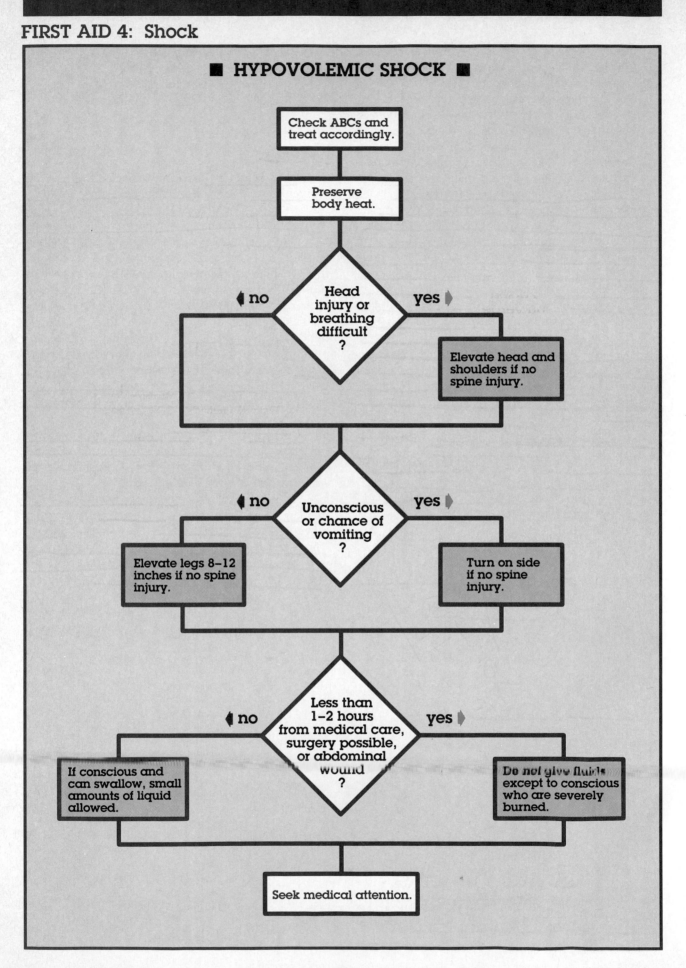

Check ABCs and treat accordingly.

Preserve body heat.

Head injury or breathing difficult?

no →

yes ▶

Elevate head and shoulders if no spine injury.

Unconscious or chance of vomiting?

no →

yes ▶

Elevate legs 8–12 inches if no spine injury.

Turn on side if no spine injury.

Less than 1–2 hours from medical care, surgery possible, or abdominal wound?

no →

yes ▶

If conscious and can swallow, small amounts of liquid allowed.

Do not give fluids except to conscious who are severely burned.

Seek medical attention.

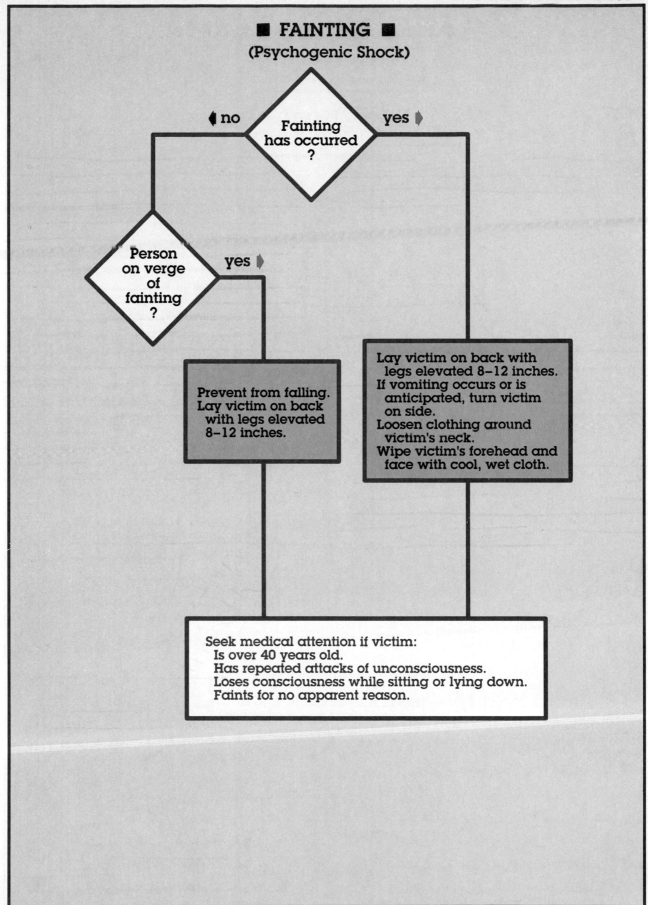

■ FAINTING ■
(Psychogenic Shock)

Fainting has occurred?

no → **Person on verge of fainting?**

yes →

Prevent from falling. Lay victim on back with legs elevated 8–12 inches.

yes →

**Lay victim on back with legs elevated 8–12 inches.
If vomiting occurs or is anticipated, turn victim on side.
Loosen clothing around victim's neck.
Wipe victim's forehead and face with cool, wet cloth.**

**Seek medical attention if victim:
Is over 40 years old.
Has repeated attacks of unconsciousness.
Loses consciousness while sitting or lying down.
Faints for no apparent reason.**

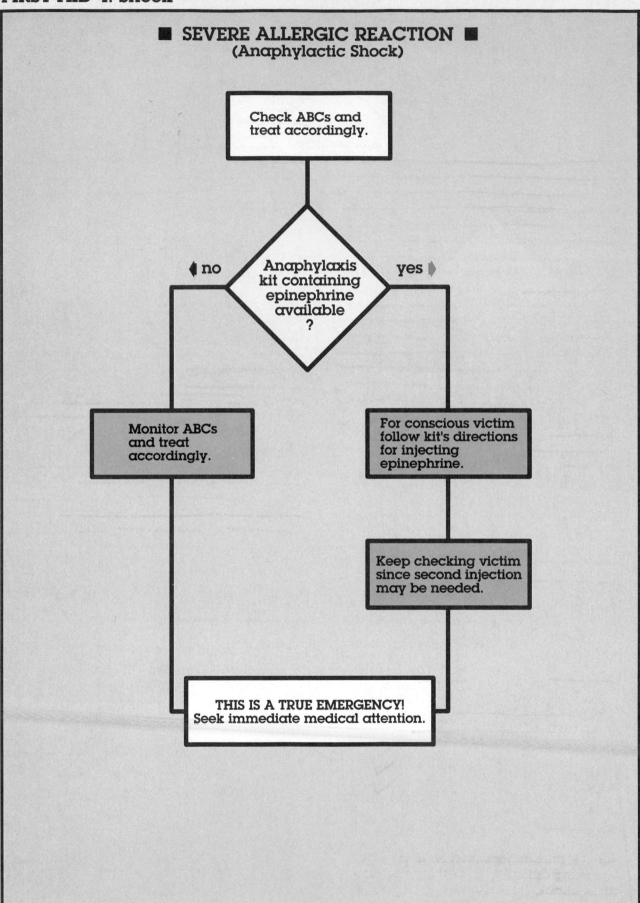

■ SEVERE ALLERGIC REACTION ■
(Anaphylactic Shock)

Check ABCs and treat accordingly.

Anaphylaxis kit containing epinephrine available ?

◄ no   yes ►

Monitor ABCs and treat accordingly.

For conscious victim follow kit's directions for injecting epinephrine.

Keep checking victim since second injection may be needed.

THIS IS A TRUE EMERGENCY!
Seek immediate medical attention.

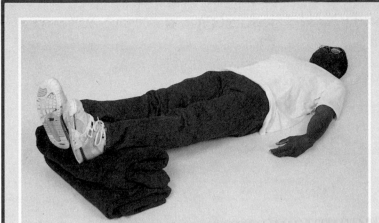

Usual shock position. Elevate the legs 8-12 inches. Do not lift the foot of bed or stretcher.

EXCEPTIONS:

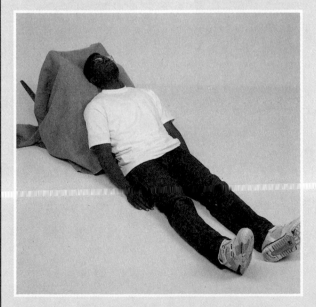

Elevate the head for injuries or stroke.

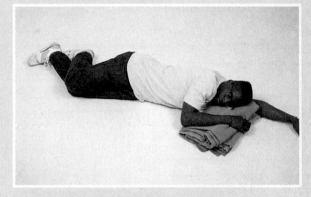

Lay an unconcious, semiconcious, or vomiting victim on his or her side.

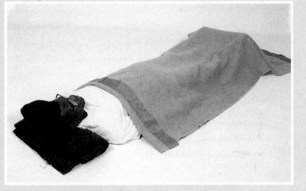

Use a semisitting position for those with breathing difficulties, chest injuries, or a heart attack.

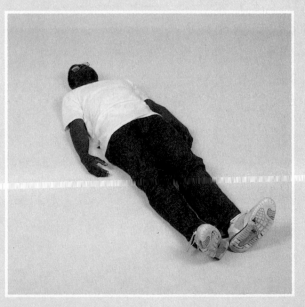

Keep victim flat if a neck or spine injury is suspected or victim has leg fractures.

(handwritten top margin) heart pump
Right into heart left side into arteries

Arteries carries oxygenated blood then the body.

5

Bleeding and Wounds

■ **External Bleeding** ■ **Internal Bleeding** ■ **Wounds** ■
■ **Tetanus** ■ **Amputations** ■ **Animal Bites** ■

(handwritten) Cardiovascular System
heart Veins & Arteries

The average-sized adult has about six quarts of blood and can safely lose a pint during a blood donation. However, rapid blood loss of one quart or more can lead to shock and death. A child losing one pint is in extreme danger.

Blood can be lost from arteries, veins, or capillaries. Most bleeding involves more than one type of blood vessel. Blood from arteries is bright red and spurts. Arterial bleeding produces the fastest blood loss, is the most difficult to control, and is therefore the most dangerous.

Blood from a vein flows steadily and appears to be darker red. Blood oozes slowly from capillaries. Though each blood vessel contains blood differing in shades of red, an inexperienced person may have difficulty detecting the difference. The two basic types of bleeding are external and internal.

External Bleeding

Bleeding is classified as external when it involves visible blood coming from an open wound. In most cases, bleeding stops after 5 to 10 minutes with proper first aid.

Types of External Bleeding

Three types of external bleeding exist: arterial, venous, and capillary.

1. **Arterial.** When completely severed, arteries often constrict and seal themselves off. However, if an artery is merely torn or punctured, it will probably continue to bleed. Arterial bleeding is the most serious type of external bleeding. The blood loss from the wound is often rapid and profuse, as blood spurts from the wound. Blood from an artery is bright red in color because it is rich in oxygen.

Arterial bleeding is less likely to clot than other types of bleeding because a blood clot can form only when there is a slow flow or no flow at all. Therefore, arterial bleeding is dangerous, and some external means of control must be used to stop the flow. Unless a very large artery has been

severed, it is unlikely that a person will bleed to death before the flow can be controlled, however.

2. **Venous.** Blood from a vein flows steadily and is bluish-red. This type of bleeding may be profuse, but it is easier to control than arterial bleeding. Veins are usually located closer to the body surface than are arteries. Most veins collapse when they are cut; however, bleeding from deep veins can be as copious and as hard to control as arterial bleeding.

3. **Capillary.** Blood oozes from capillaries. Capillary bleeding is the most common type of blood loss. It is usually not serious and is easily controlled. It is characterized by a general seeping from the tissues, the blood dripping steadily from the wound or gradually forming a puddle in it. Quite often, this type of bleeding will more or less control itself by clotting spontaneously.

In hemophilia, the tendency to bleed, as well as the inability to clot, may be so great as to threaten life. Bleeding in a person with this condition is difficult to control. Hospitalization is required. First aid measures include firm compression on the bleeding site and immediate transport to a medical facility.

First Aid

Several methods can control or stop bleeding. They appear below in the order to be tried:

1. **Direct pressure.** Most external bleeding can be controlled by direct pressure over the wound. Steps in applying direct pressure:
   a. Place a sterile gauze dressing directly over the wound and press against it. If a sterile gauze dressing is not available, use a handkerchief, towel, or any available clean cloth.
   b. If possible, wear latex or vinyl gloves, or use other methods (e.g., extra layers of gauze, plastic wrap) for protection from the victim's blood. Afterwards, wash your hands with soap and water. When gauze dressings, latex gloves, or other protective barriers are not available and speed is important, put your bare hand and/or fingers on the wound and press to stop the blood flow.

(handwritten bottom) Arteries → arterioles → capillaries → venules → veins

■ BLEEDING ■

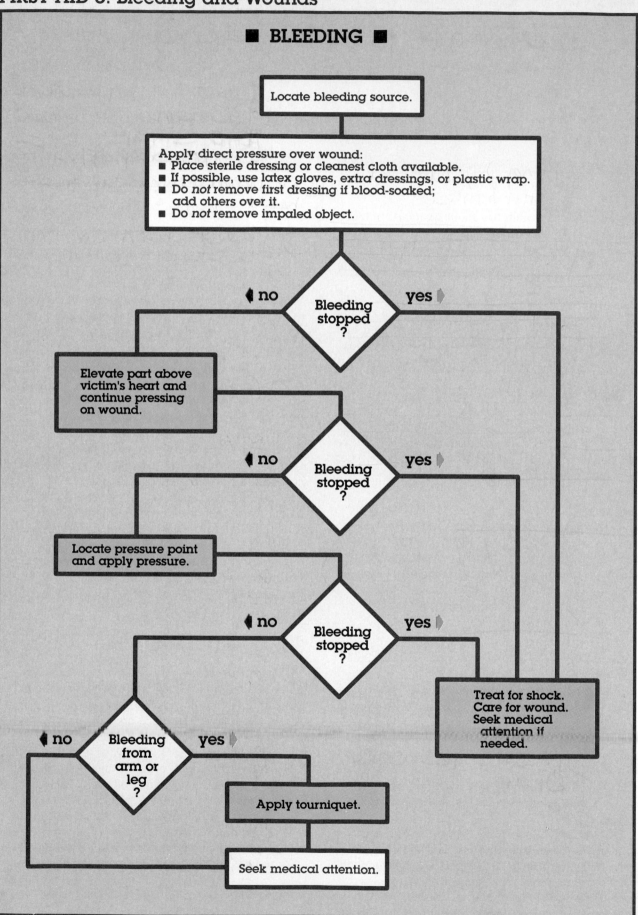

Locate bleeding source.

Apply direct pressure over wound:
- Place sterile dressing or cleanest cloth available.
- If possible, use latex gloves, extra dressings, or plastic wrap.
- Do *not* remove first dressing if blood-soaked; add others over it.
- Do *not* remove impaled object.

Bleeding stopped?

no → Elevate part above victim's heart and continue pressing on wound.

Bleeding stopped?

no → Locate pressure point and apply pressure.

Bleeding stopped?

no → Bleeding from arm or leg?

yes → Treat for shock. Care for wound. Seek medical attention if needed.

yes → Apply tourniquet.

Seek medical attention.

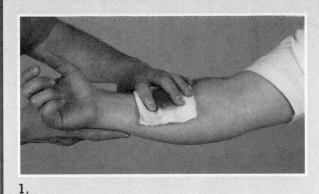

1.

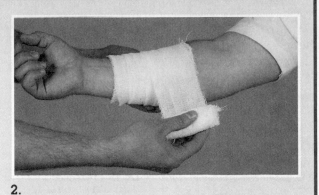

2.

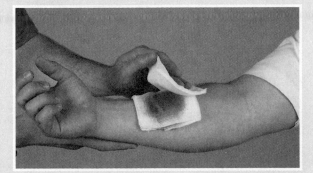

3.

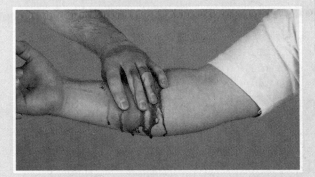

4.

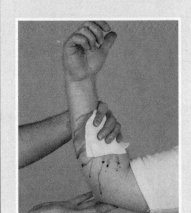

5.

1. Direct pressure. Use dressing.

2. Pressure bandage.

3. If dressing is blood-soaked, add more on top.

4. For severe bleeding, don't waste time looking for a dressing.

5. Combine direct pressure and elevation.

6. Combine direct pressure with a pressure point at (a) brachial or (b) femoral artery.

Use a tourniquet only as a last resort! Tourniquets are rarely needed.

impervious

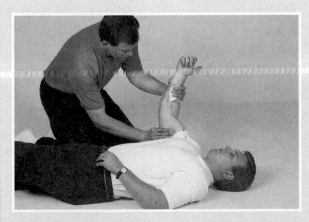

6a. Brachial

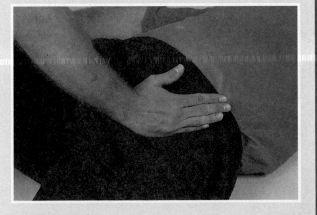

6b. Femoral

c. Apply a pressure bandage over the gauze dressing and wound to free yourself to perform other first aid. The dressing is best held in place with a roller bandage wrapped tightly over the dressing and above and below the wound site.

d. Do *not* remove a dressing once it is in place because bleeding may start again. If a dressing becomes blood-soaked, apply another dressing on top of the blood-soaked one and hold them both in place.

e. If bleeding does not stop, apply more pressure.

f. After bleeding has stopped, maintain pressure with a bandage.

2. *Elevation.* If bleeding persists, continue applying direct pressure and elevate the extremity above the heart level. Elevation alone will not stop bleeding. Gravity helps reduce blood pressure and thus slows bleeding to allow clotting. Do *not* elevate a broken extremity.

3. *Pressure points.* If bleeding still continues, apply pressure at a pressure point while still applying direct pressure. A wound may be supplied by more than one major blood vessel, so using the pressure point alone is rarely enough to control severe bleeding.

A pressure point exists where an artery is near the skin's surface, and where it passes close to a bone against which it can be compressed. Two locations on both sides of the body are usually used to control most external bleeding cases. These are the brachial point in the arm and the femoral point in the groin.

Using pressure points requires a skillful first aider. Unless the exact location of the pulse point is known, the pressure point technique is useless.

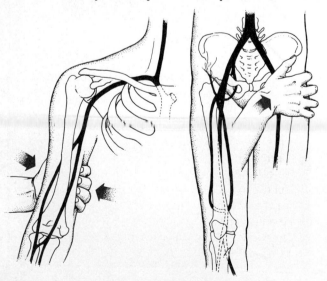

Proper hand positions for applying brachial and femoral pressure

4. *Tourniquet.* Tourniquets are rarely, if ever, necessary. Use a tourniquet only as a last resort to save a life when all other methods have failed. A tourniquet can damage nerves and blood vessels and may cause loss of an arm or leg. If used, apply wide, flat materials—never rope or wire, and do *not* loosen it.

Internal Bleeding

Internal bleeding occurs when the skin is unbroken, and is not usually visible.

Signs and Symptoms
- Blood from the mouth (vomit, sputum) or rectum, or blood in the urine
- Nonmenstrual bleeding from the vagina
- Bruise or contusion
- Rapid pulse
- Cold and moist skin
- Dilated pupils
- Nausea and vomiting
- Painful, tender, rigid, bruised abdomen
- Fractured ribs or bruises on chest

First Aid
For severe internal bleeding:
- Monitor breathing and pulse.
- Expect vomiting. Do *not* give any liquids. If vomiting occurs, keep the victim lying on his or her side for drainage.
- Treat for shock by raising the victim's legs 8–12 inches and keeping the victim warm.
- Seek immediate medical attention.

For bruises:
- Apply an ice pack. Protect the victim's skin from frostbite by having a cloth between the ice and the skin.
- Elevate the injured part if it is not broken.
- If an arm or leg is involved, apply an elastic bandage. Do *not* apply it too tightly.

Wounds

Wounds are divided into two types: closed or open. An open wound has a break in the skin's surface with visible bleeding. A closed wound involves damage beneath the skin's surface. The skin remains unbroken, and no blood is seen.

Open Wounds

These types of wounds have damaged skin, involve visible bleeding, and could become infected.

At times, a first aider may face significant amounts of blood and other body fluids. Many first aiders become concerned about the possibility of becoming infected with the hepatitis B or AIDS virus in such situations.

Here are some facts about hepatitis B and AIDS:

- Hepatitis B virus causes serious liver disease and appears to be related to liver cancer. The virus is very infectious.
- AIDS is a universally fatal disease that cripples the immune system, leaving the victim susceptible to illnesses the body can usually fight off, such as pneumonia, meningitis, and a cancer called Kaposi's sarcoma. At present, there is no cure for AIDS.

In any situation involving body fluids, there is a small but real risk of infection.

Use these precautions whenever possible while giving first aid:

1. Keep open wounds covered with dressings to prevent both the victim and first aider from coming in contact with each other's blood.

2. All first aid kits should have several pairs of latex or vinyl rubber gloves. Use these gloves in every situation involving blood or other body fluids.

3. If latex or vinyl gloves are not available, use the most waterproof material available (e.g., plastic wrap) or extra gauze dressings to form a barrier between body fluids and the skin.

4. Use face masks with a one-way valve for protection when doing mouth-to-mouth resuscitation. Every first aid kit should have one. While saliva is not considered a high risk, there may be blood in the mouth.

During clean-up, use these precautions:

1. Wash in hot, soapy water, while vigorously scrubbing the skin and rinse well.

2. Wash all clothing and other items that have blood or other body fluids on them in hot, soapy water.

3. Clean reusable items with a solution of one part liquid chlorine bleach to nine parts of water and rinse well.

Some people are concerned about becoming infected while participating in cardiopulmonary resuscitation training. The American Heart Association, the American Red Cross, and the Centers for Disease Control say the risk of acquiring any infectious disease by CPR manikin practice appears to be very minimal.

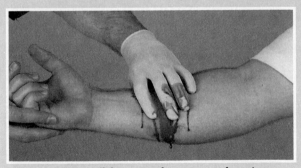

Whenever possible, use gloves as a barrier.

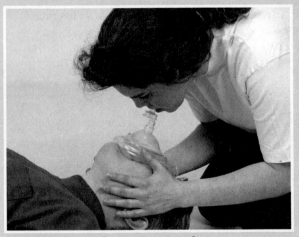

Pocket face mask, one-way valve

Types of Open Wounds

- **Abrasion.** Scraped skin resulting in partial loss of the skin surface. It has little bleeding but can be very painful and serious if it covers a large area or if foreign matter becomes embedded in it.
- **Incision.** The wound is smooth-edged and bleeds freely. The amount of bleeding depends upon the depth, location, and size of the wound. There may be severe damage to muscles, nerves, and tendons if the wound is deep.
- **Laceration.** A skin cut with jagged, irregular edges. It can bleed freely.
- **Puncture.** This is a stab from a pointed object. The entrance wound is usually small. Special treatment of the puncture wound may be required when the object causing the injury remains impaled in the wound.
- **Avulsion.** This is the tearing of a patch of skin or other tissue that is not totally torn from the body and leaves a loose, hanging flap. Avulsions can involve such parts as ears, fingers, and hands.

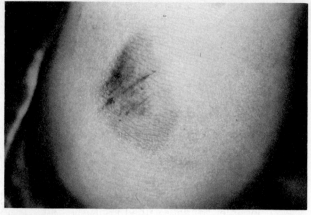

Abrasion

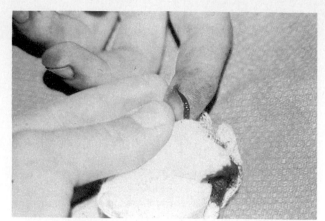

Laceration

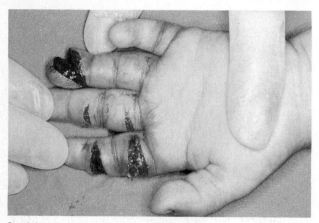

Incision

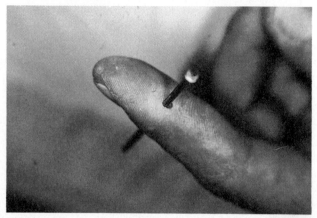

Puncture

TABLE 5-1 Types of Open Wounds

Type	Cause(s)	Signs and Symptoms	First Aid
Abrasion (scrape)	Rubbing or scraping	Only skin surface affected	Remove all debris.
		Little bleeding	Wash away from wound with soap and water.
Incision (cut)	Sharp objects	Smooth edges of wound	Control bleeding.
		Severe bleeding	Wash wound.
Laceration (tearing)	Blunt object tearing skin	Veins and arteries can be affected	Control bleeding.
		Severe bleeding Danger of infection	Wash wound.
Puncture (stab)	Sharp pointed object piercing skin	Wound is narrow and deep into veins and arteries Embedded objects Danger of infection	Do not remove impaled objects.
Avulsion (torn off)	Machinery, Explosives	Tissue torn off or left hanging	Control bleeding.
		Severe bleeding	Take avulsed part to medical facility.

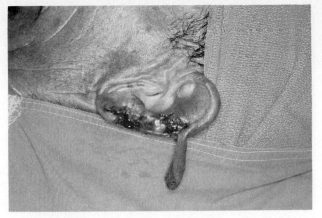

Avulsion

- **_Amputation._** This involves the cutting or tearing off of a body part such as fingers, toes, hands, feet, arms, or legs. See page 71 for more information.

First Aid

- Remove any clothing covering the wound.
- Protect against exposure to AIDS or hepatitis by wearing latex or vinyl gloves or using other methods of protection (e.g., extra layers of dressings, plastic material).
- Control bleeding by applying pressure while using a dry sterile dressing or clean cloth over the entire wound. Refer to the proper steps above and under the topic of bleeding.
- Do *not* remove an impaled (penetrating) object.
- Save amputated part(s); using the procedure on page 72.

Cleaning wounds

For minor wounds (not seen by a physician):

- Wash your hands in a vigorous scrubbing action, using soap and water.
- Using a sterile gauze pad or a clean cloth saturated with soap and water, gently wash away from the wound edges. Hydrogen peroxide (3 percent solution) helps to bubble away old blood and clots—*not* to disinfect the wound or destroy bacteria, as many think. Foreign bodies (e.g., dirt, gravel) should be removed to avoid infection and a tattoo look after the skin heals.
- Flush the wound with large amounts of water and dry it with a sterile gauze.
- Rubbing alcohol might be used as an antiseptic on the undamaged skin around the wound, *not* in the wound.
- Do not put mercurochrome, merthiolate, or iodine on a wound. They kill few bacteria, can damage the skin, and many people are allergic to them.

- Cover the wound with a sterile gauze dressing and bandage. Dressings are most needed during the first 24 hours after an injury. A "band-aid" type of dressing is useful on small cuts. The dressing should *not* be airtight because it might trap moisture given off by the skin, which would encourage bacteria growth. One of the "nonstickable" dressings works well for abrasions.
- Dressings and bandages are two different kinds of first aid supplies. *Dressings* are applied over the wound to control bleeding and prevent contamination. *Bandages* hold the dressings in place. A dressing should be sterile or as clean as possible; bandages need not be.
- If using an antibiotic skin-wound ointment, apply a small amount over the wound and cover with a sterile dressing. The antibiotic can be applied several times daily. Many antibiotic skin-wound protectants are available.
- If a wound bleeds after a dressing is applied and the dressing becomes stuck, leave it on as long as the wound is healing. Pulling the scab loose to change the dressing retards healing and increases the chance of infection. If a dressing must be removed, soak it in warm water or hydrogen peroxide to help soften the scab and make removal easier.
- If a dressing becomes wet, change it. A wet dressing provides an excellent place for bacteria. Dirty dressings should be changed for a better appearance.

For severe wounds, to be seen by a physician the first aider should:

- Remove clothing covering the wound.
- Control bleeding as described previously.
- Prevent contamination by applying a dry, sterile dressing. Do *not* wash the wound. Leave wound cleaning to a physician. If in a remote situation with medical care many hours away, clean the wound if possible, making certain that bleeding is controlled.

Closed Wounds

A bruise (contusion) results when a blunt object strikes the body. The skin is not broken and no blood appears on the skin's surface. This is the only type of closed wound.

Signs and symptoms include: discoloration, swelling, pain, redness, and loss of use.

First Aid

- Control bleeding by applying ice and an elastic bandage immediately to the injury. Cold constricts blood vessels and thus slows bleeding. Compression over the area also helps decrease bleeding.

- Suspect and check for a fracture.
- Elevate the injured part above the victim's heart level to decrease swelling and pain.

Wounds Requiring Medical Attention

At some point in your life, you will probably have to make a decision about obtaining medical assistance for a wounded victim. To help in this decision, look for the following signs:

- Arterial bleeding
- Uncontrolled bleeding
- Deep incisions, lacerations, or avulsions that:

  1. Go into the muscle or bone

  2. Are located on a body part that bends (e.g., elbows or knees)

  3. Tend to gape widely

  4. Are located on the thumb or palm of hand (because nerves may be affected)

- Large or deep punctures
- Large embedded objects or deeply embedded objects of any size
- Foreign matter left in wound
- Human and animal bites
- Wounds where a scar would be noticeable. Stitched cuts usually heal with less scarring than unstitched ones.
- Eyelid cuts (to prevent later drooping)
- Slit lips (easily scarred)
- Internal bleeding
- Any wound that a first aider is *not* certain how to treat

Stitches

If stitches are needed they should be made by a physician within six to eight hours of the injury. Stitching wounds allows faster healing, reduces infection, and reduces scarring.

Wounds *not* usually requiring stitches include:

1. Those in which the skin's cut edges tend to fall together

2. Cuts less than one inch long that are not deep

Gaping wounds may be closed by using a "butterfly" bandage if all of the following are found:

1. The wound is less than eight hours old;

2. The wound is very clean; and

3. It is impossible to get to a physician because of distance.

Infection

All wounds, large or small, present one common danger—infection. Serious wounds also present the danger of severe bleeding.

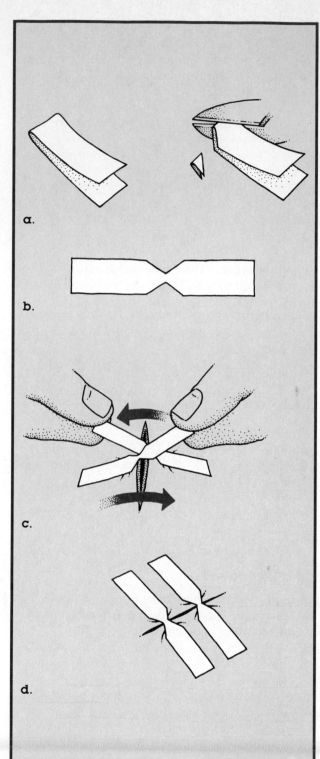

a.

b.

c.

d.

Butterfly bandage **a.** Fold a piece of tape and cut off both corners at the fold. **b.** The straightened tape reveals the "butterfly." **c.** Pull two butterfly bandages together to close and hold the wound edges together. **d.** Butterfly bandages holding edges together. Cover the butterflies and wound with a sterile dressing.

Microorganisms grow in abundance on the skin and are found especially on the hands because our hands touch so many things. Once an infection begins, damage can be extensive, so prevention is the best way to avoid this problem.

Every wound, regardless of size, should be washed immediately with soap and water. If the wound is deep, it may be best to leave the cleaning to trained medical personnel, who will use an antiseptic agent, such as Betadine, and will irrigate the wound with a sterile saline solution. Early cleansing can reduce the number of germs in and around the wound so that the body's natural defenses can ward off infection.

Because infection is a danger in all wounds, a tetanus shot is often given especially a wound caused by a dirty object.

It is important to know how to recognize and treat an infected wound. Most infected wounds swell and become reddened. They may give off a sensation of heat and develop a throbbing pain and a pus discharge.

An infection that is not treated soon enough could cause more serious symptoms affecting other areas of the body. For example, the person with an infection may develop a fever. Lymph nodes near the infection may swell. If the infection is in the hand, lymph nodes in the armpit may swell. If the infection is in the leg, lymph nodes in the groin may swell. If the infection is in the head, lymph nodes in the neck may swell. Then one or more red streaks may develop, leading from the wound toward the heart. This is a serious sign that the infection is spreading and could cause death.

In the early stages of an infection, a physician may allow the following home treatment: applying warm, wet compresses; elevating the injured part; and taking antibiotics.

Some wounds are more likely to become infected than others. Special care should be given a wound received from a bite—either human or animal. Wounds of the hands and feet are susceptible to infection. Any head wound, especially of the scalp, has a high likelihood of infection. Puncture wounds that are difficult to clean have a high incidence of infection, as do wounds made by dirty objects.

Do *not* use Mercurochrome™ and Merthiolate™, since they do not kill all of the bacteria. They can damage the skin, and many people are allergic to them.

If you feel you must use an antiseptic, use rubbing alcohol (isopropyl). Apply it only on the undamaged skin around the wound, not in the wound.

Most minor wounds need only cleaning and a dressing placed over the wound. If an antibiotic skin ointment is used, wash the wound first, then cover the wound with a small amount and a sterile dressing. The antibiotic ointment can be replaced up to three times daily.

Tetanus

Tetanus is caused by a toxin produced by a bacterium. The bacterium forms a spore that can survive in a variety of environments for years. It has been found in soil and air samples throughout the world, on human skin, and in human and animal feces.

The bacterium by itself does not cause tetanus. But when it enters a wound that contains little oxygen (e.g., a puncture wound), it can produce a toxin, which is a powerful poison. The toxin travels through the nervous system to the brain and spinal cord. It then causes contractions of certain muscle groups (particularly in the jaw). There is no known antidote to the toxin once it enters the nervous system.

The World Health Organization reports 50,000 deaths each year from tetanus, but some authorities estimate that the disease may kill as many as one million people each year. Because of good medical care in the United States, about 100 deaths a year are reported.

Vaccination can completely prevent the disease. Everyone needs a series of vaccinations to prepare the immune system to defend against the toxin. Then a booster shot once every 10 years is sufficient to jog the immune system's memory.

People who are wounded a long time after their last vaccination (e.g., 10 years) or those who did not receive all the recommended vaccinations early in life may not be able to defend themselves adequately against the tetanus toxin. In such cases, physicians can administer solutions of tetanus antibodies.

Vaccination can completely prevent the disease. Everyone needs a series of vaccinations periodically to prepare the immune system to defend against the toxin. If a wound is contaminated with material beneath the skin and is not exposed to the air, and if the victim has never had a tetanus shot, or has not had a booster shot within the past five years, a booster shot is advised to keep the immunity level high. Whenever in doubt, check with a physician about the need for a tetanus shot.

Amputations

An amputation can be one of the more gruesome wounds seen.

Types of Amputations

Amputations can be classified according to the type of injury (crushing or guillotine) and the extent of injury (partial or complete). A crushing amputation, which is the more common type, has a poor chance of reattachment. A guillotine-type of amputation has a much better chance because it is clean-cut. Microsurgical techniques can allow amputated parts to sometimes be replaced so they function normally or nearly normally.

A complete amputation may not involve heavy blood loss. This is because blood vessels tend to go into a spasm, recede into the injured body parts, and shrink in diameter, resulting in a surprisingly small blood loss. More blood is seen in a partial amputation.

First Aid

- Apply direct pressure to the bleeding site and elevate any involved extremity. Pressure on the supplying main artery (brachial or femoral) can also help in cases of severe bleeding. Tourniquets are rarely needed or used.
- Recover the amputated body part. It is best to take the amputated part to the hospital with the victim. However, in multicasualty cases, in reduced lighting conditions, or when untrained people transport the victim, someone may be requested to locate and take the missing body part to the hospital after the victim's departure. If possible, use clean water to rinse off debris—do *not* scrub.

    Studies indicate that amputated body parts without oxygen or cooling for more than six hours without cooling have little chance of survival; 24 hours is probably the maximum time allowable for an adequately cooled part.
- Care for the amputated body part by following these procedures:

    1. Rinse the part with clean water to remove any contamination—do *not* scrub.

    2. Wrap the amputated part with a dry sterile gauze or other available dry, clean cloth. The use of a wet or moist wrapping next to the skin and tissue of an amputated part can cause water logging and tissue softening, thus affecting the chances of successful reattachment. Therefore, do *not* wrap the part in a moistened or damp material.

    3. If a plastic bag or waterproof container (e.g., cup or glass) is available, put the wrapped amputated part in it.

    4. Place the bag or container with the wrapped amputated part on a bed of ice, but do *not* bury it. Reattaching frostbitten parts is usually unsuccessful.

    5. Transport the part immediately to the hospital.
- If the injured part is still partially attached to the stump by a tendon or small skin "bridge," the first aid is essentially the same. Control bleeding. Wrap the part in a dry sterile dressing and place a cold pack on it. The part can still be wrapped and ice can be placed on it after it is repositioned in the normal position. Do *not* cut the "bridge" attaching the injured part.

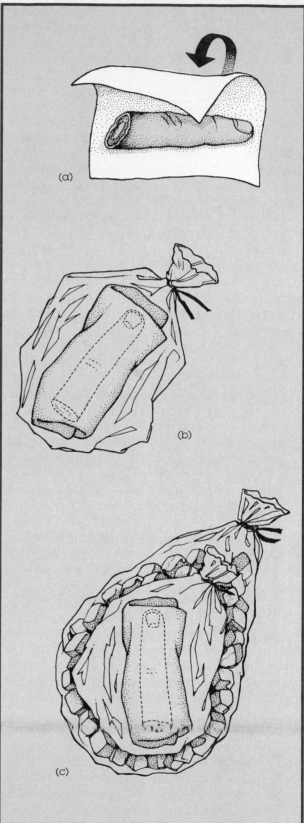

Care of an Amputated Part a. Wrap amputated body part in dry, sterile gauze. **b.** Place in plastic bag or other type of waterproof container. **c.** Place on bed of ice; do *not* bury it.

■ AMPUTATION ■

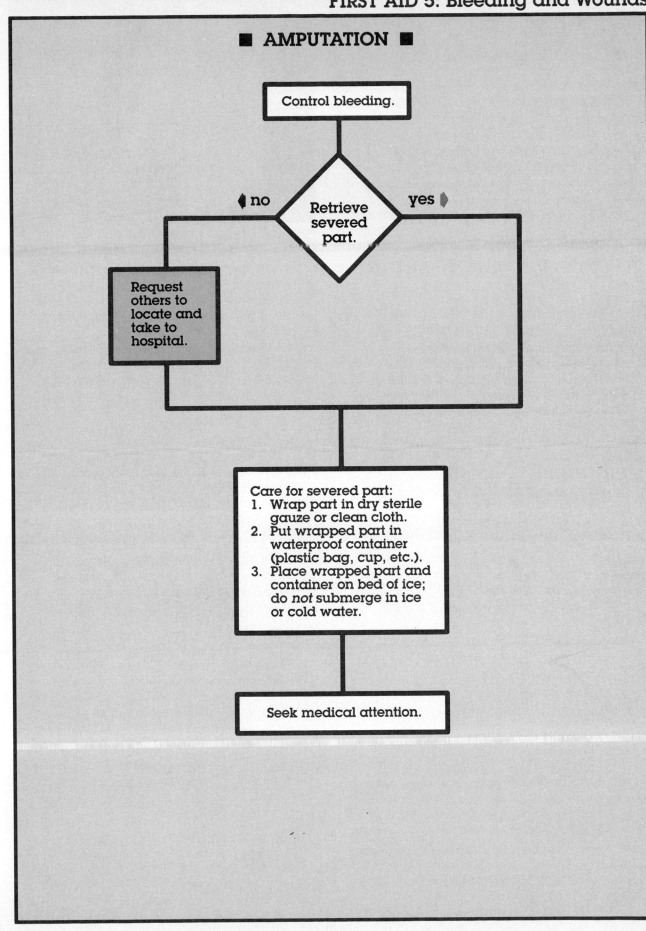

Control bleeding.

Retrieve severed part.

no → Request others to locate and take to hospital.

yes →

Care for severed part:
1. Wrap part in dry sterile gauze or clean cloth.
2. Put wrapped part in waterproof container (plastic bag, cup, etc.).
3. Place wrapped part and container on bed of ice; do *not* submerge in ice or cold water.

Seek medical attention.

Animal Bites

Animal bites rarely cause lethal bleeding, but they can produce significant damage. Sixty to 90 percent of the animal bites in the United States come from dogs. The annual number of dog bites has been estimated to be between one to two million cases.

Animal bites of all kinds account for about one percent of all hospital emergency department visits. About one bite in 10 needs stitches, but all bites require complete cleaning, which may be impossible by a first aider.

A dog's mouth may carry more than 60 different species of bacteria, some of which are very dangerous to humans (e.g., rabies). Human, cat, and other animal bites are equally contaminated and dangerous.

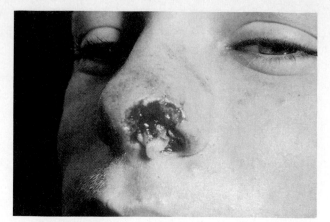

Dog Bite: Collie

First Aid

From a first aid standpoint, the main concerns regarding animal bites are bleeding, rabies, and infection.

- If the wound is not bleeding heavily, wash it with soap and water. Washing should take five to 10 minutes. Scrubbing can traumatize tissues, so avoid it whenever possible. Allowing a wound to bleed a little helps remove bacteria left in the tissues.
- Rinse the wound thoroughly with running water.
- Control bleeding with direct pressure, and if an extremity is involved and the bleeding con-

tinues, use elevation along with the direct pressure.
- Cover with a sterile dressing, but do *not* seal the wound tightly with tape or butterfly bandages.
- Seek medical attention because of the danger of infection, need for further cleaning, the possible need for a tetanus shot and stitches to close the wound.

Rabies

Although many people are still concerned about the possibility of getting rabies from dogs, 96 percent of

Avoiding Dog Bites

With an estimated 1 to 2 million Americans bitten by dogs each year, everyone should attempt to avoid being bitten. The U.S. postal system offers advice about dogs to its carriers which could be of use to others:

1. **Observe the area.** Take a quick glance at all places a dog could be—under parked cars or hedges, on the porch, etc.

2. **Size up the situation.** Is the dog asleep, barking, growling, nonchalant, large, small, etc?

3. **Avoid showing signs of fear.** A dog is more apt to bite if he knows you are afraid of him.

4. **Don't startle a dog.** If he is asleep, make some kind of nonstartling noise, such as a whistle. Do this before you are close to him, while you still have time for an "out."

5. **Never assume a dog won't bite.** You may encounter a certain dog for days or weeks without incident, but one day he may decide to bite you.

6. **Keep your eyes on the dog.** A dog is basically a coward and a sneak, and is more likely to bite you when you aren't looking.

7. **Make friends.** Talk in a friendly tone of voice, call his name if you know it, but don't attempt to pet him.

8. **Stand your ground.** If a dog comes toward you, turn and face him; if you have a satchel, hold it in front of you and back slowly away, making sure you don't stumble and fall. By all means, never turn and run.

9. **Never walk between a dog and its master,** and never walk toward children when a dog is present, because it may take action to defend them.

the rabies cases seen in the United States come from skunks, raccoons, and bats. During a recent year, about 100 rabid dogs were reported nationally, and those dogs did not always bite someone.

Only one or two cases of human rabies occur in the United States each year, and they generally originate outside the country. Since there is no cure for rabies, few victims survive it. In fact, only two cases of survival have been reported in medical history. A virus found in warm-blooded animals causes rabies and spreads from one animal to another, usually through a bite or by licking involving saliva from an infected animal.

Bites from animals that are not warm-blooded (e.g., snakes, reptiles) do not carry the danger of rabies. However, such bites can become infected and should be washed well and watched for signs of infection.

What to Do in Case of a Bite

- Try to locate the animal's owner or in the case of a wild animal find its location. Call the EMS, police, or animal control to capture it. Do *not* try to capture the animal yourself, and keep away from it. The health department will observe the captured animal for possible rabies. When the animal cannot be found or identified, the bitten victim must usually go through a series of rabies shots (vaccination).
- Do *not* kill the animal. If it is killed, protect the head and brain from damage so they can be examined for rabies. If it is dead, transport the animal intact to prevent exposure to the potentially infected tissues or saliva. If necessary, the animal's remains can be refrigerated (avoid freezing).
- Give first aid as described above and seek medical attention for a possible series of vaccine inoculations and stitches to close the wound.

Central nervous system — they'll jerk.

Human Bites

Human bites can cause a very severe injury—more often than animal bites do. The human mouth contains a wide range of bacteria and the likelihood of infection is greater from a human bite than from other warm-blooded animals.

Types of Human Bites

There are two kinds of human bites:

1. *True bites.* These occur when any part of the body's flesh is deliberately caught between teeth. These bites happen during fights between children and between adults and in cases involving abuse of children, spouses, and elders.

2. *Fight bites.* These occur when the victim cuts his or her knuckles on another person's teeth. Though these injuries usually result from a deliberate action (e.g., during a fight), unintentional injury can happen during sports and play (e.g., basketball).

First Aid

First aid involves:

- Thoroughly washing the wound with soap and water
- Applying a dry, sterile dressing and seeking medical attention

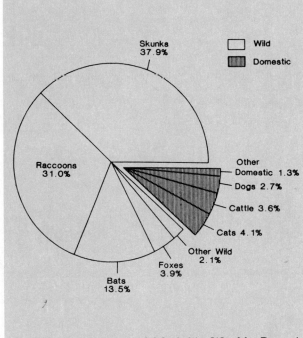

Source: Morbidity and Mortality Weekly Report *published by the Centers for Disease Control.*

Distribution of rabies cases in animals, United States, 1988

■ ANIMAL BITES ■

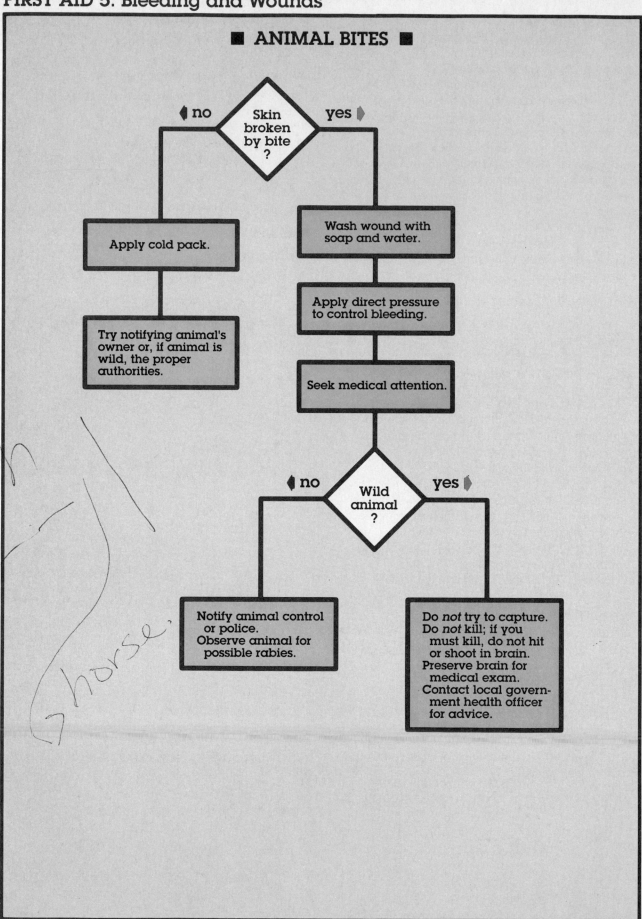

Skin broken by bite?

◀ no   yes ▶

Apply cold pack.

Try notifying animal's owner or, if animal is wild, the proper authorities.

Wash wound with soap and water.

Apply direct pressure to control bleeding.

Seek medical attention.

Wild animal?

◀ no   yes ▶

**Notify animal control or police.
Observe animal for possible rabies.**

**Do *not* try to capture.
Do *not* kill; if you must kill, do not hit or shoot in brain.
Preserve brain for medical exam.
Contact local government health officer for advice.**

6

Specific Body Area Injuries

■ Head Injuries ■ Eye Injuries ■ Nosebleeds ■ Dental Injuries ■ Chest Injuries ■
■ Abdominal Injuries ■ Finger and Toe Injuries ■ Fishhook Removal ■
■ Ring Removal ■ Blisters ■

Head Injuries

Scalp Wounds

Scalp wounds bleed profusely because of the scalp's rich blood supply. Look in the wound for skull bone or brain exposure and indentation of the skull.

- Control bleeding by gently applying direct pressure with a dry sterile dressing. If it becomes blood-filled, do *not* remove it but add another dressing on top of the first one.
- If a depressed skull fracture is suspected, apply pressure around the edges of the wound rather than at its center.
- Elevate the head and shoulders to help control bleeding.
- Do *not* remove an impaled object; instead, immobilize it in place with bulky dressings.

Skull Fracture

A skull fracture is a break or crack in the cranium (bony case surrounding the brain). Skull fractures may be open or closed, as with other bone fractures.

Signs and symptoms

- Pain at the point of injury
- Deformity of the skull
- Bleeding from ears and/or nose
- Leakage of clear or pink watery fluid dripping from the nose or ear. This watery fluid is known as cerebrospinal fluid (CSF). CSF can be detected by having the suspected fluid drip onto a handkerchief, pillowcase, or other cloth. CSF will form a pink ring resembling a target around the blood; this is also called the "halo sign."
- Discoloration under the eyes ("raccoon eyes")
- Discoloration behind an ear (Battle's sign)
- Unequal pupils
- Profuse scalp bleeding if skin is broken. A scalp wound may expose skull or brain tissue.

First aid for skull fractures is similar to that for a victim with a scalp wound (see above) or a brain contusion (see page 82).

Concussion

A concussion comes from a blow to the head that results in a violent jar or shaking to the brain, causing an immediate change in brain function, including possible loss of consciousness.

Signs and Symptoms

- Loss of consciousness
- Severe headache
- Memory loss (amnesia)
- Seeing stars
- Dizziness
- Weakness
- Double vision

Degrees of Concussion

Categorizing concussion helps the first aider to decide how to manage the victim. Concussions may be categorized as follows:

TABLE 6-1 Concussion Guidelines

Type	Description	Guidelines
Mild	Momentary or no loss of consciousness	Delay return to activity until medical evaluation has been made.
Moderate	Unconscious for less than five minutes	Avoid vigorous activity for a few days or longer. Resume activity only when associated symptoms of headache, visual disturbances, etc. have been resolved.
Severe	Unconscious for more than five minutes	Avoid rigorous activity for one month or longer. Clearance from a neurosurgeon is advised.

A **mild** concussion involves no loss of consciousness, but a disturbance of neurological function.

A **moderate** concussion involves a loss of consciousness for less than five minutes, usually with the inability to remember events after being injured.

In a **severe** concussion, the loss of consciousness lasts more than five minutes and eye movements wander.

Contusion

Contusions are more serious than concussions. Both can be produced by hits or blows to the head. Contusions involve bruising and swelling of the brain, with blood vessels within the brain rupturing and bleeding. Inside the skull, there is no way for the blood to escape and no room for it to accumulate.

Signs and Symptoms

- Similar to those of a concussion but more severe
- Unconsciousness
- Paralysis or weakness
- Unequal pupil size
- Vomiting and nausea
- Blurred vision
- Amnesia or memory lapses
- Headache

First Aid for Concussions and Contusions

Any head injury may be accompanied by a spinal injury. If you suspect a spinal injury, keep the head, neck, and spine in the same alignment you found originally.

For unconscious victims

- Assume that all unconscious victims of head injury have a spinal neck injury. Open the airway by the jaw thrust method to check for breathing. Do *not* bend the neck. Give rescue breathing if needed.
- Stabilize the victim's head and neck as you found them, using your hands along both sides of the head and/or placing blankets and other soft yet rigid materials alongside the head and neck.
- Check for severe bleeding. Cover any bleeding with a sterile dressing. Do *not* stop the flow of blood or fluid from the ears. Stopping it could put pressure on the brain. Do *not* remove any object embedded in the skull.
- If there are no signs of a neck or spinal injury, try to place the victim in the coma position (on victim's side, knees bent, head supported on one arm).

For conscious victims

- Check for spinal injury by noting arm or leg weakness or paralysis; if you get little or no reaction when you pinch the feet and hands, there may be a spinal injury. Stabilize the head and neck as they were found, to prevent movement.
- Do *not* block the escape of cerebrospinal fluid since it may add more pressure to the brain.
- Ask the victim what day it is, where he or she is, and personal questions such as birthday and home address. If the victim cannot answer these questions, there may be a significant

Head Injury Follow-Up

If any of the following signs appear within 48 hours of a head injury, seek medical attention:

- **Headache.** Expect a headache. If it lasts more than one or two days or increases in severity, however, seek medical advice.
- **Nausea, vomiting.** If nausea lasts more than two hours, seek medical advice. Vomiting once or twice, especially in children, may be expected after a head injury. Vomiting does not tell anything about the severity of the injury. However, if vomiting begins again hours after one or two episodes have ceased, consult a physician.
- **Drowsiness.** Allow a victim to sleep, but wake the victim at least every hour to check the state of consciousness and sense of orientation by asking his or her name, address, telephone number, and an

information-processing question (e.g., adding or multiplying numbers). If the victim cannot answer correctly or appears confused or disoriented, call a physician.
- **Vision problems.** If the victim "sees double," if the eyes fail to move together, or if one pupil appears to be larger than the other, seek medical advice.
- **Mobility.** If the victim cannot use his or her arms or legs as well as previously or is unsteady in walking, medical care should be sought.
- **Speech.** If the victim slurs his or her speech or is unable to talk, a doctor should be consulted.
- **Seizures or convulsions.** If the victim has a violent involuntary contraction (spasm) or series of contractions of the skeletal muscles, seek medical assistance.

problem. Another useful test is to give a list of five or six numbers and ask the victim to repeat them back in that order. Lists of objects can also be used as short-term memory tests. Failing on these short-term memory tests indicates a concussion.

- Keep victim in a semisitting position; do *not* elevate the legs since this increase blood pressure in the head.
- Do *not* give the victim anything to eat or drink.

Eye Injuries

Penetrating Injuries

Most penetrating eye injuries are fairly obvious. Suspect penetration any time you see a lid laceration or cut. Often first aiders concentrate upon the lid injury and neglect the penetrating eye injury. A penetrating injury requires immediate ophthalmological attention.

- Do *not* remove foreign bodies impaled in the eye.
- Protect the eye with a paper cup or cardboard cone to prevent the object from being driven farther into the eye.
- Cover the undamaged eye with a patch in order to stop movement of the damaged eye due to sympathetic eye movement.

Blows to the Eye*

Apply an ice cold compress immediately for about 15 minutes to reduce pain and swelling. A black eye or blurred vision could signal internal eye damage. See an ophthalmologist immediately.

Cuts of the Eye and Lid*

- Bandage both eyes lightly and seek medical help immediately.
- Do *not* attempt to wash out the eye or remove an object stuck in the eye.
- Never apply hard pressure to the injured eye or eyelid.

Chemical Injury*

- Flood the eye with warm water immediately. Use your fingers to keep the eye open as wide as possible. Hold head under a faucet or pour water into the eye from any clean container for at least 15 minutes, continuously and gently. Roll the eyeball as much as possible to

Source: American Academy of Ophthalmology; used with permission.

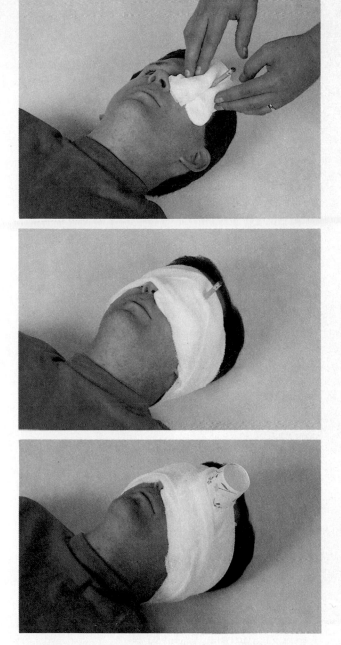

Bandaging penetrating eye injury (paper cup)

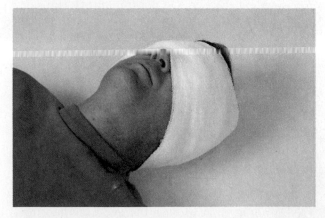

Bandaging both eyes stops eye movement

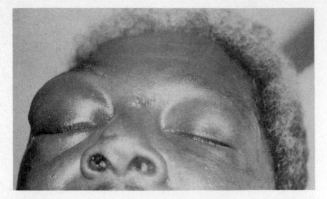

Blow to the eye

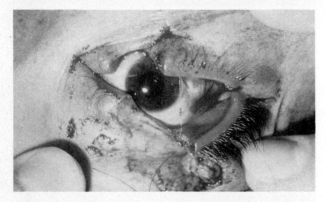

Lacerated eyelid

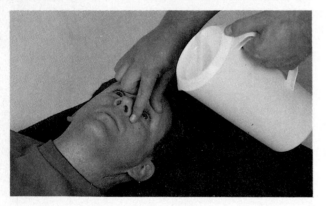

Flushing eye for chemical burn

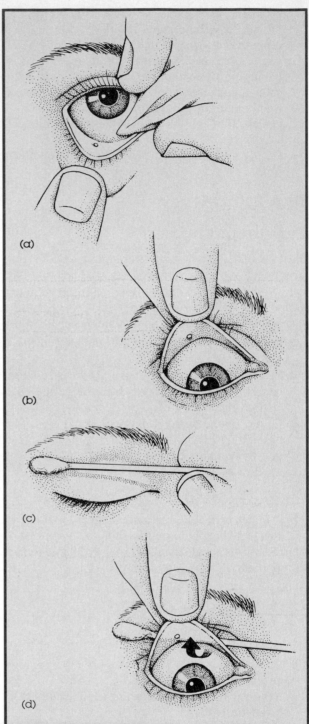

(a)

(b)

(c)

(d)

Everted Eyelid a. If tears or gentle flushing do not remove object, gently pull lower lid down. Remove an object by gently flushing with lukewarm water or a wet sterile gauze. **b.** If no object is seen inside lower lid, check the upper lid. **c.** Tell the person to look down. Pull gently downward on upper eyelashes. Lay a swab or matchstick across the top of the lid. **d.** Fold the lid over the swab or matchstick. Remove an object by gently flushing with lukewarm water or a wet sterile gauze.

wash out the eye. Do *not* use an eye cup.

- Loosely bandage both eyes. Seek medical help immediately after these steps are taken.

Alkalis cause greater concern than acids since they penetrate deeper and continue to damage longer. No matter how well the eye is irrigated, some alkali will always remain, often for weeks, to cause tissue damage. A first aider cannot use enough water on these injuries.

Avulsion of the Eye

A blow to the face can avulse an eye from its socket.

- Do *not* attempt to push the eye back into the socket.

- Cover the extruded eye loosely with a sterile dressing that has been moistened with clean water. Then cover the eye with a paper cup, using the same procedures for an impaled object in the eye.
- Cover the uninjured eye with a patch to prevent sympathetic eye movement in the damaged eye.

Foreign Bodies

Foreign bodies in the eye are the most frequent of eye injuries. They can be very painful. Tearing is very common, as it is the body's way of attempting to remove the object.

- Do *not* rub any speck or particle that is in the eye. Lift the upper lid over the lower lid, allowing the lashes to brush the speck off the inside of the upper lid. Blink a few times and let the eye move the particle out. If the speck remains, keep the eye closed and seek medical help.
- Try flushing the object out by rinsing the eye gently with warm water. You may have to help hold the eye open and tell the victim to move the eye as it is rinsed. If the object is on the white part of the eye, have the victim look down while rinsing the eye with water.
- If rinsing does not work, the object is probably stuck under the upper or lower lid. Examine the lower lid by pulling it down gently. If you see the object, flush the eye with water. To examine the upper lid, grasp the lashes of the upper lid, place a match stick or swab across the upper lid and roll the lid upward over the stick or swab. If you see the object, remove it with a moistened sterile gauze.

Start

Light Burns

These injuries can result from looking at ultraviolet light (e.g., sunlight, arc welding, bright snow). Severe pain occurs one to six hours after exposure.

- Cover both eyes with cold, moist compresses and prevent light from reaching the victim's eyes by having him or her rest in a darkened room.
- An analgesic for pain may be needed.
- Call an ophthalmologist for advice.

Contact Lenses

Determine if the victim is wearing contact lenses by asking, by checking on a driver's license, or by looking for them on the eyeball, using a light shining on the eye from the side. In cases of chemical eye burns, lenses should be immediately removed. Usually the victim can effectively remove the lenses.

Nosebleeds

Severe nosebleed frightens the victim and often challenges the first aider's skill. Most nosebleeds are self-limited and seldom require medical attention. However, in cases of accompanying head or neck injuries, stabilize the head and neck for protection. In some cases enough blood could be lost to cause shock.

Types of Nosebleeds

- *Anterior* (front of nose). The most common (90 percent); bleeds out of one nostril.
- *Posterior* (back of nose). Massive bleeding backward into the mouth or down the back of the throat; bleeding starts on one side, then comes out of both nostrils and down the throat; serious and requires medical attention.

First Aid

Most anterior (front of nose) nosebleeds can be stopped by these simple procedures:

- Reassure and keep the victim quiet. Though a large amount of blood may appear to have been lost, most nosebleeds are not serious.
- Keep the victim in a sitting position to reduce blood pressure.
- Keep the victim's head tilted slightly forward so that the blood can run out the front of the nose, not down the back of the throat, which causes either choking or nausea and vomiting. The vomit could be inhaled into the lungs.

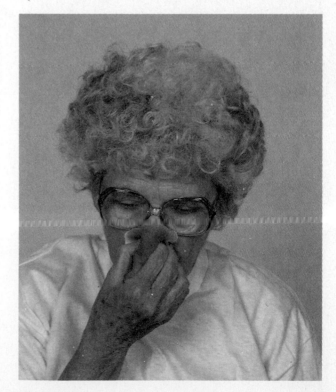
Nosebleed

■ HEAD INJURIES ■

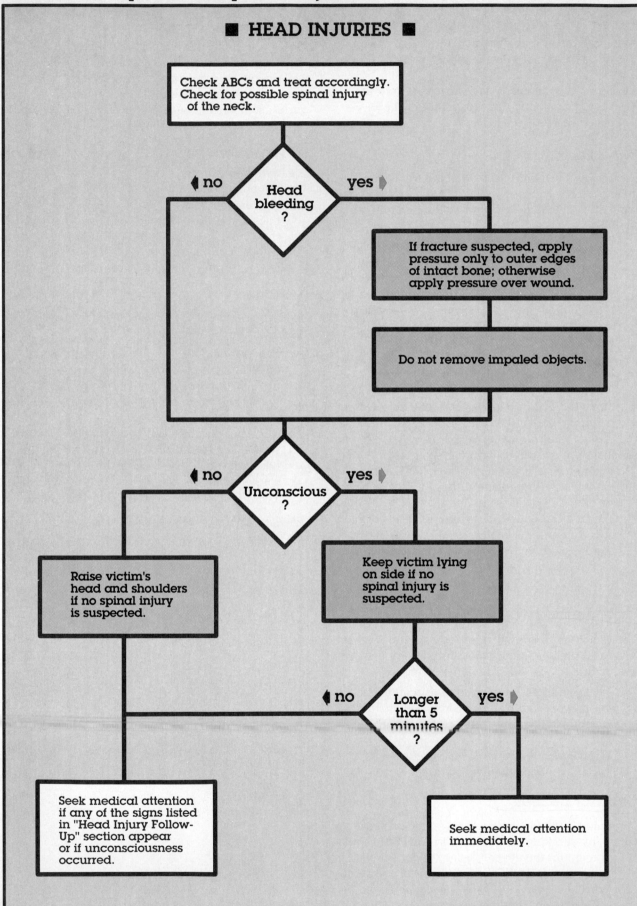

Check ABCs and treat accordingly. Check for possible spinal injury of the neck.

Head bleeding?

no → yes

If fracture suspected, apply pressure only to outer edges of intact bone; otherwise apply pressure over wound.

Do not remove impaled objects.

Unconscious?

no → yes

Raise victim's head and shoulders if no spinal injury is suspected.

Keep victim lying on side if no spinal injury is suspected.

Longer than 5 minutes?

no → yes

Seek medical attention if any of the signs listed in "Head Injury Follow-Up" section appear or if unconsciousness occurred.

Seek medical attention immediately.

■ EYE INJURIES ■

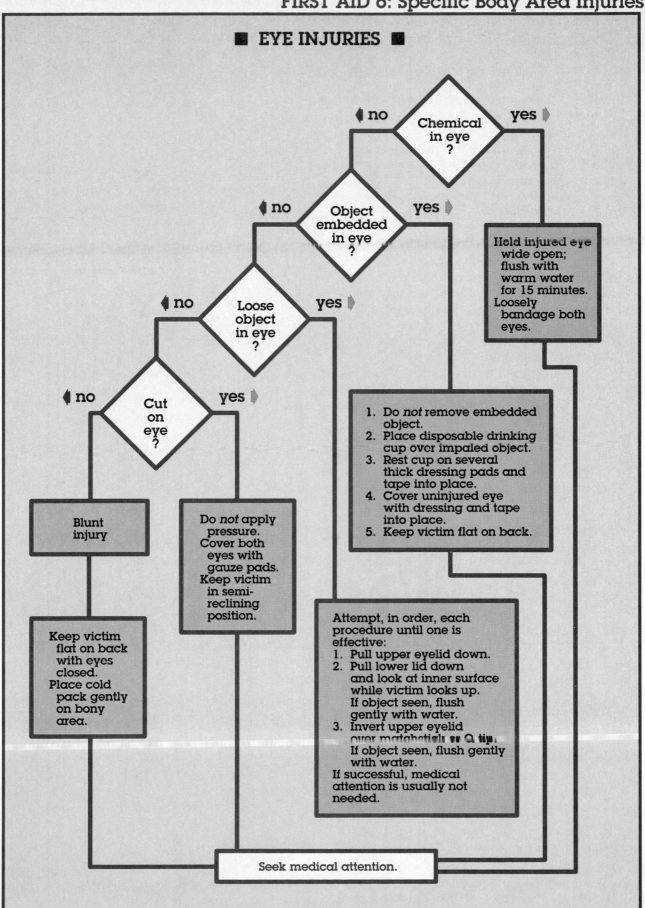

no ◄   Chemical in eye ?   ► **yes**

no ◄   Object embedded in eye ?   ► **yes**

no ◄   Loose object in eye ?   ► **yes**

no ◄   Cut on eye ?   ► **yes**

Hold injured eye wide open; flush with warm water for 15 minutes. Loosely bandage both eyes.

1. Do *not* remove embedded object.
2. Place disposable drinking cup over impaled object.
3. Rest cup on several thick dressing pads and tape into place.
4. Cover uninjured eye with dressing and tape into place.
5. Keep victim flat on back.

Blunt injury

Do *not* apply pressure. Cover both eyes with gauze pads. Keep victim in semi-reclining position.

Keep victim flat on back with eyes closed. Place cold pack gently on bony area.

Attempt, in order, each procedure until one is effective:
1. Pull upper eyelid down.
2. Pull lower lid down and look at inner surface while victim looks up. If object seen, flush gently with water.
3. Invert upper eyelid over matchstick or Q tip. If object seen, flush gently with water.
If successful, medical attention is usually not needed.

Seek medical attention.

- If a foreign object in the nose is suspected, look into the nose, but do *not* probe with a finger or swab.
- With thumb and forefinger, apply steady pressure to both nostrils for five minutes before releasing. Remind the victim to breathe through his or her mouth and to spit out any accumulated blood.
- If bleeding persists, have the victim gently blow the nose to remove any clots and excess blood, and to minimize sneezing. This allows new clots to form. Then, press the nostrils again for five minutes.
- Some experts recommend gently placing inside the bleeding nostril a cotton ball that has been soaked in hydrogen peroxide, a nasal decongestant, or plain water. Sometimes lack of time and/or materials prevent using this procedure.
- Some authorities suggest placing a roll of gauze (diameter of a pencil in size) between the upper lip and teeth and pressing against it with your fingers to stop the blood flow.
- Apply ice over the nose to help control bleeding.
- If the victim is unconscious, place the victim on his or her side to prevent inhaling of blood and attempt the procedures in the above list.
- Seek medical attention if any of the following occurs:

    1. The nostril pinching does *not* stop the bleeding after a second attempt.

    2. Signs and symptoms suggest a posterior source of bleeding.

    3. The victim has high blood pressure, is taking anticoagulants (blood thinners) or large doses of aspirin.

    4. Bleeding occurs after a blow to the nose (suspect a broken nose).

Most nosebleed victims never need medical care since nosebleeds are self-limited, and the victim can control the bleeding.

Dental Injuries

The following first aid procedures provide temporary relief for dental emergencies, but it is important to consult with a dentist as soon as possible.

Objects Wedged Between Teeth

- Attempt to remove the object with dental floss. Guide the floss in carefully so the gum tissue is not injured.
- Do *not* use a sharp or pointed tool to remove the object. If unsuccessful, take the victim to a dentist.

Care After a Nosebleed

After a nosebleed has stopped, suggest to the victim:

1. Sneeze through an open mouth, if there is a need to sneeze.

2. Avoid bending over or too much physical exertion.

3. Elevate the head with two pillows when lying down.

4. Keep the nostrils moist by applying a little petroleum jelly just inside the nostril for a week; increase the humidity in the bedroom during the winter months with a cold-mist humidifier.

5. Avoid picking or rubbing the nose.

6. Avoid hot drinks and alcoholic beverages for a week.

7. Avoid smoking or taking aspirin for a week.

Bitten Lip or Tongue

Apply direct pressure to the bleeding area with a sterile gauze or clean cloth. If the lip is swollen, apply a cold compress. Take the victim to a hospital emergency room if the bleeding persists or if the bite is severe.

Knocked-Out Tooth

More than 2 million teeth are accidentally knocked out in the United States each year. More than 90 percent of them can be saved with the proper treatment.

- When a permanent tooth is completely knocked out, save it and take it, along with the victim, to the dentist immediately. With proper first aid procedures, the tooth may be successfully reimplanted in the socket.
- Do *not* put the tooth in mouthwash or alcohol or scrub it with abrasives or chemicals. And do *not* touch the root of the tooth.

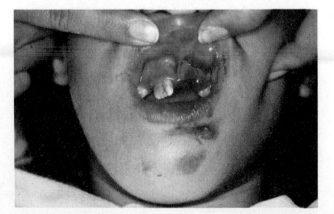

Tooth avulsion

Place the tooth in a cup of cold whole milk. Avoid low fat or powdered milk or milk by-products such as yogurt.

- Take the victim and tooth to a dentist immediately (within 30 minutes). Some experts recommend that the tooth be placed in the victim's mouth to keep it moist until dental treatment is available. This method, though convenient, presents the risk, especially in children, of the tooth's being accidentally swallowed.
- A partially extracted tooth can be pushed into place without rinsing the tooth. Then seek a dentist so the loose tooth can be stabilized.
- If in remote areas with no dentist nearby, replant a knocked out tooth by first running

cool water over it to clean away debris (do *not* scrub the tooth), and then by gently repositioning it in the socket, using adjacent teeth as a guide. Push the tooth so the top is even with the adjacent teeth. Successful replanting occurs best within 30 minutes of the accident. See a dentist as soon as possible.

[handwritten: , only if you have running water nearby]

Broken Tooth

- Immediate attention is necessary when a tooth breaks since it may need to be extracted. Attempt to clean any dirt, blood, and debris from the injured area with a sterile gauze or clean cloth and warm water.

TABLE 6-2 Dental Emergency Procedures

Toothache	Rinse the mouth vigorously with warm water to clean out debris. Use dental floss to remove any food that might be trapped between the teeth. (*Do not place aspirin on the aching tooth or gum tissues.*) See your dentist as soon as possible.
Orthodontic problems (braces and retainers)	If a wire is causing irritation, cover end of the wire with a small cotton ball, beeswax, or a piece of gauze, until you can get to the dentist.
	If a wire is embedded in the cheek, tongue, or gum tissue, do not attempt to remove it. Go to your dentist immediately.
	If an appliance becomes loose or a piece of it breaks off, take the appliance and the piece and go to the dentist.
Knocked-out tooth	If the tooth is dirty, rinse it gently in running water. *Do not scrub it.*
	Gently insert and hold the tooth in its socket. If this is not possible, place the tooth in a container of milk or cool water.
	Go immediately to your dentist (within 30 minutes, if possible). Don't forget to bring the tooth.
Broken tooth	Gently clean dirt or debris from the injured area with warm water. Place cold compresses on the face, in the area of the injured tooth, to minimize swelling.
	Go to the dentist immediately.
Bitten tongue or lip	Apply direct pressure to the bleeding area with a clean cloth. If swelling is present, apply cold compresses. If bleeding does not stop, go to a hospital emergency room.
Objects wedged between teeth	Try to remove the object with dental floss. Guide the floss carefully to avoid cutting the gums. If not successful in removing the object, go to the dentist. Do not try to remove the object with a sharp or pointed instrument.
Possible fractured jaw	Immobilize the jaw by any means (handkerchief, necktie, towel). If swelling is present, apply cold compresses. Call your dentist or go immediately to a hospital emergency room.

Source: Copyright by the American Dental Association; reprinted by permission.

■ NOSEBLEEDS ■

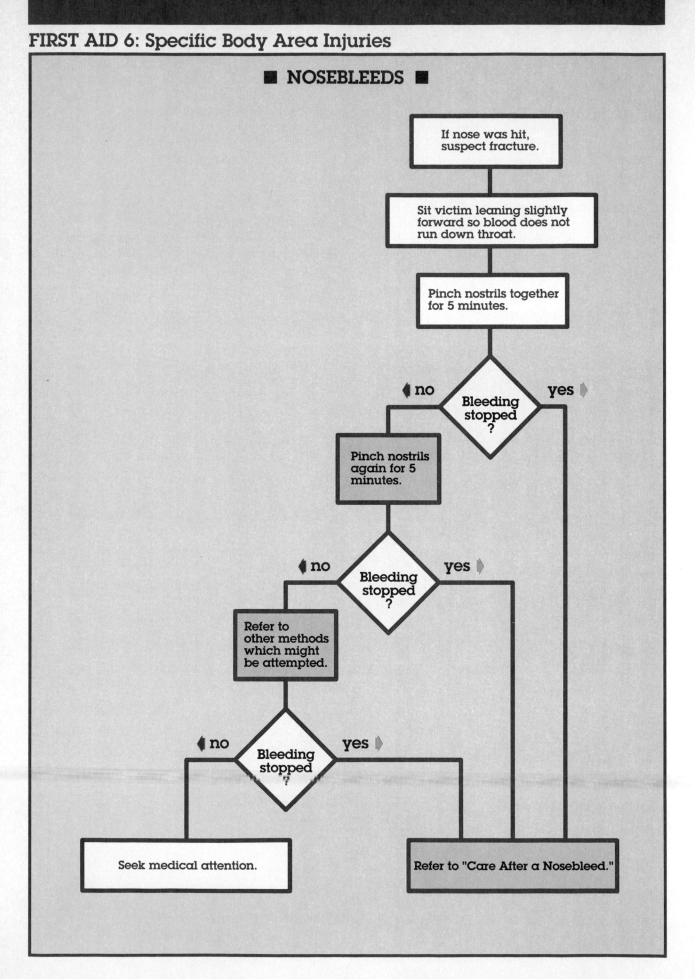

If nose was hit, suspect fracture.

Sit victim leaning slightly forward so blood does not run down throat.

Pinch nostrils together for 5 minutes.

Bleeding stopped?

no — Pinch nostrils again for 5 minutes.

yes

Bleeding stopped?

no — Refer to other methods which might be attempted.

yes

Bleeding stopped?

no — Seek medical attention.

yes — Refer to "Care After a Nosebleed."

■ DENTAL INJURIES ■

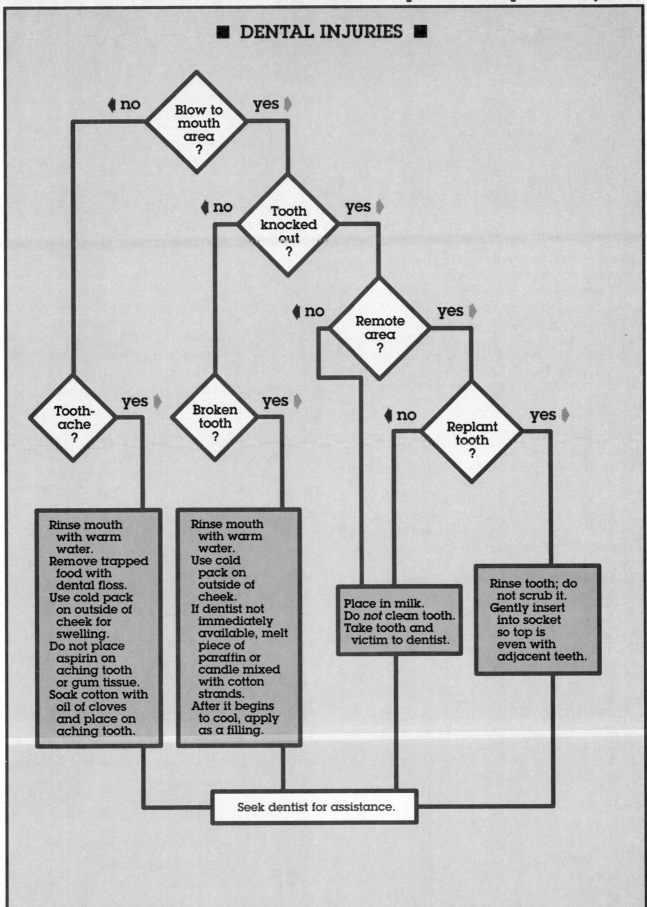

no ◀ **Blow to mouth area ?** ▶ yes

no ◀ **Tooth knocked out ?** ▶ yes

no ◀ **Remote area ?** ▶ yes

Tooth-ache ? ▶ yes

Broken tooth ? ▶ yes

no ◀ **Replant tooth ?** ▶ yes

Rinse mouth with warm water.
Remove trapped food with dental floss.
Use cold pack on outside of cheek for swelling.
Do not place aspirin on aching tooth or gum tissue.
Soak cotton with oil of cloves and place on aching tooth.

Rinse mouth with warm water.
Use cold pack on outside of cheek.
If dentist not immediately available, melt piece of paraffin or candle mixed with cotton strands.
After it begins to cool, apply as a filling.

Place in milk.
Do *not* clean tooth.
Take tooth and victim to dentist.

Rinse tooth; do not scrub it.
Gently insert into socket so top is even with adjacent teeth.

Seek dentist for assistance.

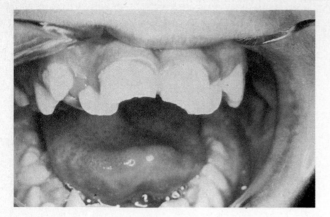
Broken teeth

- Apply a cold compress on the face next to the injured tooth to minimize swelling.
- If a jaw fracture is suspected, immobilize the jaw by any available means—place a scarf, handkerchief, tie, or towel over and under the chin, and tie the ends on top of the victim's head. In either case, immediately take the victim to an oral surgeon or hospital emergency room.

Toothache

- Rinse the mouth vigorously with warm water to clean out debris.
- Use dental floss to remove any food that might be trapped between the teeth.
- Do *not* place aspirin on the aching tooth or gum tissues.
- If a cavity is present, insert a small cotton ball soaked in oil of cloves (eugenol). Do *not* cover a cavity with cotton if there is any pus discharge or facial swelling. See a dentist as soon as possible.

Although temporary relief can be provided in most dental emergencies, by all means, when in doubt, consult a dentist as soon as possible.

Chest Injuries

Chest wounds may be either **open** or **closed. Open chest wounds** are caused by penetrating objects. **Closed chest wounds** result from blunt blows.

Signs and Symptoms

Important signs of chest injuries include:

- Pain at the injury site
- Breathing difficulty
- Blueness of the lips and/or fingernail beds, indicating oxygen deficiency (cyanosis)
- Coughing or spitting up blood
- Bruising or an open chest wound
- Failure of one or both sides of the chest to expand normally when inhaling

Types of Chest Injuries and First Aid

Rib fracture. The upper four ribs are rarely fractured because they are protected by the collarbone and shoulder blade. The lower two ribs are hard to fracture because they are attached on only one end and have the freedom to move (therefore known as "floating ribs").

The victim of a rib fracture can usually point out the injury's exact location. Deep breathing, coughing, or movement is usually quite painful. There may or may not be a rib deformity, bruise, or laceration of the area. Shortness of breath, severe coughing, or coughing up blood all indicate a major injury rather than a simple rib fracture.

Do *not* bind, strap, or tape a rib fracture. Such wrapping predisposes the victim to pneumonia. Instead, the victim can hold a pillow against the injured area. Instruct the victim to take deep breaths to prevent pneumonia.

Flail chest. A rib fracture involving three or more adjacent ribs that are broken in more than one place is known as a **flail chest** and represents a serious injury. The chest wall may move in the opposite direction to the rest of the chest wall during breathing (called **paradoxical breathing**). Stabilize the ribs by holding a pillow against them to improve breathing. Place the victim in a semisitting position, inclined to the injured side to assist breathing.

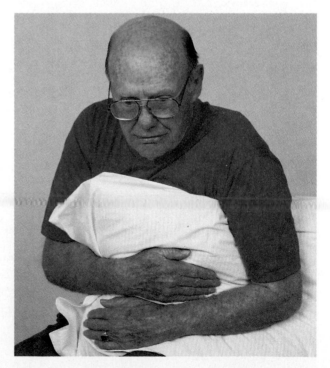
Pillow over broken ribs

■ CHEST INJURIES ■

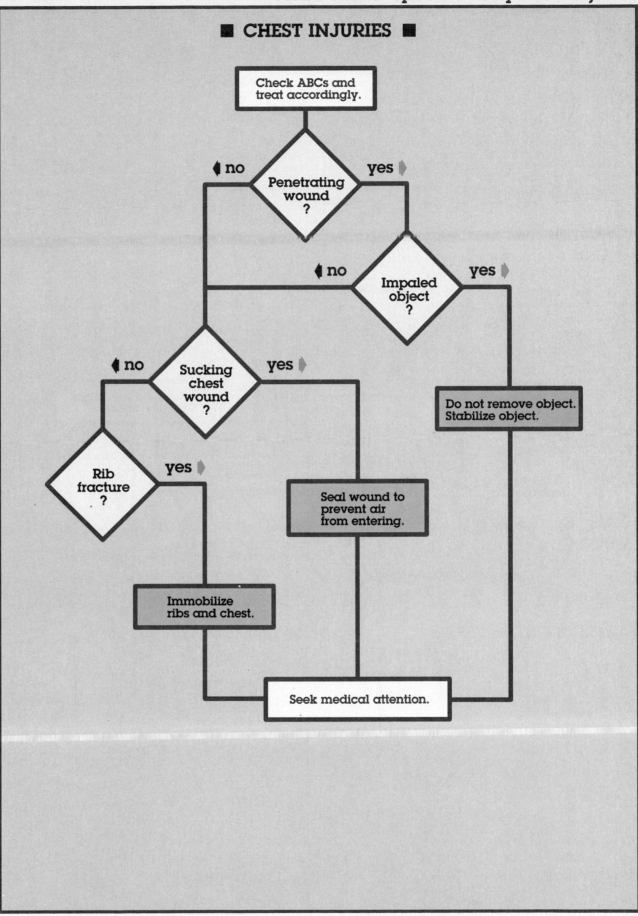

Check ABCs and treat accordingly.

Penetrating wound ?
- no
- yes

Impaled object ?
- no
- yes

Do not remove object. Stabilize object.

Sucking chest wound ?
- no
- yes

Seal wound to prevent air from entering.

Rib fracture ?
- yes

Immobilize ribs and chest.

Seek medical attention.

■ ABDOMINAL INJURIES ■

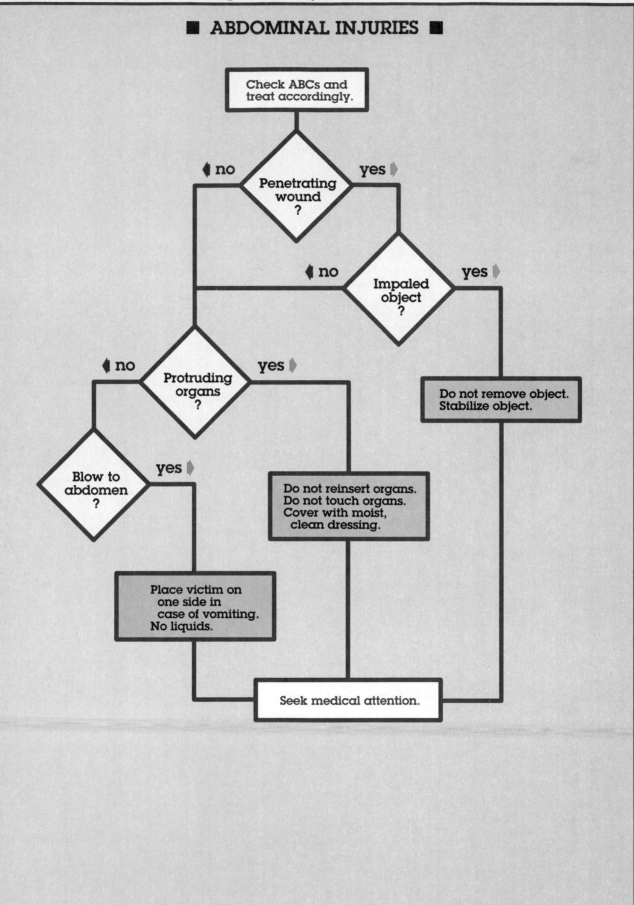

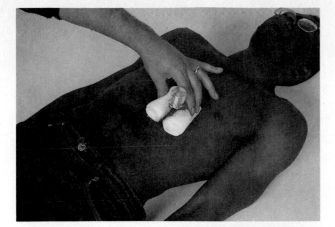

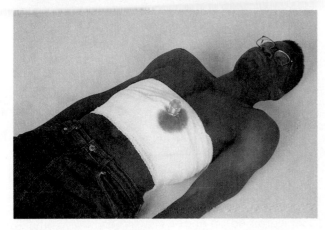

Stabilizing impaled object

Penetrating wound. This wound must be closed quickly to prevent outside air from entering the chest cavity. Do *not* remove or attempt to remove an impaled object because bleeding and air in the chest cavity can occur. Stabilize the object in place with bulky dressings and pads.

A **sucking chest wound** can result when a chest wound allows air to pass into and out of the chest with each respiration. Have the victim take a breath and let it out; then seal the wound with anything available to stop air from entering the chest cavity. A household plastic wrap folded several times works well, or you can use your hand. Be sure that the wrap is several inches wider than the wound. Place a dressing over the plastic wrap, and tape it in place, leaving one corner untaped. This creates a flutter valve that prevents air from being trapped in the chest cavity. If the victim has trouble breathing, remove the plastic cover to let all air escape, then reapply. *Don't do, may cause collapsed lung.*

Abdominal Injuries

Abdominal injuries may be **open** or **closed**. **Open injuries** occur when a foreign object enters the abdomen, resulting in external bleeding. **Closed injuries** result from a severe blow that shows no open wound or bleeding on the outside of the body.

Hollow organ (e.g., stomach, intestines) ruptures spill their contents into the abdominal cavity, causing inflammation. Solid organ (e.g., liver, pancreas) ruptures result in severe bleeding.

Signs and Symptoms

- Pain in the abdomen, which may involve cramping
- Legs drawn up to the chest
- Skin wounds and penetrations
- Nausea and vomiting
- Protruding organs
- Blood in the urine or stool
- Guarding abdomen
- Rapid pulse
- Moist, cold skin

Types of Abdominal Injuries and First Aid

Blunt wound. Internal organ bruising and damage can result from a severe blow to the abdomen. Place the victim on one side in a comfortable position, and expect vomiting. Do *not* give liquids or food. If you are hours from medical assistance, allow victim to suck on a clean cloth soaked in water to relieve a dry mouth.

Penetrating injuries. Expect internal organs to be damaged. If the penetrating object is still in place, leave it in and bandage around it to control external bleeding and to stabilize the object. Do *not* remove the object. Place the victim on his or her side.

Protruding organs. If any of the abdominal organs lie outside the abdominal cavity, do *not* try to reinsert

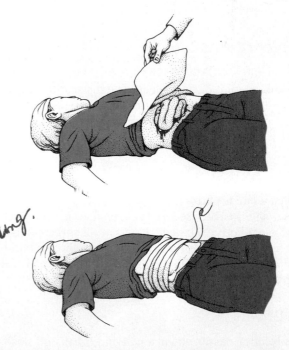

Protruding organs. Do not reinsert them. Cover them with a moist sterile dressing.

them inside the abdomen because this introduces infection and could damage the intestine. Cover any extruding organs with a sterile dressing if you have one; otherwise, use a clean cloth. Do *not* cover the organs tightly or with any material that clings or disintegrates when wet. Since ambulances carry sterile saline (saltwater), which is the best solution to pour on the dressing to keep the protruding organs from drying out, it is usually best to wait for the ambulance to arrive. Place the victim on his or her side. In remote locations, the cleanest available water might be used to keep the organs from drying out.

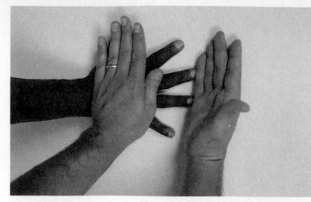

Hammer test

Finger and Toe Injuries

Hands and feet are marvels of complexity that are able to sustain considerable abuse. Nevertheless, fingers and toes are often injured.

Fractures

The presence of swelling and tenderness help identify a fractured finger. However, one of the most useful ways to tell if a finger might be broken is by using the "hammer" test. In this test the victim holds the fingers in full extension. The first aider firmly hammers the ends of the victim's fingers toward the victim's hand, transmitting the force down the shaft of the finger's bones and producing pain if a fracture is present. If this hammering produces additional pain, suspect a broken bone. Immobilize the finger by either taping the injured finger to an adjacent finger or by following the procedures described on page 231.

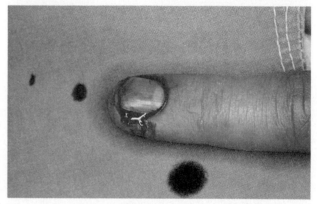

Door slammed on finger

Dislocations

The victim of a dislocated finger should never attempt to pull the joint back in place. The dislocation should be reduced by a physician after x-rays are taken to see that no other injury is involved. Care for the finger as you would a fracture.

Nail Avulsion

When a nail is partly torn loose, do not trim away the loose nail. Instead, secure the damaged nail in place with an adhesive bandage. If part or all of the nail has been completely torn away, apply an adhesive bandage coated with antibiotic ointment. A new nail will appear about a month or so later.

Splinters

If a splinter passes under a nail and breaks off flush, remove the embedded part by grasping its end with tweezers after cutting a V-shaped notch in the nail to

gain access to the splinter. Remove a splinter in the skin by teasing it out with a sterile needle until the end can be grasped with tweezers or fingers.

Bleeding and Wounds

Standard first aid (see Chapter 5) should be applied. Take finger and toe wounds seriously because nerve and tendon damage can accompany lacerations and other types of wounds.

Amputations

Fingers and toes are the body parts most often amputated. Standard first aid (see Chapter 5) should be applied. Note that, while fingers can often be reattached, toes cannot.

Bandaging/Splinting

Place an injured hand into what is called the "position of function" (finger joints flexed as you would when comfortably holding a baseball). A wad of bulky dressings and cloths is then placed in the palm of the hand. Apply to the palm side of the hand and secure with a roller bandage either a padded board splint or about 40 pages of folded newspapers. See page 231.

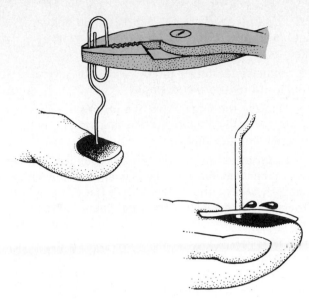

Making a hole in a fingernail

Bleeding Under a Fingernail

Blood can collect under a fingernail after any direct blow to the fingernail. The accumulated blood under the nail causes severe pain.

First Aid

- Immerse the end of the finger in ice water or apply an ice pack against the injured nail while elevating the hand.
- Relieve the severe pain by one of two methods:

  1. Using a rotary action, drill through the nail with the sharp point of a knife. This method can produce pain.

  2. Straighten the end of a metal (noncoated) wire paper clip. Hold the paper clip by pliers and heat the paper clip until red-hot (best done with a match). Press the glowing end of the clip to the nail so it melts through. Little pressure is needed. The nail has no nerves, so this causes no pain.
- Apply a dressing to absorb the draining blood and to protect the injured nail.

Fishhook Removal

Tape an embedded fishhook in place and do *not* try to remove it if injury to a nearby body part (e.g., eye) or an underlying structure (e.g., blood vessel or nerve) is possible, or if the victim is uncooperative.

If only the point and not the barb of a fishhook penetrates the skin, remove the fishhook by backing it out. Then treat the wound like a puncture wound and seek medical attention for a possible tetanus shot.

However, if the hook's barb has entered the skin, follow these procedures:

1. If medical care is near, transport the victim and have a physician remove the hook.

2. If in a remote area far from medical care, remove the hook by either the pliers method or the fishline method.

Pliers Method ("push and cut")

This method should be undertaken with extreme care because it can produce further injury that is even more severe if the hook is pushed into blood vessels, nerves, or tendons.

- Pliers must have tempered jaws that can cut through a hook. The proper kind of pliers is usually unavailable or the barb is buried too deeply to be pushed through. Test the pliers by first cutting a similar fishhook.
- Use cold or hard pressure around the hook to provide temporary numbness.
- Push the embedded hook further in, in a shallow curve, until the point and barb come out through the skin.
- Cut the barb off and back the hook out the way it came in.
- After removing the hook, treat the wound and seek medical attention for a possible tetanus shot.

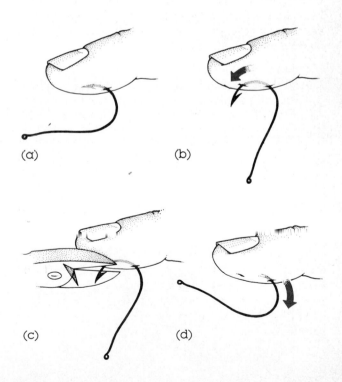

(a)   (b)

(c)   (d)

Fishhook removal: pliers method

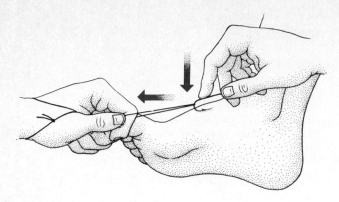

Fishhook removal: fishline method

Fishline Method ("push and pull")

- Loop a piece of fishline over the bend or curve of the embedded hook.
- Stabilize the victim's hooked body area.
- Use cold or hard pressure around the hook to provide temporary numbness.
- With one hand, press down on the hook's shank and eye while the other hand sharply jerks the fishline that is over the hook's bend or curve. The jerk movement should be parallel to the skin's surface. The hook will neatly come out of the same hole it entered, causing little pain.
- After removing the hook, treat the wound and seek medical attention for a possible tetanus shot.

Ring Removal

Sometimes a finger is too swollen for a ring to be removed. Ring strangulation can be a serious problem if it cuts off circulation long enough. Gangrene may result within four or five hours. Try one or more of the following methods:

1. Lubricate the finger with grease, oil, butter, petroleum jelly, or some other slippery substance, then try to remove the ring.

2. Immerse the finger in cold water for several minutes to reduce the swelling.

3. Massage the finger from the tip to the hand to move the swelling; lubricate the finger again and try removing the ring.

4. Slide several inches of thin string under the ring toward the hand. Push the string under the ring with a match stick or toothpick. Then wrap the string tightly around the finger below the ring, going toward the fingernail and away from the ring. Each wrap should be right next to the one before. While holding the wrapping snugly in place with the fingers of one hand, grasp the upper end of the string with the other hand. Pull the string downward over the ring. The ring may slide over the string. Repeat the procedure several times to get the ring off.

5. Start about an inch from the ring edge and smoothly wind string around the finger, going toward the ring with one strand touching the next. Continue winding smoothly and tightly right up to the edge of the ring. The advantage of this method is that it tends to push the swelling toward the hand. Slip the string end under the ring with a match stick or toothpick. Slowly unwind the string on the hand side of the ring. You should then be able to gently twist the ring off the finger over the wound and string.

6. Cut the narrowest part of the ring with a ring saw, jeweler's saw, ring cutter, or fine hacksaw blade. Protect the exposed portions of the finger.

7. Inflate an ordinary balloon (preferably a slender, tube-shaped one) about three-fourths full. Tie the end. Insert the victim's swollen finger into the end of the balloon so that the balloon rolls back evenly around the finger. In about 15 minutes, the finger should return to its normal size and the ring can be removed.

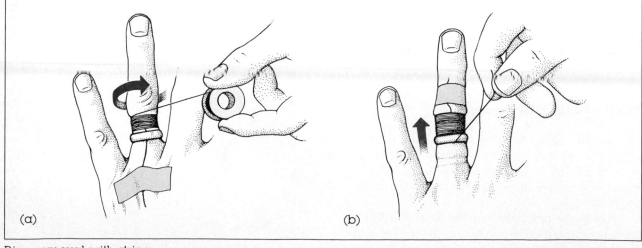

(a)   (b)

Ring removal with string

■ FISHHOOK REMOVAL ■

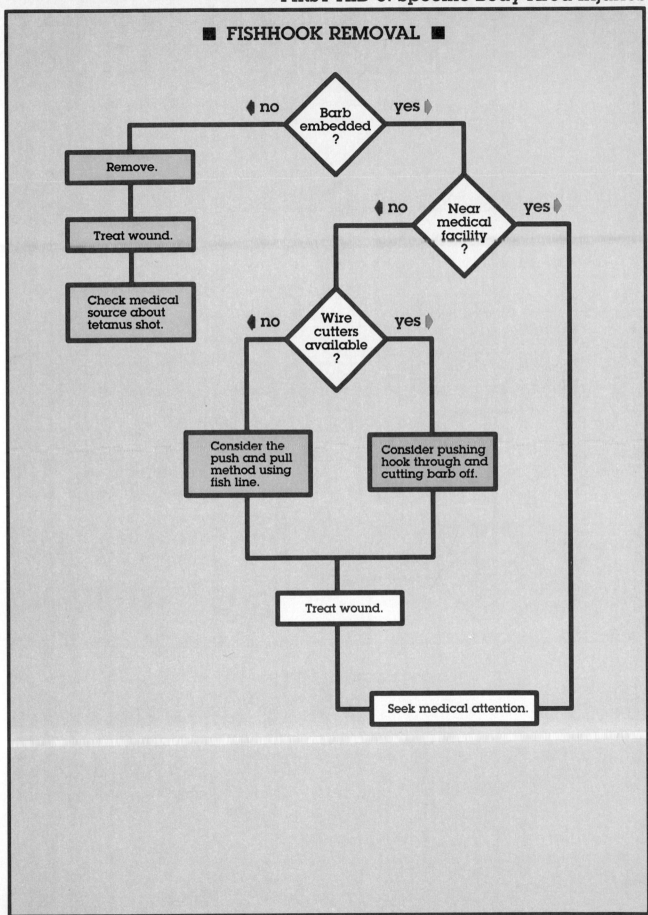

■ BLISTERS ■

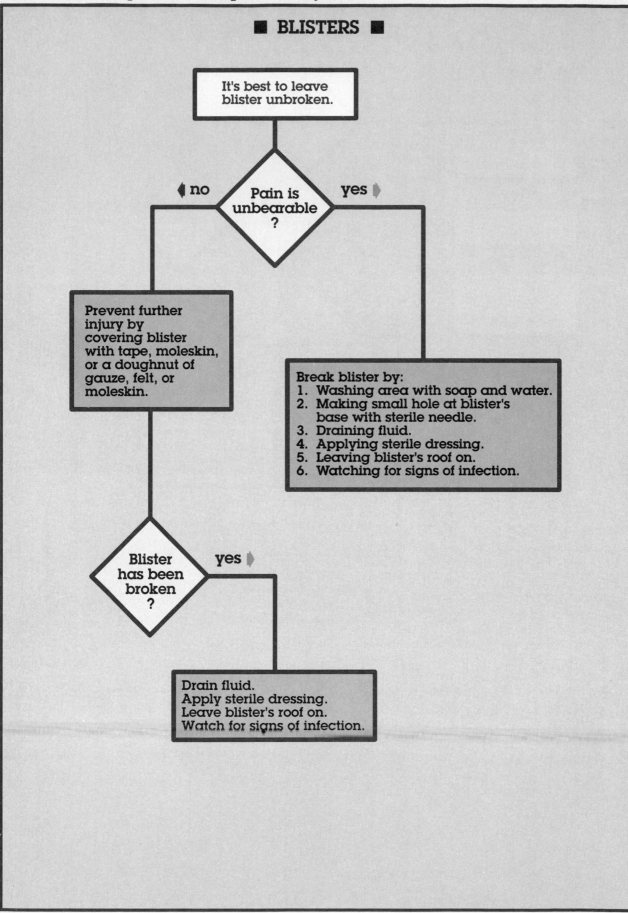

It's best to leave blister unbroken.

Pain is unbearable?

no → Prevent further injury by covering blister with tape, moleskin, or a doughnut of gauze, felt, or moleskin.

yes → Break blister by:
1. Washing area with soap and water.
2. Making small hole at blister's base with sterile needle.
3. Draining fluid.
4. Applying sterile dressing.
5. Leaving blister's roof on.
6. Watching for signs of infection.

Blister has been broken?

yes → Drain fluid.
Apply sterile dressing.
Leave blister's roof on.
Watch for signs of infection.

Blisters

A blister is a collection of fluid in a "bubble" under the outer layer of skin. It results from excessive rubbing or friction. (This section does not apply to blisters from burns, frostbite, or contact with a poisonous plant.)

Signs and Symptoms

- Fluid collection under the skin's outer layer
- Pain resulting from touch or pressure
- Swelling and redness around the blister

First Aid

After a blister forms, prevent further injury and reduce pain from pressure by covering small blisters with an adhesive bandage. A large blister should be covered with a porous, plastic-coated gauze pad (which allows the area to breathe) or a stack of gauze pads cut in a doughnut shape to dissipate pressure from the blister. Whenever possible, do *not* break a blister.

When a blister must be broken because of pain:

- Wash the area with soap and warm water. Dry and swab the area with 70% rubbing alcohol.
- Make several small holes at the base of the blister with a sterilized needle. Sterilize the needle by either soaking it in rubbing alcohol or holding it until it gets red over the top of a match flame. Let it cool before using.
- Drain the fluid by gently pressing the blister's top. Do *not* remove the blister's roof. In some cases, the blister may have to be drained several times in the first 24 hours. Apply an antibiotic ointment over the site and cover with a sterile dressing to protect the area from further irritation. After several days, "unroof" any dead skin by using tweezers to lift the skin, and cut it away with scissors. Reapply antibiotic ointment and a sterile gauze dressing.
- If a blister has ruptured and its roof is gone, apply antibiotic ointment, a sterile gauze dressing, and stacked sterile dressings cut in a doughnut shape. All ruptured blisters should be cleaned with soap and water to prevent infection.
- Check daily for signs of infection (redness or pus). See a doctor if the blister becomes infected. If not infected, blisters usually heal in three to seven days.

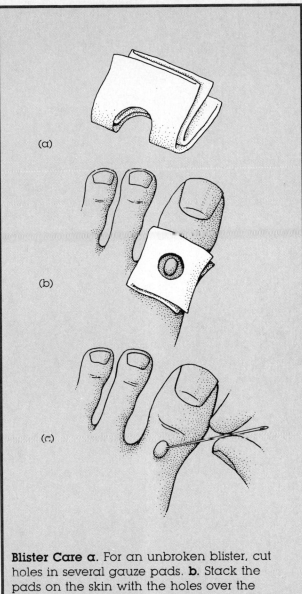

(a)

(b)

(c)

Blister Care a. For an unbroken blister, cut holes in several gauze pads. **b.** Stack the pads on the skin with the holes over the blister. Loosely tape an uncut gauze pad over the top. **c.** If blister is painful or likely to break, puncture the blister's edge with a sterilized needle. Drain all the fluid. Tape a sterile or clean gauze pad or cloth over the flattened blister.

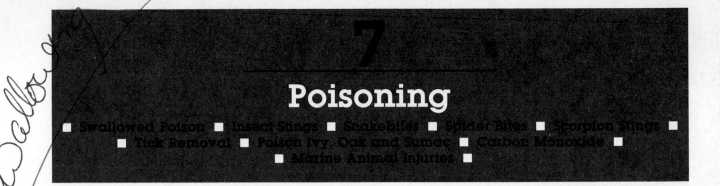

7

Poisoning

■ Swallowed Poison ■ Insect Stings ■ Snakebites ■ Spider Bites ■ Scorpion Stings ■
■ Tick Removal ■ Poison Ivy, Oak and Sumac ■ Carbon Monoxide ■
■ Marine Animal Injuries ■

A poison is a relatively small amount of any substance (solid, liquid, or gas) that when swallowed, inhaled, absorbed, or injected can by its chemical action damage tissue or adversely change organ function and thus can affect health or cause death.

Swallowed Poison

Deaths by swallowing poison have dramatically decreased in recent years, particularly in children under age five. Despite this reduction, nonfatal poisoning remains a major cause of hospital admissions and emergency room care. For every poisoning death among children under the age of five, 80,000 to 90,000 nonfatal cases are seen in emergency rooms and about 20,000 children are hospitalized.

Swallowed poisons usually remain in the stomach only a short time, and the stomach absorbs only small amounts. Most absorption takes place after the poison passes into the small intestine. Suspect poisoning in any person who is suddenly ill with abdominal pain, nausea, and/or vomiting.

Signs and Symptoms

■ Abdominal pain and cramping
■ Nausea or vomiting
■ Diarrhea
■ Burns, odor, stains around and in mouth
■ Drowsiness or unconsciousness
■ Poison containers or plants nearby

First Aid

■ Determine the critical information, which includes:

  1. *Who?* Age and size of the victim
  2. *What?* Type of poison swallowed
  3. *How much?* A taste, half a bottle, etc.
  4. *How?* Circumstances
  5. *When?* Time taken

■ Contact the poison control center, hospital emergency department, or a physician immediately. Some poisons produce little damage until hours later, while others do

damage immediately. More than 70 percent of poisonings can be treated through instructions taken over the telephone. Otherwise, victims should be transported to a medical facility.

■ Check respirations and pulse often, if victim is unconscious.
■ Unless a medical authority advises it, do *not* automatically give water or milk to dilute except when the victim has swallowed caustics or corrosives (e.g., acids and alkalis). Reasons include the fact that fluids may dissolve tablets or capsules more rapidly, and may fill up the stomach, thus forcing poison into the small intestines where absorption is faster.
■ Do *not* induce vomiting unless a medical authority advises it. Inducing vomiting removes 30–50 percent of the poison from the stomach. Inducing vomiting must be done within 30 minutes of swallowing or before the poison leaves the stomach.

A medical authority will usually say *never* induce vomiting for:

■ A victim with seizures
■ An unconscious or drowsy victim
■ A woman in the late stages of pregnancy
■ A person with a history of advanced heart disease or who is likely to suffer a heart attack
■ A person who has swallowed corrosives (strong acids and alkalis)
■ A victim who has swallowed petroleum products (e.g., gasoline, lighter fluid, furniture polish)
■ A person who has swallowed strychnine
■ A child less than 6 months old

Do *not* use salt water to induce vomiting because it is dangerous and can kill children. Do *not* gag the victim by sticking a finger down his or her throat since it is usually ineffective in causing vomiting (only in 15 percent of cases does it work) and it wastes time.

Many poisons induce vomiting for some victims; others require syrup of ipecac. It can be purchased without a prescription, and is easily given, effective, and relatively safe.

■ SWALLOWED POISON ■

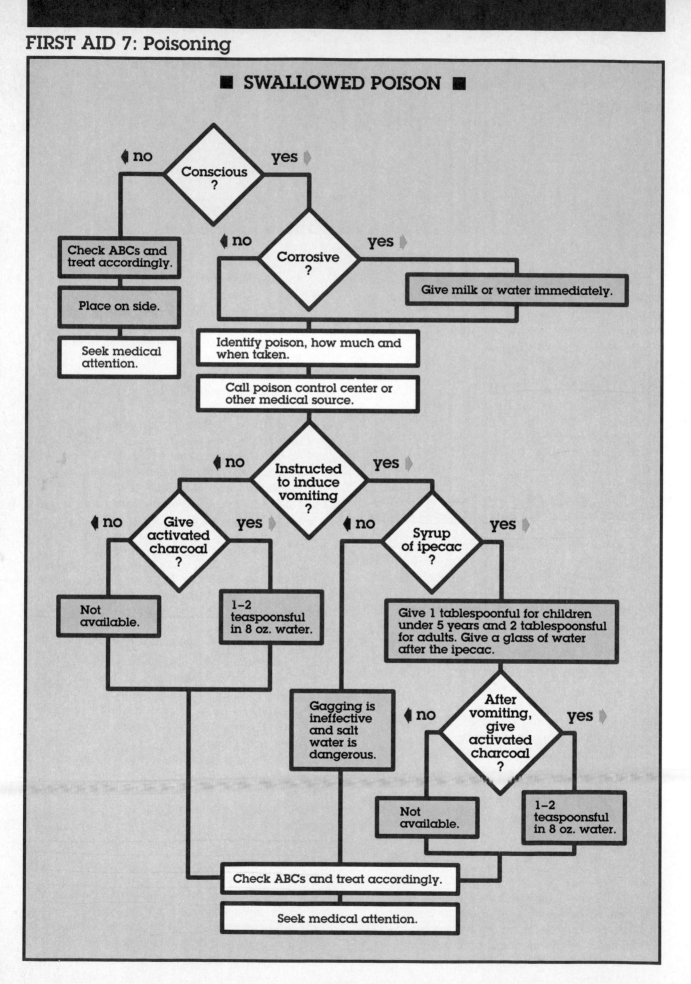

How to Poison-Proof Your Home

1. Keep all medicines (including over-the-counter products), cleaning products, automotive care products and plants out of reach of children. Store them up high or in locked cabinets.

2. Use products with child-resistant packaging and always replace the cap properly. But don't rely on the packaging alone to protect your child.

3. Use medicines wisely. Follow label or prescription instructions carefully. Give prescription medicine only to the person for whom it was prescribed. Discard outdated medications safely—flush them down the toilet, rinse out the container and bury it deep in the trash.

4. Avoid transferring poisonous products from their original containers. If you must do this, carefully copy all information from the original label—product name, expiration date, contents—and attach it to the new container. And never put poisonous substances into a container that once held food, such as a soda bottle. Even an adult may mistake the contents for an edible product.

5. Store harmful products away from food, and store external medications separately from internal medications to lessen the chance of someone mistaking one for the other.

6. Do not refer to medicine as "candy" when talking to children—they may take you literally. And don't take medicine in front of the children. Their imitative behavior may lead to tragedy.

7. Keep a one-ounce bottle of syrup of ipecac to induce vomiting for each child in the house, but don't administer it without professional medical advice. (Syrup of ipecac is available from your pharmacist.) Keep the number of your local poison control center, hospital emergency room or family doctor posted near the phone.

Source: National Safety Council, Family Safety & Health.

If instructed by a medical authority to induce vomiting by using syrup of ipecac, give:

- Adults: 2 tablespoons with 2–3 glasses of warm water
- Children: 1 tablespoon with 1–2 glasses of warm water
- Infants: 1–2 teaspoons with 1 bottle or glass of warm water (when possible, infants should be given ipecac in a medical facility)

Syrup of ipecac may take up to 20 minutes to work. Vomiting occurs in 97 percent of all people and a second dose is seldom needed. However, repeat the initial dosage once if the victim does not vomit after 20 minutes.

- Activated charcoal can be given after the victim has stopped vomiting. This substance handles the remaining poison in the stomach since syrup of ipecac removes only 30–50 percent of swallowed poisons. Activated charcoal acts like a sponge and binds the poison within the digestive system. Substances such as burned toast, fireplace ashes, and charcoal briquettes are all ineffective. Most pharmacies do not routinely carry charcoal activated by heating in carbon dioxide. First aiders seldom give it since a victim can usually arrive at a medical facility within minutes.
- Save poison containers, plants, and vomit to help medical personnel identify the poison and prescribe appropriate treatment.
- Position unconscious victims on their side and do *not* give anything by mouth.
- Do *not* follow a container label's first aid procedures or recommended antidotes without getting confirmation from a medical authority since many labels are wrong.

Insect Stings

For a severely allergic person, a single sting may be fatal within minutes. Although accounts exist of individuals who have survived some 2,000 stings, 500

Avoiding Insect Stings

Here are some ways to avoid being stung:

1. Have a nonallergic person destroy any insect nests that appear around the home or yard.

2. Do not go barefoot or wear sandals outdoors.

3. Wear close-fitting clothes that won't trap an insect. Long-sleeved shirts, long pants, and gloves provide protection. They should be light-weight for comfort on hot days.

4. Do not look or smell like a flower. Brightly colored clothing, perfumed lotions, aftershaves, shampoos, and cosmetics can attract insects.

5. Be alert while eating outdoors since food and garbage attract insects.

6. If you find yourself close to an insect, do not swat or run since such actions can trigger an attack. Retreat slowly, or if retreat is impossible, lie face down and cover your head with your arms.

TABLE 7-1 Facts About Troublesome Insects

Description	Habitat	Problem	Severity	Treatment	Protection
Chigger Oval with red velvety covering. Sometimes almost colorless. Larva has six legs. Harmless adult has eight and resembles a small spider. Very tiny—about 1/20-inch long.	Found in low damp places covered with vegetation: shaded woods, high grass or weeds, fruit orchards. Also lawns and golf courses. From Canada to Argentina.	Attaches itself to the skin by inserting mouthparts into a hair follicle. Injects a digestive fluid that causes cells to disintegrate. Then feeds on cell parts. It does not suck blood.	Itching from secreted enzymes results several hours after contact. Small red welts appear. Secondary infection often follows. Degree of irritation varies with individuals.	Lather with soap and rinse several times to remove chiggers. If welts have formed, dab antiseptic on area. Severe lesions may require antihistamine ointment.	Apply proper repellent to clothing, particularly near uncovered areas such as wrists and ankles. Apply to skin. Spray or dust infested areas (lawns, plants) with suitable chemicals.
Bedbug Flat oval body with short broad head and six legs. Adult is reddish brown. Young are yellowish white. Unpleasant pungent odor. From 1/8- to 1/4-inch in length.	Hides in crevices, mattresses, under loose wallpaper during day. At night travels considerable distance to find victims. Widely distributed throughout the world.	Punctures the skin with piercing organs and sucks blood. Local inflammation and welts result from anticoagulant enzyme that bug secretes from salivary glands while feeding.	Affects people differently. Some have marked swelling and considerable irritation; others aren't bothered. Sometimes transmits serious diseases.	Apply antiseptic to prevent possible infection. Bug usually bites sleeping victim, gorges itself completely in 3 to 5 minutes and departs. It's rarely necessary to remove one.	Spray beds, mattresses, bed springs, and baseboards with insecticide. Bugs live in large groups. They migrate to new homes on water pipes and clothing.
Brown Recluse Spider Oval body with eight legs. Light yellow to medium dark brown. Has distinctive mark shaped like a fiddle on its back. Body from 3/8- to 1/2-inch long, 1/4-inch wide, 3/4-inch from toe-to-toe.	Prefers dark places where it's seldom disturbed. Outdoors: old trash piles, debris, and rough ground. Indoors: attics, storerooms, closets. Found in southern and midwestern United States.	Bites produce an almost painless sting that may not be noticed, at first. Shy, it bites only when annoyed or surprised. Left alone, it won't bite. Victim rarely sees the spider.	In 2 to 8 hours pain may be noticed, followed by blisters, swelling, hemorrhage, or ulceration. Some people experience rash, nausea, jaundice, chills, fever, cramps, or joint pain.	Summon doctor. Bite may require hospitalization for a few days. Full healing may take from 6 to 8 weeks. Weak adults and children have been known to die.	Use caution when cleaning secluded areas in the home or using machinery usually left idle. Check firewood, inside shoes, packed clothing and bedrolls—frequent hideaways.
Black Widow Spider Color varies from dark brown to glossy black. Densely covered with short microscopic hairs. Red or yellow hourglass marking on the underside of the female's abdomen. Male does not have this mark and is not poisonous. Overall length with legs extended is 1 1/2 inch. Body is 1/4-inch wide.	Found with eggs and web. Outside: in vacant rodent holes, under stones, logs, in long grass, hollow stumps, and brush piles. Inside: in dark corners of barns, garages, piles of stone, wood. Most bites occur in outhouses. Found in southern Canada, throughout United States, except Alaska.	Bites cause local redness. Two tiny red spots may appear. Pain follows almost immediately. Larger muscles become rigid. Body temperature rises slightly. Profuse perspiration and tendency toward nausea follow. It's usually difficult to breathe or talk. May cause constipation, urine retention.	Venom is more dangerous than a rattlesnake's but is given in much smaller amounts. About 5% of bite cases result in death. Death is from asphyxiation due to respiratory paralysis. More dangerous for children; to adults its worst feature is pain. Convulsions result in some cases.	Use an antiseptic such as alcohol or hydrogen peroxide on the bitten area to prevent secondary infection. Keep victim quiet and call a doctor. Do not treat as you would a snakebite since this will only increase the pain and chance of infection; bleeding will not remove the venom.	Wear gloves when working in areas where there might be spiders. Destroy any egg sacs you find. Spray insecticide in any area where spiders are usually found, especially under privy seats. Check them out regularly. General cleanliness, paint, and light discourage spiders.
Tick Oval with small head; the body is not divided into definite segments. Grey or brown. Measures from 1/4 to 3/4 inch when mature.	Found in all United States areas and in parts of southern Canada, on low shrubs, grass, and trees. Carried around by both wild and domestic animals.	Attaches itself to the skin and sucks blood. After removal there is danger of infection, especially if the mouthparts are left in the wound.	Sometimes carries and spreads Rocky Mountain spotted fever, Lyme disease, Colorado tick fever. In a few rare cases, causes paralysis until removed.	Gently remove with tweezers so none of the mouthparts are left in skin. Wash with soap and water; apply antiseptic.	Cover exposed parts of body when in tick-infested areas. Use proper repellent. Remove ticks attached to clothes, body. Check neck and hair. Bathe.

TABLE 7–1 Facts About Troublesome Insects (continued)

Description	Habitat	Problem	Severity	Treatment	Protection
Scorpion Crablike appearance with claw-like pincers. Fleshy post-abdomen or "tail" has five segments, ending in a bulbous sac and stinger. Two poisonous types: solid straw yellow or yellow with irregular black stripes on back. From 2 1/2 to 4 inches long.	Spends days under loose stones, bark, boards, floors of outhouses. Burrows in the sand. Roams freely at night. Crawls under doors into homes. Lethal types are found only in the warm desert-like climate of Arizona and adjacent areas.	Stings by thrusting its tail forward over its head. Swelling or discoloration of the area indicates a nondangerous, though painful, sting. A dangerously toxic sting doesn't change the appearance of the area, which does become hypersensitive.	Excessive salivation and facial contortions may follow. Temperature rises to over 104°F. Tongue becomes sluggish. Convulsions, in waves of increasing intensity, may lead to death from nervous exhaustion. First 3 hours most critical.	Apply constriction. Keep victim quiet and call a doctor immediately. Do not cut the skin or give pain killers. They increase the killing power of the venom. Antitoxin, readily available to doctors, has proved to be very effective.	Apply a petroleum distillate to any dwelling places that cannot be destroyed. Cats are considered effective predators, as are ducks and chickens, though the latter are more likely to be stung and killed. Don't go barefoot at night.
Bee Winged body with yellow and black stripes. Covered with branched or feathery hairs. Makes a buzzing sound. Different species vary from 1/2 to 1 inch in length.	Lives in aerial or underground nests or hives. Widely distributed throughout the world wherever there are flowering plants—from the polar regions to the equator.	Stings with tail when annoyed. Burning and itching with localized swelling occur. Usually leaves venom sac in victim. It takes between 2 and 3 minutes to inject all the venom.	If a person is allergic, more serious reactions occur—nausea, shock, unconsciousness. Swelling may occur in another part of the body. Death may result.	Gently scrape (don't pluck) the stinger so venom sac won't be squeezed. Wash with soap and antiseptic. If swelling occurs, contact doctor. Keep victim warm while resting.	Have exterminator destroy nests and hives. Avoid wearing sweet fragrances and bright clothing. Keep food covered. Move slowly or stand still in the vicinity of bees.
Mosquito Small dark fragile body with transparent wings and elongated mouth-parts. From 1/8- to 1/4-inch long.	Found in temperate climates throughout the world where the water necessary for breeding is available.	Bites and sucks blood. Itching and localized swelling result. Bite may turn red. Only the female is equipped to bite.	Sometimes transmits yellow fever, malaria, encephalitis, and other diseases. Scratching can cause secondary infections.	Don't scratch. Lather with soap and rinse to avoid infection. Apply antiseptic to relieve itching.	Destroy available breeding water to check multiplication. Place nets on windows and beds. Use proper repellent.
Tarantula Large dark "spider" with a furry covering. From 6 to 7 inches in toe-to-toe diameter.	Found in southwestern United States. The tropical varieties are poisonous.	Bites produce pin-prick sensation with negligible effect. It will not bite unless teased.	Usually no more dangerous than a pin prick. Has only local effects.	Wash and apply antiseptic to prevent the possibility of secondary infection.	Harmless to man, the tarantula is beneficial since it destroys harmful insects.

Source: *National Safety Council,* Family Safety, *Spring 1980, pp. 20–21.*

or more stings will kill most people who are not allergic to stinging insects.

Some experts report that 1 percent of all children and 4 percent of adults have such an allergy. An estimated 50–100 sting-related deaths occur yearly. The number of cases may actually be higher but not reported as involving insect stings because they are mistaken for heart attacks or naturally caused death.

Signs and Symptoms

- *Usual reactions.* Momentary pain, redness around sting site, itching, heat
- *Worrisome reactions.* Skin flush, hives, localized swelling of lips or tongue, "tickle" in throat, wheezing, abdominal cramps, diarrhea
- *Life-threatening reactions.* Bluish or grayish skin color (cyanosis), seizures, unconsciousness, inability to breathe due to swelling of vocal cords

One of the difficulties that first aiders and medical personnel encounter in dealing with stings is the lack of uniformity in victims' responses. One sting is not necessarily equivalent to another, even within the same species, because the amount of venom injected varies from sting to sting.

A person who goes into anaphylactic shock after being stung by a hornet may respond to a bee sting with only a small amount of swelling. One person may have local reactions involving an entire limb, while the more typical response is a small circle of redness and

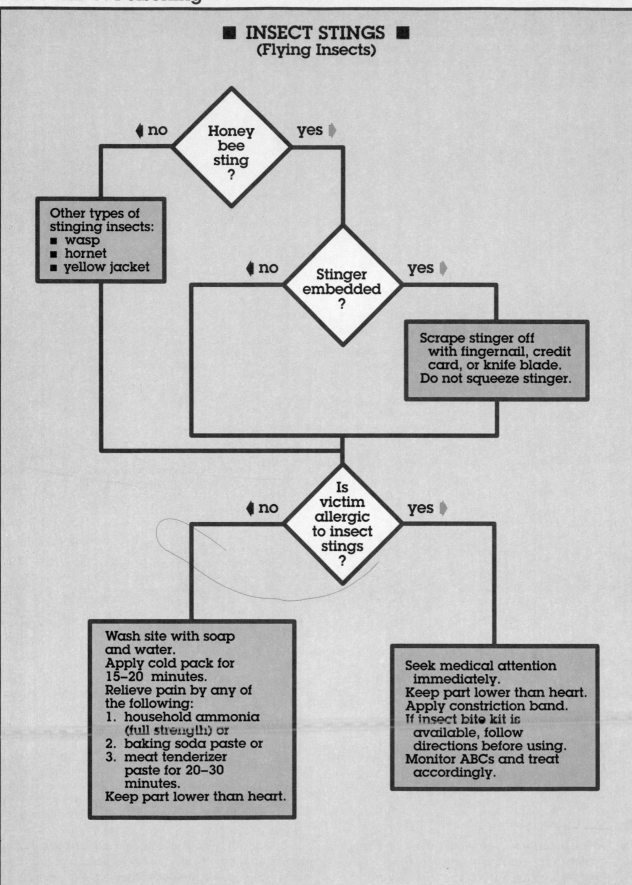

■ INSECT STINGS ■
(Flying Insects)

Honey bee sting?
- no →
- yes →

Other types of stinging insects:
- ■ wasp
- ■ hornet
- ■ yellow jacket

Stinger embedded?
- no →
- yes →

Scrape stinger off with fingernail, credit card, or knife blade. Do not squeeze stinger.

Is victim allergic to insect stings?
- no →
- yes →

Wash site with soap and water.
Apply cold pack for 15–20 minutes.
Relieve pain by any of the following:
1. household ammonia (full strength) or
2. baking soda paste or
3. meat tenderizer paste for 20–30 minutes.
Keep part lower than heart.

Seek medical attention immediately.
Keep part lower than heart.
Apply constriction band.
If insect bite kit is available, follow directions before using.
Monitor ABCs and treat accordingly.

swelling that disappears without incident within days. In beekeepers, for whom stings are an accepted occupational hazard, the response is likely to be even less than in most other people, because they have become tolerant to the toxins in the venom. There seems to be no easy way to predict which way a person may react. However, most people who get stung have local reactions: redness, swelling, and pain.

The most dangerous single stings in nonallergic individuals are those inside the throat, which may result from ingesting an insect that has dropped into a can of soft drink or from inhaling one that zooms into the victim's open mouth. Swallowing a yellowjacket that stings the pharynx on the way down can cause life-threatening swelling in that area. It's not an allergic problem, but the swelling in the airway can cause respiratory obstruction.

Massive multiple stings from the common honeybee are rare. It might happen, however, if a person stumbles into a hive, or if a truck carrying a load of hives has an accident. With the approach of the Africanized bees (killer bees) from South and Central America, the number of multiple sting cases is likely to increase. The venom of the Africanized bee is no more potent than that of the European type; however, they have earned their nickname by their aggressiveness.

The rule of thumb is that the sooner symptoms develop after the sting, the more serious the reaction will be. People with known allergies to stings should have epinephrine injection devices. After receiving an injection, a sting-allergic person should immediately seek medical help because he or she will likely require more epinephrine within 30 minutes.

First Aid

Those who have had a reaction to an insect sting should be instructed in self-treatment so they can protect themselves from severe reactions. They should also be advised to purchase a medical alert bracelet or necklace identifying them as insect-allergic.

- Carefully examine the sting site for a stinger embedded in the skin. The bee is the only stinging insect that leaves its stinger behind. If the stinger is still embedded, it needs to be removed, because it will continue to inject poison for two or three minutes unless removed. Do *not* pull at the stinger directly with tweezers or fingers because it has a sac at the exposed end that can pump more venom into the victim. Instead scrape the sac away cleanly with a long fingernail, credit card, scissor edge or knife blade.
- Wash the sting site thoroughly.
- Apply an ice pack over the sting site to slow absorption of the venom and relieve pain.
- Several items may help relieve the pain and itching. One is calamine lotion and another is

Fire Ant Bites

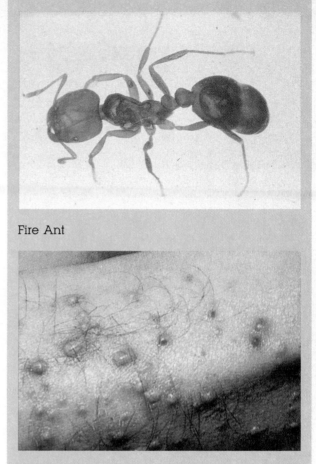

Fire Ant

Fire Ant Bite

Five fire ant species are found in the United States. Particular concern has centered on the imported species, which is more aggressive than the native fire ant. Imported fire ants have become widely distributed in the southern states, from Texas to North Carolina. They have become the most common stinging ants in North America.

The ant bites its victim by securing itself to the skin with its mandibles, causing pain. Then, using its head as a pivot, the ant swings the abdomen in an arc, repeatedly stinging its victim with an abdominal stinger.

The South American fire ants range in color from red to dark brown. They are about 1/8–1/4" long, and usually live in foot-high, dome-shaped mounds.

a paste made of meat tenderizer and water. A paste of baking soda and water or using full-strength household ammonia may also help. An antihistamine may prevent some local symptoms if given early, but it works too slowly to counteract a life-threatening allergic reaction.

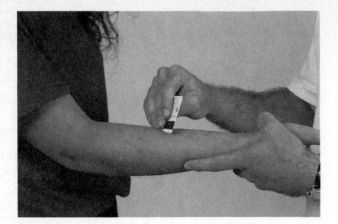

Scraping stinger away with credit card

- Observe victims for at least 30 minutes for signs of an allergic reaction (anaphylactic shock). For those who are highly allergic, a dose of epinephrine (adrenalin) is the only effective life-saving treatment. It is given subcutaneously at the sting site. A physician can prescribe an emergency kit that includes a prefilled syringe of epinephrine or a spring-loaded device that automatically triggers the injection of epinephrine by a quick thrust into the thigh or large muscle. The spring-loaded device is useful for those reluctant to use a syringe with a visible needle. The allergic person should take the kit whenever going places where stinging insects are known to exist. Refer to the section on anaphylactic shock for more about kits containing epinephrine. Since epinephrine is short-acting, the victim must be watched closely for signs of returning anaphylactic shock, and another dose of epinephrine should be injected as often as every 15 minutes if needed. Epinephrine should *not* be used to treat a sting unless the victim has an allergic reaction. Epinephrine has a limited shelf life of one to three years, or until it has turned brown.
- Some kits contain an antihistamine. It is *not* an effective emergency treatment and is included in the kit to reduce later symptoms after the epinephrine treatment.
- Some physicians provide their sting-senstitive patients with an inhaler containing epinephrine, and instruct them in its use.

Snakebites

Throughout the world about 50,000 people die each year from snakebite. In the United States, of the 40,000 to 50,000 annually bitten, about 8,000 are bitten by poisonous snakes. Amazingly, only a dozen Americans die each year.

Of the many different snake species, only four in the United States are poisonous: rattlesnake (accounts for about 65 percent of all venomous snakebites and nearly all the deaths in the United States), copperhead (30 percent of all venomous snakebites), water moccasin (9 percent of all venomous snakebites), and coral snake (1 percent of all venomous snakebites).

The first three are known as pit vipers. They have three common characteristics:

- Triangular, flat head wider than its neck
- Elliptical pupils (i.e., cat's eye)
- Heat-sensitive "pit" located between each eye and nostril

The coral snake is small and very colorful, with a series of bright red, yellow, and black bands around its body. Every other band is yellow. A black snout also marks the coral snake.

Imported snakes, found in zoos, schools, snake farms, and amateur and professional collections, account for at least 15 bites a year.

Pit Vipers

(rattlesnake, copperhead, water moccasin)

Signs and Symptoms

- Severe burning pain at the bite site
- Two small puncture wounds about 1/2 inch apart (some cases may have only one fang mark)

Snakebite Prevention

1. Avoid handling poisonous snakes.

2. Stay away from stone walls and wood piles, because they are known habitats of poisonous snakes.

3. Be careful about placing your hands and feet on or into places you cannot see, such as ledges, holes, and deserted buildings.

4. Walk on cleared paths.

5. Wear protective clothing (boots, high shoes, long pants, long-sleeved shirts, and gloves) when placing your extremities in possible snake habitats.

6. Don't sit on or step over logs until you closely scrutinize the area.

7. Don't handle a dead poisonous snake, because the reflex action of the fangs can still inflict a wound up to 45 minutes after the snake is killed.

8. Don't surprise or corner a snake. Use a walking stick to prod uncleared ground, and make noise so a snake can sense you coming.

—The National Recreation and Park Association

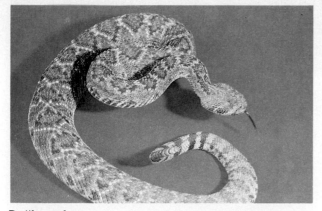

Rattlesnake

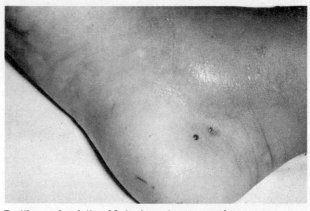

Rattlesnake bite. Note two fang marks.

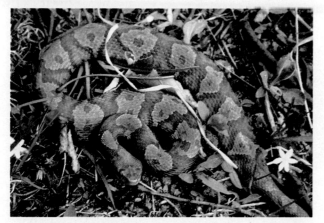

Copperhead snake

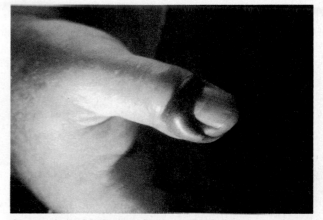

Copperhead bite two hours after bite.

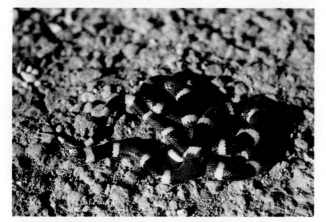

Coral snake. America's most poisonous snake.

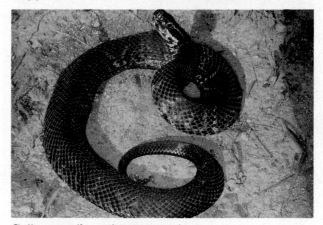

Cottonmouth water moccasin

- Swelling (happens within 5 minutes and can involve an entire extremity)
- Discoloration and blood-filled blisters
- In severe cases: nausea, vomiting, sweating, weakness
- No venom injection occurs in about 25 percent of all poisonous snakebites, only fang and tooth wounds

First Aid

Most snakebites occur within a few hours of a medical facility where antivenin is available. Bites showing no sign of venom injection require only a possible tetanus shot and care of the bite wounds.

Controversy exists about proper first aid procedures for snakebite. The following list represents the most widely accepted first aid procedures:

- Keep the victim quiet. Do *not* allow victim to increase the heart rate—if possible, transport the victim by carrying. If alone, walk very slowly to help.
- Get victim away from snake. Snakes have been known to bite more than once.
- Identify the snake species since snakes vary in

■ SNAKEBITES ■

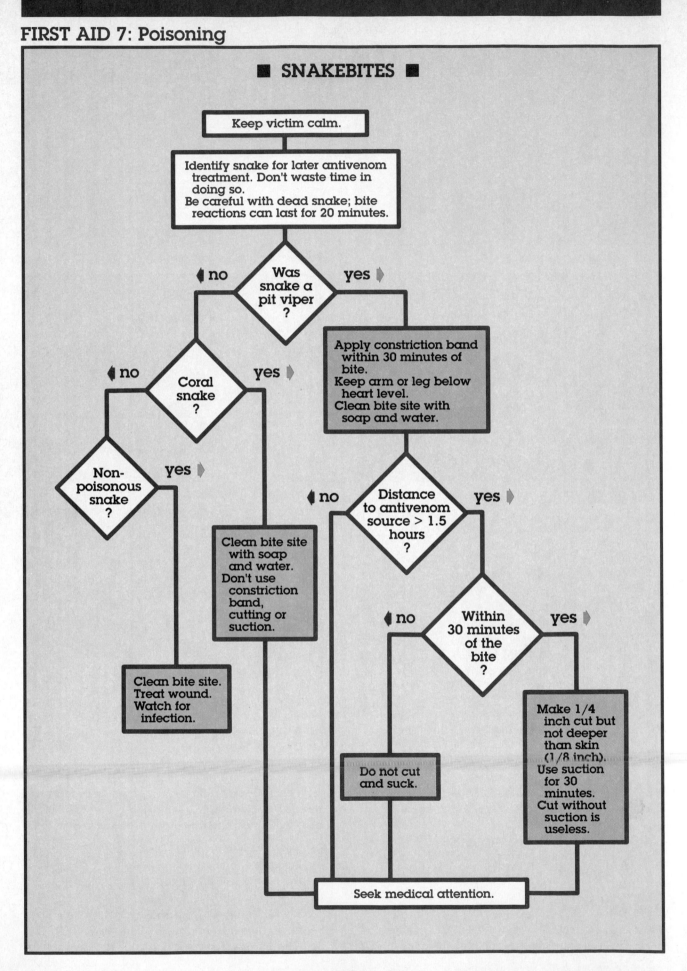

Keep victim calm.

Identify snake for later antivenom treatment. Don't waste time in doing so.
Be careful with dead snake; bite reactions can last for 20 minutes.

Was snake a pit viper ?

no

yes

Coral snake ?

no

yes

Apply constriction band within 30 minutes of bite.
Keep arm or leg below heart level.
Clean bite site with soap and water.

Non-poisonous snake ?

yes

Clean bite site with soap and water.
Don't use constriction band, cutting or suction.

Distance to antivenom source > 1.5 hours ?

no

yes

Clean bite site.
Treat wound.
Watch for infection.

Within 30 minutes of the bite ?

no

yes

Do not cut and suck.

Make 1/4 inch cut but not deeper than skin (1/8 inch).
Use suction for 30 minutes.
Cut without suction is useless.

Seek medical attention.

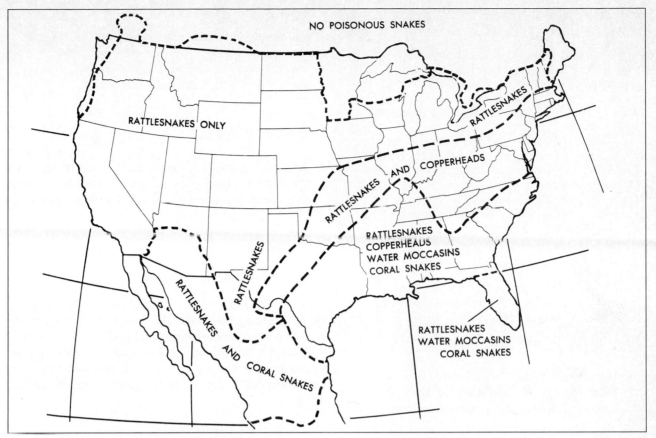

Location of poisonous snakes in North America

their toxicity. This helps in determining the amount of antivenin required for treating the victim. Some experts suggest taking the dead snake with the victim to the medical facility. Be careful around a decapitated snake head since head reactions persist for 20 or more minutes.

■ Gently wash the bitten area with soap and water.

■ Apply a constriction band just above the bite area if it can be done within 30 minutes of the bite, to limit the spread of venom. Do *not* tie it too tightly—test tightness by passing a finger under the band. Do *not* apply a band around a finger. If swelling appears, loosen the band but do *not* take it off. The band can usually stay safely on for about one hour.

■ Every 15 minutes keep track of swelling on the victim's skin with a pen and write down the time the mark was made. This shows how rapidly swelling has moved.

■ If more than a few hours from a medical facility with antivenin, or if the snake was large and the skin is swelling rapidly, you should cut and suck immediately. *This procedure is seldom needed because most bites happen within a short distance from medical care.*

If done within three minutes of the bite, 10–20 percent of the venom can be removed, and a lesser amount if done within 30 minutes of the bite. Do *not* cut and suck if 30 minutes has passed since the bite.

The cuts over the puncture wounds (fang marks) should be about 1/4 inch in length and deep enough to go through the skin, allowing fat to be visible (about 1/8 inch). Do *not* cut deeper because of tendons, nerves, or blood vessels. Do *not* use cross-cuts, but a single cut along the long axis of the limb. Do *not* make cuts on the head, neck, or trunk. Use a strong suctioning device for 30 minutes. Cutting over the fang marks without suction is ineffective. Do *not* cut over an area of advancing swelling. Use mouth suction if no suctioning device is available. Rinse the mouth between suctions.

■ Quickly transport all snakebite victims to a medical facility for antivenin.

Heaviest Venomous Snake

The heaviest venomous snake is the Eastern diamondback rattlesnake, found in the southeastern United States. A specimen 7'9" in length weighed 34 lbs. Less reliable weights up to 40 lbs. and lengths up to 8 feet 9 inches have been reported.

—*Guinness Book of World Records*

The most venomous snake is the sea snake *Hydrophis belcheri,* which has a venom 100 times as toxic as that of the Australian taipan. The snake abounds around Ashmore Reef in the Timor Sea, off the coast of northwestern Australia.

The most venomous land snake is the small-scaled or fierce snake (*Parademansia microlepidotus*) of southwestern Queensland and northeastern South Australia and Tasmania. One specimen yielded 0.00385 oz. of venom after milking, a quantity sufficient to kill at least 125,000 mice.

It is estimated that between 30,000 and 40,000 people (excluding Chinese and Russians) die from snakebite each year, 75% of them in densely populated India. Burma has the highest mortality rate, with 15.4 deaths per 100,000 population per annum.

—*Guinness Book of World Records*

- Do *not* use cold on a snakebite. It does more harm than good. Cold does not decrease the enzyme activity, and it may cause frostbite.

Coral

(not a pit viper)

The coral snake is America's most poisonous snake. This snake has short fangs and "chews" its venom into the victim.

Signs and Symptoms

(apparent after about 1 hour)

- Bite usually happens on a small part of the body (e.g., finger, toe) because of the coral's small mouth and teeth.
- One or more punctures or scratchlike wounds
- Few or no local signs (e.g., swelling, discoloration, pain)
- Dizziness, drooling, blurred or double vision, drooping eyelids, drowsiness, nausea, vomiting

First Aid

- Keep victim calm.
- Gently clean bite site with warm soap and water.
- Do *not* apply a constriction band or cut the victim's skin.
- Transport the victim to a medical facility for antivenin.

Nonpoisonous Snakes

Nonpoisonous snakes leave a horseshoe shape of tooth marks on victim's skin.

First Aid

- Gently clean the bitten area with warm soap and water.
- Care for the bite as a minor wound.
- Consult with a medical authority.

Spider Bites

Nearly all spiders are venomous; that is how they paralyze and kill their prey. However, very few spiders have fangs long enough to bite humans. Exceptions include the black widow, brown recluse, and tarantula spiders. Two spiders, the black widow and the brown recluse, can be deadly.

Black Widow Spider

The black widow spider is found throughout the world. A red spot (often in the shape of an hourglass) on the abdomen identifies the female—she is the one that bites. Females have a glossy black body. By volume, black widow spider venom is more deadly than the rattlesnake's, but it is injected in much smaller amounts.

Signs and Symptoms

Determining whether a person has been bitten by a black widow spider is difficult.

- A sharp pinprick of the spider's bite may be felt, although some victims are not even aware of the bite. In no more than 15 minutes a dull, numbing pain develops in the bitten area.
- Faint red bite marks appear.
- Muscle stiffness and cramps occur next, usually affecting the abdomen when the bite is in the lower part of the body or legs, and affecting the shoulders, back, or chest when the bite is on the upper body or arms.

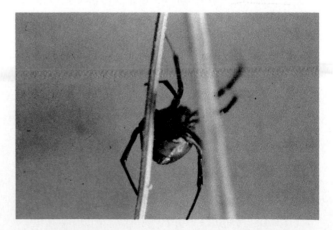

Black widow spider. Note red hourglass configuration on abdomen.

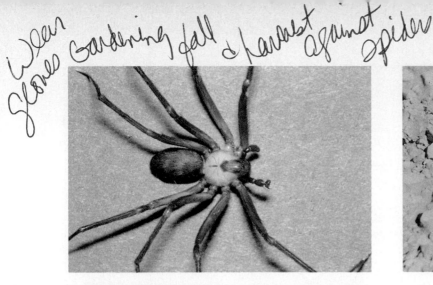

Brown recluse spider. Note violin or fiddle configuration on back.

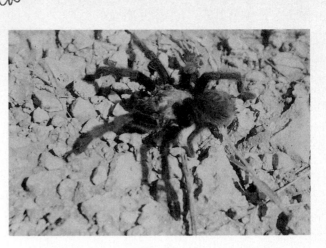

Tarantula

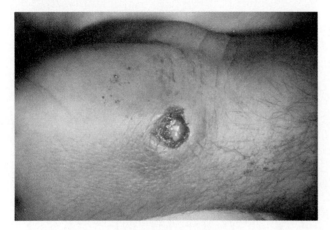

Brown recluse spider bite

- Headache, chills, fever, heavy sweating, dizziness, nausea, vomiting, and severe abdominal pain afflict the victim.

First Aid

Even without treatment, most healthy adults survive, and few people have died. However, black widow bites can threaten the lives of children and the elderly.

- If possible, catch the spider to confirm its identity. Even if the body is crushed, save it for identification.
- Clean the bitten area with alcohol. Do *not* apply a constricting band because the black widow venom's action is swift, and there is little to be gained by trying to slow absorption with a constriction band.
- Place an ice pack over the bite to relieve pain.
- Keep the victim quiet and monitor breathing.
- Seek immediate medical attention. There is an antivenin for black widow bites. It brings relief of symptoms within one to three hours, especially if given as soon as possible after the victim was bitten. Antivenin use is usually reserved for small children, the elderly, and those with severe bites.

Brown Recluse Spider

The brown recluse spider has a brown, possibly purplish, violin-shaped figure on its back. Brown recluse bites are rarely fatal, except for hypersensitive people, children, the elderly, and those with chronic health problems.

Signs and Symptoms

- The initial pain felt may be slight enough to be overlooked.
- A blister at the bite site, along with redness and swelling, appears after several hours.
- Pain, which may remain mild but can become severe, develops within two to eight hours at the bite site.
- Fever, weakness, vomiting, joint pain, and a rash may occur.
- An ulcer forms within a week. Gangrene may develop in some cases.

First Aid

- If possible, capture the spider for positive identification.
- Clean the bitten area with alcohol.
- Apply an ice pack to the bitten area.
- Seek immediate medical attention.

Tarantula Spider

More menacing-looking than black widow and brown recluse spiders, the tarantula rarely produces symptoms other than moderate pain when it bites. First aid involves cleaning the bite wound to prevent infection, placing an ice pack wrapped in a cloth on the bite area, and seeking medical attention.

Scorpion Stings

Death from scorpion stings in the United States is rare; children are at greatest risk. A scorpion's sting causes immediate pain and burning around the sting site,

■ SPIDER BITES AND SCORPION STINGS ■

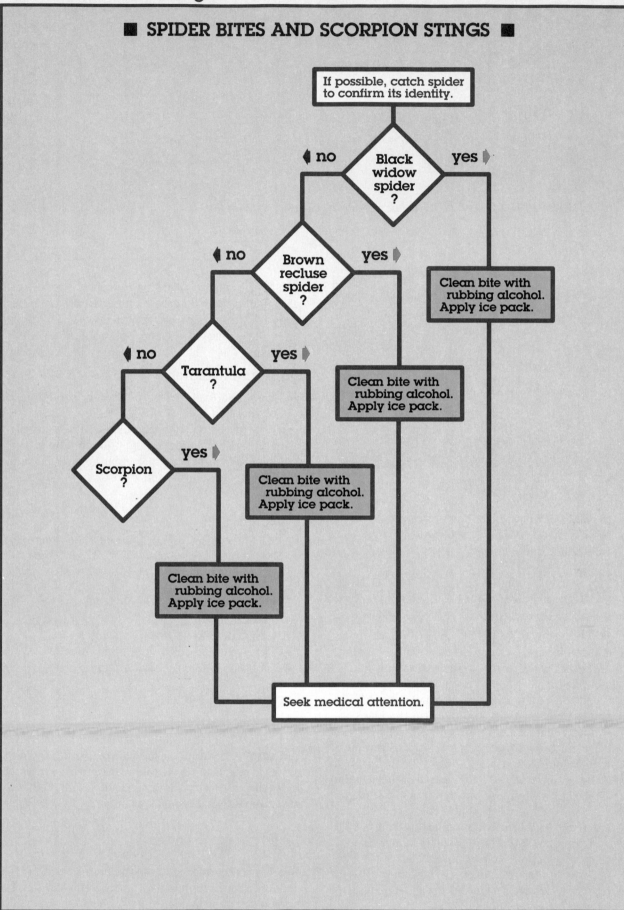

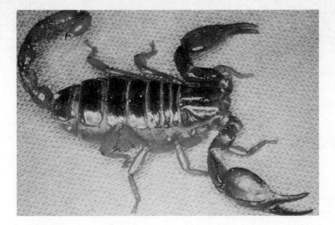

Scorpion

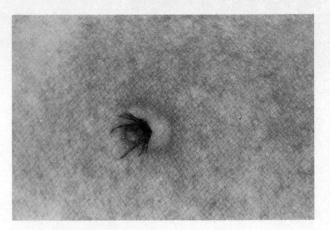

Tick embedded

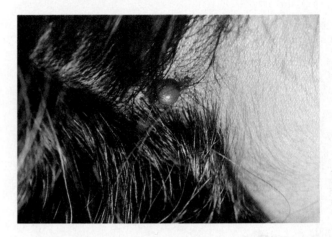

Tick embedded and engorged

followed by numbness or tingling. Severe cases may include paralysis, spasms, or respiratory difficulties. First aid consists of monitoring the ABCs and treating the victim accordingly. It is also important to clean the sting site with rubbing alcohol and then apply an ice pack over the wound.

Tick Removal

Most tick bites are harmless, though ticks can carry serious diseases (e.g., Lyme disease, Rocky Mountain spotted fever, Colorado tick fever). Ticks should be removed as soon as possible.

First Aid

- Do *not* use the following popular methods of tick removal, which have proven useless:
    1. Petroleum jelly
    2. Fingernail polish
    3. Rubbing alcohol
    4. A hot match
- Pull the tick off, employing the following methods:

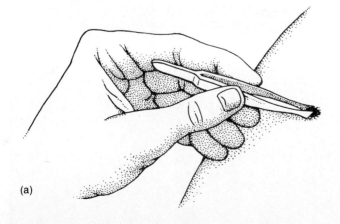

(a)

Removing a tick with tweezers

1. Use tweezers, or if you have to use your fingers, protect your skin by using a paper towel or disposable tissue. Although few people ever encounter ticks infected with a disease, the person removing the tick may become infected by germs entering through breaks in the skin.

2. Grasp the tick as close to the skin surface as possible and pull away from the skin with a steady pressure or lift the tick slightly upward and pull parallel to the skin until the tick detaches. Do *not* twist or jerk the tick since this may result in incomplete removal.

3. Wash the bite site and your hands well with soap and water. Apply alcohol to further disinfect the area. Then apply a cold pack to reduce pain. Calamine lotion might aid in relieving any itching. Keep the area clean.

Watch for signs of infection or unexplained symptoms (e.g., severe headaches, fever, or rash) which may develop 3 to 10 days later. If these symptoms appear, seek medical attention immediately.

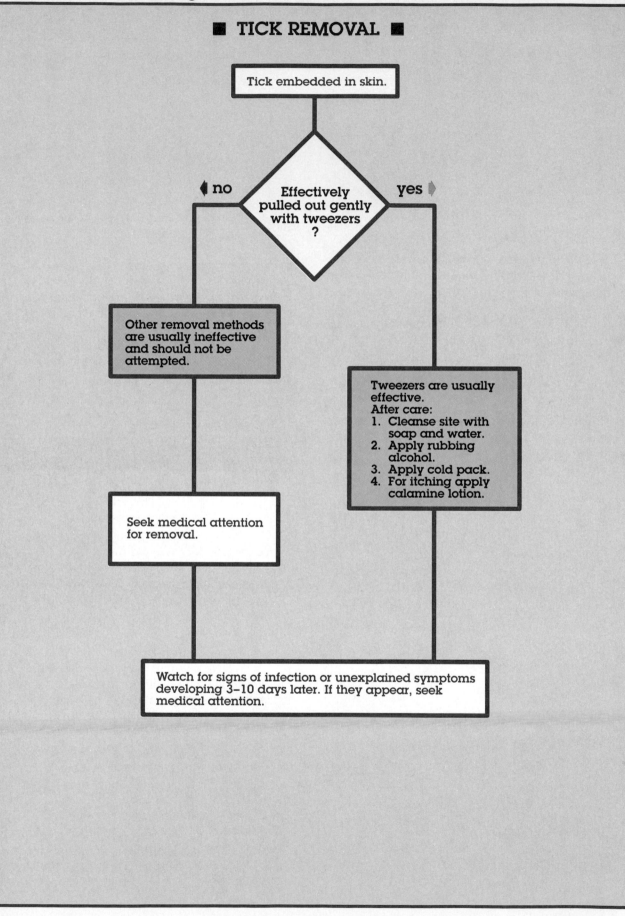

■ TICK REMOVAL ■

Tick embedded in skin.

Effectively pulled out gently with tweezers ?

no

yes

Other removal methods are usually ineffective and should not be attempted.

Tweezers are usually effective.
After care:
1. Cleanse site with soap and water.
2. Apply rubbing alcohol.
3. Apply cold pack.
4. For itching apply calamine lotion.

Seek medical attention for removal.

Watch for signs of infection or unexplained symptoms developing 3–10 days later. If they appear, seek medical attention.

Lyme Disease

Lyme Disease is the most common tick-borne disease, and its occurrence is fast-rising in almost all states. Lyme disease (named for the Connecticut town in which it was first discovered) starts out with flu-like symptoms, but can lead to arthritis and serious nerve and heart damage. Ticks carrying the disease often go undetected since they are difficult to see and are much smaller (head of a pin in size) than the common dog tick or wood tick.

Protection against ticks comes from taking these precautions:

1. Wear long-sleeved shirts and long pants (tucked into socks) whenever in wooded areas.

2. Use insect repellent containing DEET (diethyltolusmide) on clothes and exposed areas, especially arms and hands.

3. Check yourself for ticks or have someone do it for you after being in a potentially tick-infested area.

4. Immediately remove any embedded tick with tweezers.

5. Consult with a physician if any flu-like symptoms occur (chills, pain).

fur, or from smoke of burning plants. No one can develop the dermatitis by touching the fluid from blisters, since that fluid does not contain the oleoresin that comes from the juice of these poisonous plants.

Signs and Symptoms

- *Mild.* Some itching
- *Mild to moderate.* Itching and redness
- *Moderate.* Itching, redness, and swelling
- *Severe.* Itching, redness, swelling, and blisters

Severity is important but so is the amount of skin affected. The greater the skin involvement, the greater the need for medical attention. A day or two is the usual time between contact and the onset of the above signs and symptoms.

First Aid

- Those knowing that they have contacted a poisonous plant should take immediate action (within 5 minutes). That action includes rinsing with plain water or using alcohol. Most victims do not know they have contacted a poisonous plant until the next day or later when the itching and rash begin.

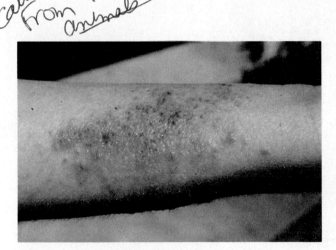

Poison ivy dermatitis

Poison Ivy, Oak, and Sumac

Poison ivy, oak, and sumac plants cause contact dermatitis or an allergic reaction in about 90 percent of all adults. Most people cannot recognize these plants. To find out whether or not a plant is poisonous upon contact, use the "black spot test." (*See* boxed information). Actually, more than 60 plants can cause an allergic reaction, but the three named above are by far the most common offenders.

Allergic people may come in contact with the juice of these plants from their clothes or shoes, from pet

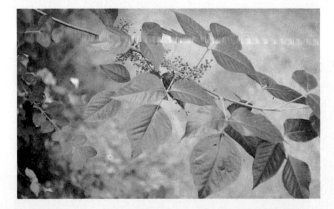

Poison ivy, found in all 48 contiguous U.S. states

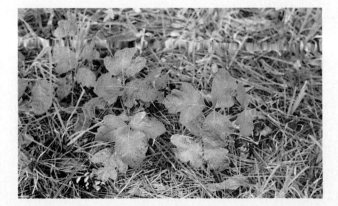

Poison oak

■ POISON IVY ■

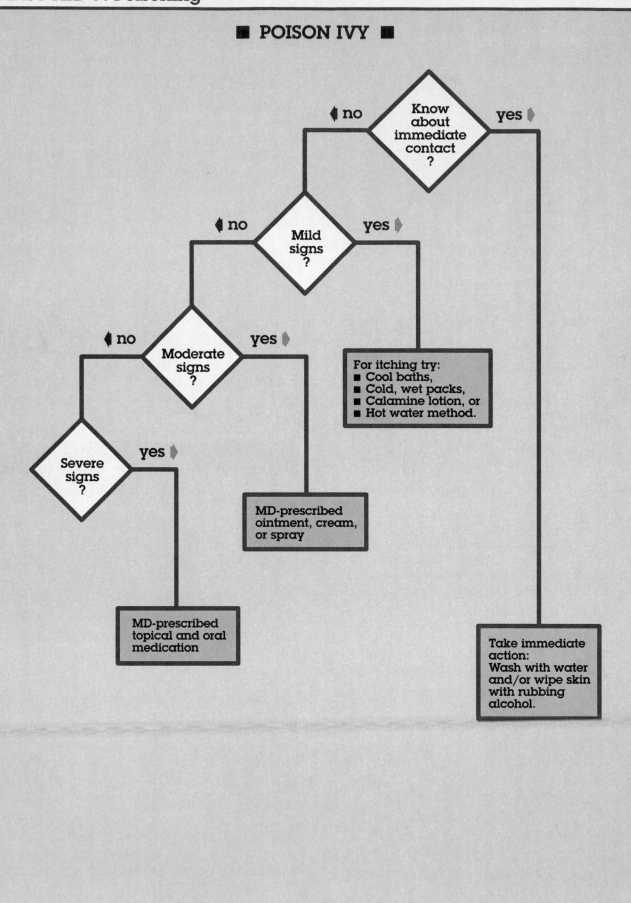

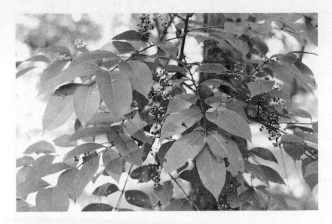

Poison sumac

- During the acute weeping and oozing stage, sodium bicarbonate (baking soda) solution should be used either as a soak, bath, or wet dressing for 30 minutes, three or four times a day. Greasy ointments should not be used during active oozing.
- Antihistamines appear to have no value either taken by mouth or in ointments and lotions. In fact, ointments and lotions could even cause their own allergic reactions on top of the poison plant eruption.
- For the various stages:

    1. *Mild.* Apply wet compresses and cool baths to help relieve itching. Calamine lotion or zinc oxide may also relieve itching. Topical over-the-counter medications are no more effective than these few simple procedures.

    2. *Mild to moderate.* Doctor-prescribed corticosteroids help. Over-the-counter (nonprescription) hydrocortisone creams, ointments and sprays in strengths of .5 percent or less offer little benefit.

    3. *Severe.* Doctor-prescribed oral corticosteriods (e.g., prednisone) may benefit victims affected most severely. Topical corticosteroid may also be applied. When using a topical cream, cover the affected area with a transparent plastic wrap and lightly bind with an elastic or self-adhering bandage.

Black Spot Test

Check a suspicious-looking plant to determine if it's poison ivy, oak, or sumac by grasping a leaf with a piece of paper and crushing it with a rock. The sap of poison ivy, oak, and sumac will turn dark brown in 10 minutes, and turn black in a day.

—Dr. Jere Guin, University of Arkansas

For severe itching, hot water—hot enough to redden the skin, but not burn it—may relieve itching. Heat releases histamine, the substance in the skin's cells that causes the intense itching. Therefore, a hot shower or bath causes intense itching as the histamine is released. This depletes the cells of histamine and the victim will then obtain up to eight hours of relief from itching.

Carbon Monoxide *Inhaled*

Victims of carbon monoxide (CO) are often unaware of its presence. The gas is invisible, tasteless, odorless and nonirritating.

Carbon monoxide produces its toxicity due to several factors. CO becomes tightly bound to hemoglobin (red blood cells) that carries oxygen. With conscious victims it takes four to five hours with ordinary air (21 percent oxygen) or 30–40 minutes with 100 percent oxygen to reverse CO's effects. When CO levels in the air are high, the level of oxygen is probably low.

Signs and Symptoms

It is difficult to tell if a person is a victim of carbon monoxide poisoning. Sometimes, a complaint of having the "flu" is really a symptom of carbon monoxide poisoning.

- Headache
- Ringing in the ears (tinnitus)
- Angina (chest pain)
- Muscle weakness
- Nausea and vomiting
- Dizziness and visual changes (blurred or double vision)
- Unconsciousness
- Breathing and cardiac failure

First Aid

- Immediately remove the victim from the toxic environment and into fresh air. Give the victim 100 percent oxygen either in an EMS ambulance or at a hospital emergency department. This will improve oxygenation and it also disassociates the linkage between the carbon monoxide and the hemoglobin.
- For a conscious victim, seek medical attention involving a blood test to determine the level of carbon monoxide.
- For an unconscious victim, place him or her on one side with the head resting on an arm. Loosen tight clothing and maintain body heat.
- Give basic life support if needed.
- Even when only mild symptoms (e.g., headache, nausea) appear, seek medical attention if carbon monoxide poisoning is suspected.

■ INHALED POISON ■

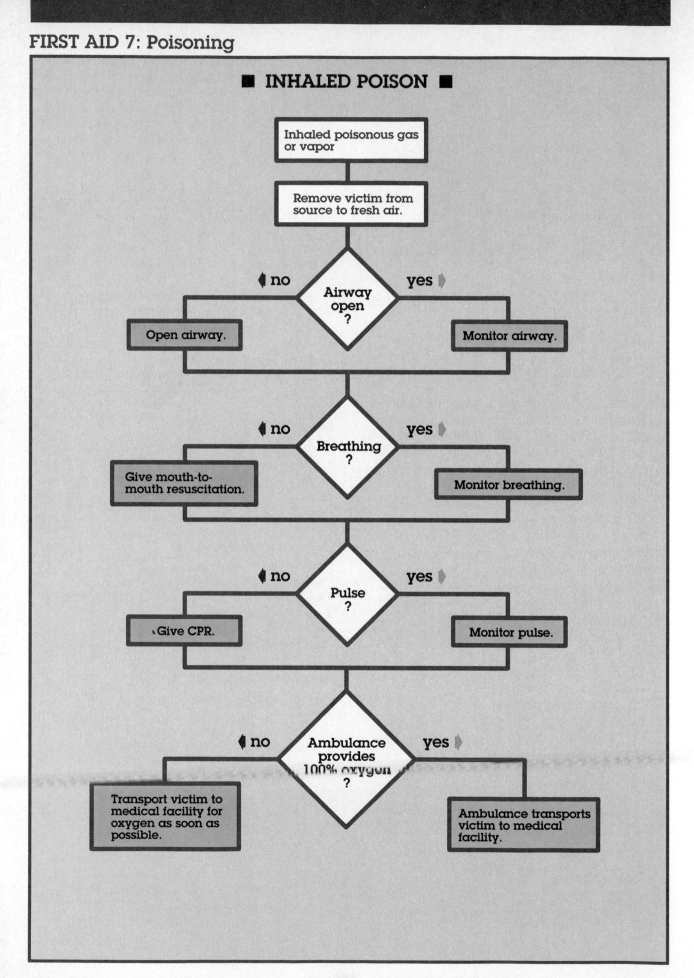

Marine Animal Injuries

Portuguese Man-of-War and Jellyfish

Each year more than one million people are stung by jellyfish, Portuguese man-of-wars, corals, and anemones that lie along the shallow ocean waters of the United States. Reactions to being stung by these ocean creatures vary from mild dermatitis to severe reactions. Most will recover without medical attention; several will need emergency medical care.

Jellyfish and Portuguese man-of-wars have long tentacles equipped with stinging devices call nematocysts. When cast ashore or onto rocks, these animals can break into thousands of pieces. These detached pieces retain their ability to sting for a long period of time, usually until they are completely dried out.

The Portuguese man-of-war sting is usually in the form of well-defined linear welts or scattered patches of welts with redness, which usually disappear within 24 hours.

The jellyfish sting produces severe muscle cramping with multiple thin lines of welts crossing the skin in a zigzag pattern. Pain usually is a burning type that lasts 10 to 30 minutes. The welts on the skin usually disappear within an hour.

First aid

Immediately remove any tentacles remaining on the skin by using a credit card, stick, or similar material other than bare skin to scrape them off. Do *not* rub the victim's skin. Wash the wound with alcohol or vinegar, or sprinkle it with meat tenderizer to prevent the nematocysts from discharging further. For symptomatic relief, apply ammonia, lemon juice, or baking soda paste.

Sting rays

Most wounds inflicted by sting rays are produced on the ankle or foot as a result of stepping on a ray. The sting is most often more like a laceration, since the large tail barb can do significant damage. The venom causes intense burning pain at the site.

First aid

For pain relief, immerse the injured part of the body in hot water for 30–60 minutes. The water must **not** be hot enough to cause a burn.

Burns

■ Heat Burns ■ Chemical Burns ■
■ Electrical Injuries ■

Heat Burns

Each year in the United States more than two million people suffer burns. Of these, 200,000 seek medical attention; about 70,000 are hospitalized, and of these about 10 percent die.

When a major burn damages or destroys the skin, it can be life-threatening until the skin heals or is resurfaced. The more severe the burn, the more life-threatening it will be. Factors contributing to the severity are the size and depth of the burn, the victim's age, the body parts affected, and any injuries or medical problems.

The temperature of the burning agent and the length of time it is in contact with the skin contribute to the extent and depth of a burn injury. For example, holding your finger under a faucet at 156°F will cause a third-degree (full-thickness) burn in little more than a second. It would take five minutes at 120°F. A gasoline fire that ignites your clothing could burn at a temperature higher than 1,000°F.

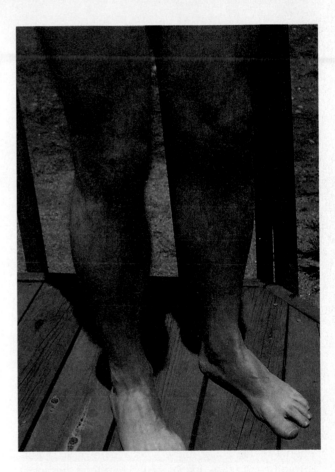

Assessing a Burn

Assess a burn after any breathing or bleeding problems have been treated. It may be difficult to accurately determine the depth of a burn during the initial stages. However, first aiders should attempt to determine both the total burned area and the depth of injury for proper first aid and for determining if medical care is needed.

How large is the burn?

Your skin will not ignite unless heated to thousands of degrees, but if your clothing ignites (or your skin is kept in contact with the heat source, such as scalding water, a hot iron, or a radiator), large areas of the skin will become involved in the injury. To *accurately* determine the extent of a burn, first remove the victim's clothing and, in the case of a flame injury, the soot and debris from the burned area.

A quick method of assessing the extent of a burn is known as the "Rule of Nines," which expresses the extent of a burn as a percentage of the total body surface. A hand and an arm are defined as 9 percent of

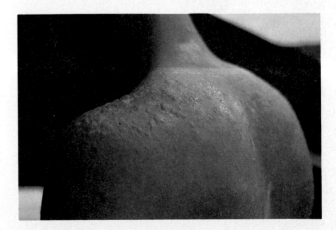

Second-degree burn—blistered shoulders

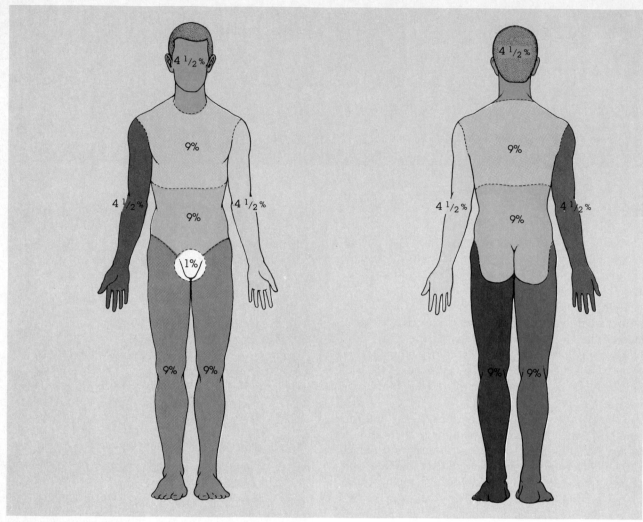

The ''Rule of Nines''

the body surface. Each leg counts as 18 percent of the body surface. The front and back torso are each valued at 18 percent with the genital area at 1 percent.

The Rule of Nines is accurate for adults, but it does not make allowances for the different proportions of a child. In small children the head accounts for 18 percent and each leg is 14 percent. Therefore, for small children the Rule of Nines must be modified.

A better method for estimating the affected surface area is to remember that the victim's hand size is about 1 percent of his or her body surface area.

How deep is the burn?

During an emergency it is difficult to determine the depth of a burn while looking at the skin surface. Make a quick assessment of burn depth to help decide whether or not to transport the victim to medical care.

First-degree burns (superficial). These burns affect the skin's outer layer (epidermis). Characteristics include redness, mild swelling, tenderness, and pain. Healing occurs without scarring, usually within a week. Often the outer edges of deeper burns are also first-degree.

Second-degree burns (partial thickness). These burns extend through the entire outer skin layer and into the inner skin layer. Blister formation, swelling, weeping of fluids, and severe pain characterize second-degree burns. These occur because the capillary blood vessels located in the dermis are damaged and give up fluid into surrounding tissues. With proper treatment, healing with little scarring should take place within three weeks.

Third-degree burns (full-thickness). These severe burns extend through all the skin layers and into the underlying fat, muscle, and bone. Discoloration (charred, white, or cherry red) and a parchmentlike appearance, in the absence of blisters or leaking tissue fluids, indicate this degree of burn. Since capillary blood vessels have been destroyed, no more fluid is brought to this area. However, injured tissue underneath may have intact capillaries and can result in swelling of the area. If you push down with your finger on the burned area, it will blanch, but there will be no capillary refill because the area is dead. The victim will not feel pain because the nerve endings have been destroyed. Any pain experienced with this burn is

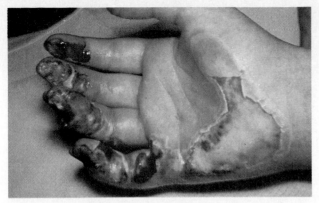

Second and third degree burns

caused by surrounding burns of lesser degrees (first- and second-degree). Any third-degree burn larger than a 50-cent piece will require medical care involving removal of the dead tissue and a skin graft to heal properly.

What parts of the body are burned?

Burns are considered to be more severe when they occur on the face (especially the mouth, nose, and eyelids), the hands, the feet, and the genitals than on other body parts. Respiratory tract burns are especially serious if associated with fumes or heat inhalation. A circumferential burn (one that goes all the way around a finger, toe, arm, leg, or chest) is considered more severe than a noncircumferential one because of the likelihood of constriction and tourniquet effect on circulation and, in some cases, breathing. All of these burns require medical care.

How old is the burned victim?

A burn is considered more serious in a child under 5 years of age and in an elderly person (over 60) than in other victims.

Does the victim have any injuries or medical problems?

Respiratory tract damage caused by heat associated with a burn remains the leading cause of death after being hospitalized. Respiratory damage may result, for example, from being forced to breathe heat or products of combustion; being burned by a flame while in a closed space; or being in an explosion. Even if there is no burn injury in these instances, there may be respiratory damage. It is rare that the upper respiratory tract or the lungs are actually burned. This is because they are constructed to cool or warm and to prepare inhaled air. The superheated air from a flame or from a hot steam explosion will be absorbed by the upper respiratory tract (the area involving the nose through to the trachea), resulting in an inflammation. Swelling results within two to twenty-four hours, restricting or even completely shutting off the airway so that air cannot reach the lungs. All respiratory injuries must receive medical care.

Burns can aggravate existing medical conditions such as diabetes, heart disease, and lung disease, as well as other medical problems. Concurrent injuries such as fractures, internal injuries, or open wounds increase the severity of the burn.

With this information and reference to Table 8.1, you can determine a burn's severity as minor, moderate, or critical.

First Aid

1. Put out the fire. Extinguish clothing fires immediately by having the victim "drop and roll," by wrapping him or her in a blanket, or by immersing the burning area in cool water.

2. Move the victim away from the heat source to avoid further injury.

TABLE 8–1 Burn Severity

Burn classification	Characteristics	
Minor burn	first-degree burn	
	second-degree burn	<15% BSA adults
	second-degree burn	<5% BSA in children/elderly persons
	third-degree burn	<2% BSA
Moderate burn	second-degree burn	15%–25% BSA in adults
	second-degree burn	10%–20% BSA in children/elderly persons
	third-degree burn	<10% BSA
Critical burn	second-degree burn	>25% BSA in adults
	second-degree burn	>20% BSA in children/elderly persons
	third-degree burn	>10% BSA
		Burns of hands, face, eyes, feet, or perineum
		Most victims with inhalation injury, electrical injury, major trauma, or significant preexisting diseases

BSA = Body surface area
Source: Adapted with permission from the American Burn Association categorization.

TABLE 8-2 First Aid for Burns

Burn	Do	Don't
First-degree (redness, mild swelling, and pain)	Apply cold water and/or dry sterile dressing.	Apply butter, oleomargarine, etc.
Second-degree (deeper; blisters develop)	Immerse in cold water, blot dry with sterile cloth for protection. Treat for shock. Obtain medical attention if severe.	Break blisters. Remove shreds of tissue. Use antiseptic preparation, ointment spray, or home remedy on severe burn.
Third-degree (deeper destruction, skin layers destroyed)	Cover with sterile cloth to protect. Treat for shock. Watch for breathing difficulty. Obtain medical attention quickly.	Remove charred clothing that is stuck to burn. Apply ice. Use home medication.
Chemical Burn	Remove by flushing with large quantities of water for at least 5 minutes. Remove surrounding clothing. Obtain medical attention.	

Source: U.S. Coast Guard.

Later Burn Care

Follow a physician's recommendations about burn care, if there are any (many burns are never seen by a doctor). The following suggestions apply to such situations:

1. Wash hands thoroughly before changing any dressing.

2. Leave unbroken blisters intact.

3. Change dressings two times a day unless told otherwise by a physician.

4. Change a dressing by:
   a. Removing old dressings. If a dressing sticks, soak it off with cool, clean water.
   b. Cleanse area gently with mild soap and water.
   c. Pat area dry with clean cloth.
   d. Apply a thin layer of antibacterial cream to the burn.
   e. Apply sterile dressings.

5. Watch for signs of infection. Call a physician if any of these appear:
   a. Increased redness, pain, tenderness, swelling, or red streaks near burn
   b. Pus
   c. Elevated temperature (fever)

6. Keep the area and dressing as clean and dry as possible.

7. Elevate the burned area, if possible, for the first 24 hours.

8. Give a pain medication if necessary.

3. Remove smoldering clothing or soak it with cold water.

4. Do *not* try to remove clothing that is stuck to the skin—cut around the clothing and do *not* pull on it since pulling will further damage the skin. If possible, remove jewelry such as rings from the burned area as soon as possible, since they retain heat, and swelling could make it difficult to remove them later. If jewelry is difficult to remove, leave the job to medical personnel with special equipment. Any valuables that are removed should be put in a safe place so they can be returned to the victim.

5. Immerse the burned area in cold water for about 10 minutes. This is effective only for the 30–45 minutes immediately after injury. Do *not* apply cold on burned areas that are larger than 20 percent of the body surface area or that are suspected third-degree burns.

6. Other types of injuries take priority over a burn (except chemical burns). With this exception, examine burned victims as though the burn injury did not exist, to prevent missing other life-threatening injuries.

7. If the eyes are burned, give them special care and protection. Rinse them *very* gently, but with copious amounts of cool, clean water. Pat them dry and cover them with a clean, dry dressing. Call an ophthalmologist at once.

8. Do *not* break any blisters.

9. Cover the burn with a dry, sterile gauze

■ HEAT BURNS ■

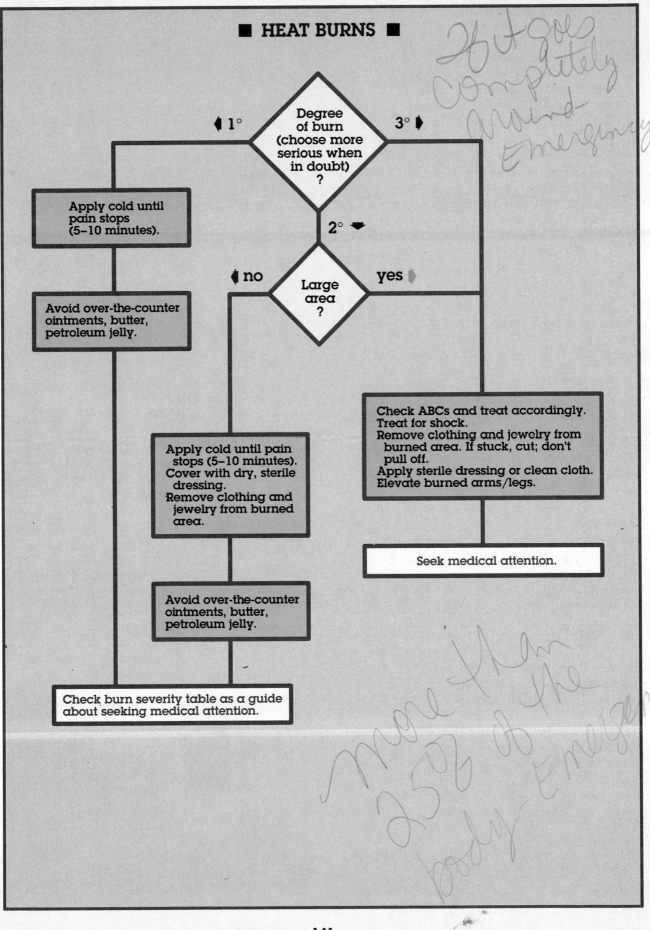

If it goes completely around - Emergency

more than 25% of the body - Emergency

dressing. Large areas may require a clean cloth (e.g., a pillowcase, towel, or sheet).

Do *not* place a moist dressing over a burn since it dries out quickly and may adhere to the burn as it dries. Also, moist dressings over a large area can induce hypothermia. Wet packs or compresses should be used only to initially cool a burn and should not serve as a dressing.

Do *not* use an occlusive dressing (its only advantage is that it does not stick to the burn) since it traps moisture, providing a good place for bacteria to grow.

10. Do *not* put any type of ointment, grease, lotion, butter, antiseptic, or home remedy on burned skin. These applications are unsterile and may lead to infection. Moreover, they can seal in the heat, resulting in further damage. Often, a physician has to scrape them off in order to give proper treatment, which can be very painful for the victim.

11. Monitor breathing and watch for respiratory distress. If the victim was burned in an enclosed space, forced to breathe products of combustion, has blackened mouth or nasal membranes, or has a face, neck or chest burn, do the following: monitor breathing; elevate the head, neck and chest; and seek medical attention.

12. Treat the victim for shock by elevating the legs 8 to 12 inches and keeping him or her warm.

13. Burn victims are susceptible to hypothermia because they lose large amounts of heat and water through the burned tissue. Keep the victim warm.

14. Using the criteria in Table 8.1, determine the burn's severity. If a specialized burn care facility can be reached in an hour, it is better to take a severely burned victim directly to that facility unless he or she is experiencing breathing or bleeding problems. In such cases, the victim should be taken to the nearest hospital emergency department.

First-degree burns

Apply cold water until the pain stops. Tap water is usually cold enough; ice is not needed.

Fast cooling decreases the size and depth of injury, and thus aids healing. Recommended times for cold applications vary from 10 to 30 minutes; some experts recommend continuing to apply cold until the pain does nor recur after cold is discontinued. However, bear in mind that excessive cold can cause frostbite. If ice is all that is available, do *not* apply it directly to the burned area; protect the skin by wrapping the ice in a cloth. Cold will stop the progression of the burn into deeper tissue, but this is only effective for 30 minutes immediately after the injury.

Second-degree burns (small area)

Apply cold as you would for a first-degree burn.

Do *not* break any blisters. They provide a protec-

tive covering against bacteria. A trained medical professional will remove large blisters and all ruptured blisters within 2-3 days of the injury.

Third-degree and large second-degree burns

1. Check immediately for an open airway, breathing, and circulation (the ABCs). Give basic life support (rescue breathing and CPR) if necessary.

2. Treat for shock by elevating the legs 8 to 12 inches and keeping the victim warm.

3. Do *not* open any blisters, since they offer an infection-free cover over the burned skin.

4. Do *not* apply cold to a third-degree or large second-degree burn. The burned victim's body heat must be conserved, since hypothermia may be induced.

5. Apply sterile dressings or, if they are not available, clean cloths.

6. Elevate burned arms or legs to reduce swelling and pain.

Chemical Burns

At least 25,000 products found in industry, agriculture, and the home can burn and cause tissue damage. A chemical continues to cause damage until it is inactivated by the tissue, is neutralized, or is diluted with water. The "burning" process may continue for long periods of time after initial contact. Alkali burns are more serious than acid burns because they penetrate deeper and remain active longer.

Toxicology training is not needed to treat all of the common chemical burns because first aid is the same for all except a few special burns for which something has to be added to neutralize the chemical.

First Aid

■ Wash with large quantities of water all liquid acids, alkalis, and caustic agents. In acid and

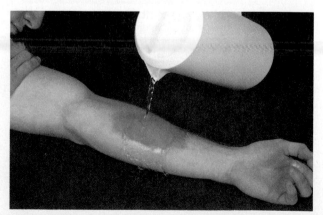

Washing/flooding chemical burns

■ CHEMICAL BURNS ■

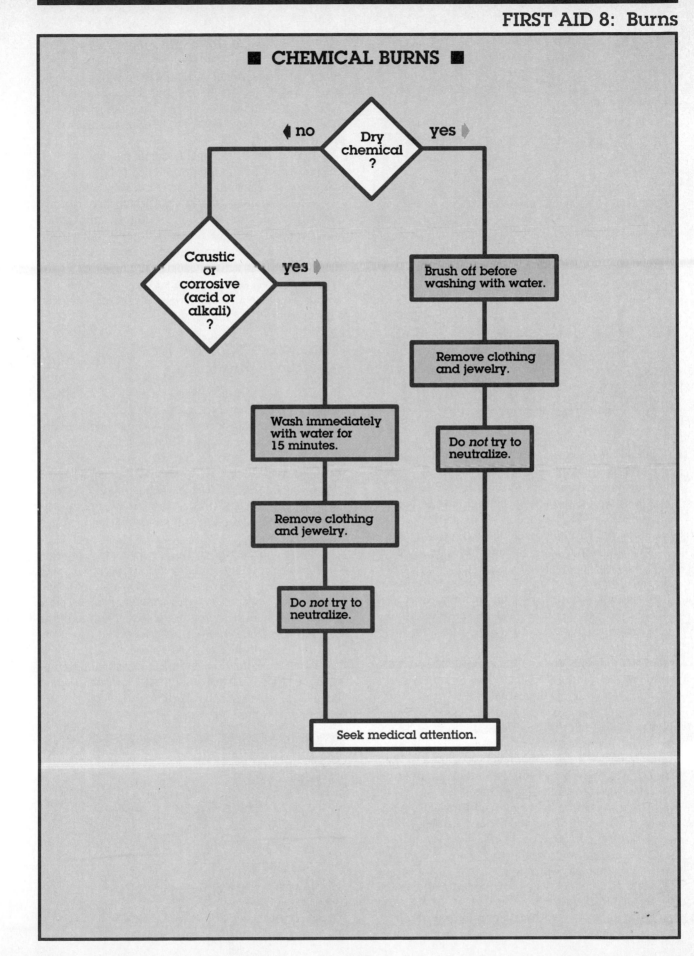

- **Dry chemical?**
  - **no** →
  - **yes** →
- **Caustic or corrosive (acid or alkali)?**
  - **yes** →

Dry chemical — yes:
- Brush off before washing with water.
- Remove clothing and jewelry.
- Do *not* try to neutralize.

Caustic or corrosive — yes:
- Wash immediately with water for 15 minutes.
- Remove clothing and jewelry.
- Do *not* try to neutralize.

- Seek medical attention.

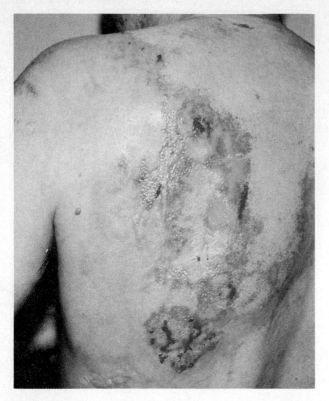

Chemical burn—sulfuric acid

alkali burns, damage is practically set within three minutes after the victim comes in contact with the chemical, so flushing the victim's burns with water in the first minutes after contact substantially reduces the damage.

- Removing contaminated clothing takes any absorbed chemicals away from the skin. Do this while washing the victim.
- Do *not* apply water under any type of pressure because pressure drives the chemical deeper into the tissue. Use a faucet or hose under low pressure and wash with a gentle flow for long periods of time.
- Brush off a dry or solid chemical substance (e.g., lime) before flushing with water. Water activates a dry chemical and will cause more damage to the skin than when it is dry.
- Do *not* attempt to neutralize a chemical because heat may be produced, resulting in more damage. Some product label directions for neutralizing may be wrong. Save the container or label for the name of the chemical.
- Call a poison control center to find out other steps you can take. Additional treatments would be the same as for any heat burn of the same extent and depth.
- If the chemical is in the eye, flood it for at least 15 minutes, using low pressure. Remove any contact lenses.
- Seek immediate medical attention for all chemical burns.

Electrical Injuries

Electrical injuries are devastating. Even with just a mild shock, a victim can suffer serious internal injuries. A current of 1,000 volts or more is considered high voltage, but even the 110 volts of household current can be deadly.

High voltage electrical currents passing through the body may disrupt the normal heart rhythm, cause cardiac arrest, burns, and other injuries.

When someone gets an electric shock, electricity enters the body at the point of contact and travels along the path of least resistance (nerves and blood vessels). The current travels rapidly, generating heat and causing destruction. Usually, the electricity exits where the body is touching a surface or is in contact with a ground (e.g., a metal object). Sometimes, a victim has more than one exit site.

Contact with Power Line (Outdoor Situations)

If electric shock comes from contact with a downed power line, the power must be turned off before a rescuer approaches anyone who may be in contact with the wire.

If the victim is in a car with a power line fallen across it, tell him or her to stay in the car until the power can be shut off. The only exception to this rule is when fire threatens the car. In this case, tell the victim to jump out of the car without making contact with the car or wire.

If you approach a victim and you feel a tingling sensation in your legs and lower body, stop. This sensation signals you are on energized ground and that an electrical current is entering through one foot, passing through your lower body, and leaving through the other foot. If this happens, raise a foot off the ground, turn around and hop to a safe place.

If you can safely reach the victim, do *not* attempt to move any wires with wood poles, tools with wood handles, or objects with a high moisture content. Do *not* attempt to move downed wires at all unless you

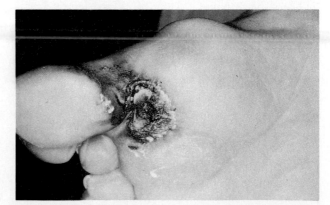

Electrical burn—toe

■ ELECTRICAL INJURIES ■

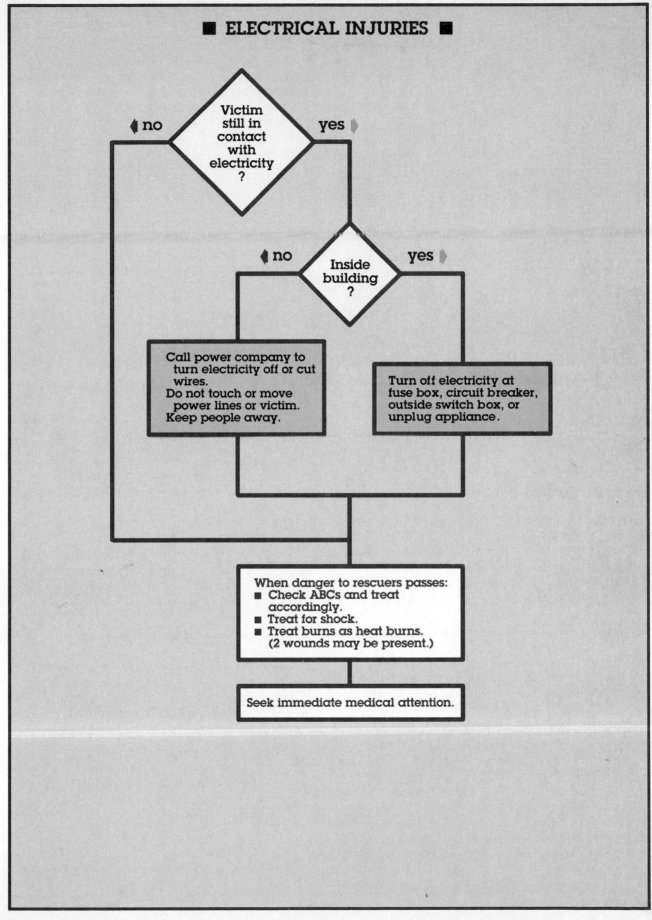

Victim still in contact with electricity ?

no → Inside building ?

yes →

no → Call power company to turn electricity off or cut wires.
Do not touch or move power lines or victim.
Keep people away.

yes → Turn off electricity at fuse box, circuit breaker, outside switch box, or unplug appliance.

When danger to rescuers passes:
■ Check ABCs and treat accordingly.
■ Treat for shock.
■ Treat burns as heat burns. (2 wounds may be present.)

Seek immediate medical attention.

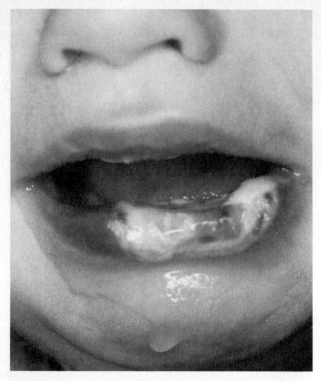
Electrical burn—chewed through electrical cord

are trained and equipped with tools able to handle the high voltage.

Wait until trained personnel with the proper equipment can cut the wires or disconnect them. Prevent bystanders from entering the danger area.

Contact Inside Buildings

Most electrical burns that occur inside are caused by faulty electrical equipment or careless use of electrical appliances. Turn off the electricity at the circuit breaker, fuse box, or outside switch box; or unplug the appliance if the plug is undamaged. Do *not* touch the appliance or the victim until the current is off.

First Aid

Once the danger to rescuers has passed, first aid can begin.

- Check the ABCs—airway, breathing, and circulation and treat accordingly.
- Check for burns and treat for shock by elevating the legs 8 to 12 inches and keeping the victim warm. Most electrical burns are third-degree burns, so cover them with a sterile dressing and elevate the affected part.

Electrical current flows quickly into the body's tissues, then exits. The surface injuries of the skin involve small surface areas (entrance and exit points); the major damage occurs deep under the skin. Any major electrical incident must be handled as if this were the case.

All victims of electrical shock should receive immediate medical attention.

The first line of defense is to know when and where you can be hit by lightning. Some parts of the day are riskier than others. According to studies, about 70% of lightning injuries and deaths occur in the afternoon, 20% between 6:00 P.M. and midnight, 10% between 7 A.M. and noon, and fewer than 1% from midnight to 6:00 A.M. Lightning is also far more common from May through September than in other months.

Armed with these facts, protect yourself when a thunderstorm threatens. Get inside a home or large building, or inside an all-metal (not convertible) vehicle. Inside a home, avoid using the telephone, except for emergencies. If you are outside, with no time to reach a safe building or an automobile, follow these rules:

- Do not stand underneath a natural lightning rod such as a tall, isolated tree in an open area.
- Avoid projecting above the surrounding landscape, as you would do if you were standing on a hilltop, in an open field, on the beach, or fishing from a small boat.
- Get out of and away from open water.
- Get away from tractors and other metal farm equipment.
- Get off and away from motorcycles, scooters, golf carts, and bicycles. Put down golf clubs.
- Stay away from wire fences, clotheslines, metal pipes, rails, and other metallic parts which could carry lightning to you from some distance away.
- Avoid standing in small, isolated sheds or other small structures in open areas.
- In a forest, seek shelter in a low area under a thick growth of small trees. In open areas, go to a low place such as a ravine or valley. Be alert for flash floods.
- If you're hopelessly isolated in a level field or prairie and you feel your hair stand on end—indicating lightning is about to strike—drop to your knees and bend forward, putting your hands on your knees. *Do not* lie flat on the ground. This will ensure that as small an area as possible is touching the ground and will minimize the danger of your body acting as a conductor.

—National Oceanic and Atmospheric Administration

Lightning Strikes

The main concern with a lightning injury is the possibility of respiratory or cardiac arrest. Many times, lightning will not strike a victim directly. Instead, it bounces off a nearby structure, then hits the victim.

First Aid

First aiders must start aggressive, vigorous resuscitation for victims of cardiac arrest. First aid begins with the ABCs. Open the airway by using the jaw thrust method in order to avoid neck hyperextension, which may injure the spinal cord.

If the victim is in cardiac arrest, start CPR. Persistent first aid is crucial for these victims. Treat for shock. Since spinal cord injuries can occur with lightning strikes, precautions should be taken for immobilizing the spine.

If more than one victim has been struck by lightning at the same time, give the highest priority to those in cardiac arrest.

Lightning-struck victims are not charged with electricity and do not represent a hazard to the first aider.

Lightning-Related deaths, 1959–1987

States where deaths attributed to lightning occur most frequently (in descending order):

1.	Florida	6.	Maryland
2.	North Carolina	7.	Louisiana
3.	Texas	8.	Arkansas
4.	Tennessee	9.	Ohio
5.	New York	10.	Pennsylvania

Places where people are killed by lightning most often (with percent of deaths):

In open fields	27%
Under trees	17%
On or near water	12%
Near tractors/ heavy equipment	6%
On golf courses	4%
At telephones	1%
Other	33%

—National Oceanic and Atmospheric Administration

Lightning-Struck

The only man in the world to be struck by lightning 7 times is former Shenandoah Park Ranger Roy C. Sullivan. His attraction for lightning began in 1942 (lost big toenail) and was resumed in July 1969 (lost eyebrows), in July 1970 (left shoulder seared), on April 16, 1972 (hair set on fire) and, finally, he hoped, on August 7, 1973: as he was driving along a bolt came out of a small, low-lying cloud, hit him on the head through his hat, set his hair on fire again, knocked him 10 feet out of his car, went through both legs, and knocked his left shoe off. He had to pour a pail of water over his head to cool off. Then, on June 5, 1976, he was struck again for the sixth time, his ankle injured. When he was struck for the *seventh* time on June 25, 1977, while fishing, he was sent to Waynesboro Hospital with chest and stomach burns. In September 1983, reportedly rejected in love, he died of a self-inflicted gunshot wound.

—Guinness Book of World Records

9

Cold- and Heat-Related Emergencies

■ Frostbite ■ Hypothermia ■ Heat Stroke ■ Heat Exhaustion ■
■ Heat Cramps ■ Heat Syncope ■

Frostbite*

Frostbite occurs when temperatures drop below freezing. Tissue is damaged in two ways: (1) actual tissue freezing, which results in the formation of ice crystals between the tissue cells; the ice crystals enlarge by extracting water from the cells, and (2) the obstruction of blood supply to the tissues; this causes "sludged" blood clots, which prevent blood from flowing to the tissues. The second way injures more than the freezing does.

Frostbite mainly affects the feet, hands, ears, and nose. These areas do not contain large heat-producing muscles and are some distance from the heat generation sources. Moreover, when the body conserves heat, the blood supply diminishes in these areas first. The most severe consequences of frostbite are gangrene and amputation. Some people are more prone to frostbite than others. Victims may also suffer from hypothermia.

Frostnip happens after long cold exposure but is not a serious problem. The condition is not usually painful. The skin becomes white or pale. First aid for frostnip consists of gently warming the affected area. This can be done with bare hands or by blowing warm air on the area.

Signs and Symptoms
(Classified by Thawing)

Types Based on the Pre-Thaw Stage

Superficial

- Skin color is white or grayish-yellow
- Pain may occur early and later subside
- Affected part may feel only very cold and numb. There may be a tingling, stinging, or aching sensation.
- Skin surface will feel hard or crusty and underlying tissue soft when depressed gently and firmly.

Source: Based on National Ski Patrol protocols; adapted with permission.

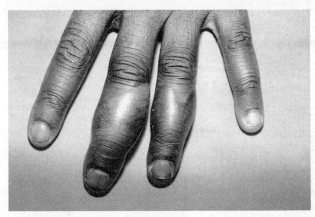

Frostbitten fingers, 6 hours after rewarming in 108°F water

Deep

- Affected part feels hard, solid, and cannot be depressed.
- Blisters appear in 12 to 36 hours.
- Affected part is cold with pale, waxy skin.
- A painfully cold part suddenly stops hurting.

Types Based on the Post-Thaw Stage

After a part has thawed, frostbite can be categorized into degrees similar to the classification of burns. First-degree frostbite is superficial, while the other three are degrees of deep frostbite.

- ***First-degree frostbite.*** Affected part is warm, swollen, and tender.
- ***Second-degree frostbite.*** Blisters form within minutes to hours after thawing and enlarge over several days.
- ***Third-degree frostbite.*** Blisters are small, contain reddish-blue or purplish fluid. Surrounding skin may have a red or blue color and may not blanch when pressure is applied.
- ***Fourth-degree frostbite.*** No blisters or swelling occurs. The part remains numb, cold, white-to-dark-purple in color.

First Aid

All frostbite injuries follow the same first aid treatment. Seek medical attention immediately. *Rewarming of*

■ FROSTBITE ■

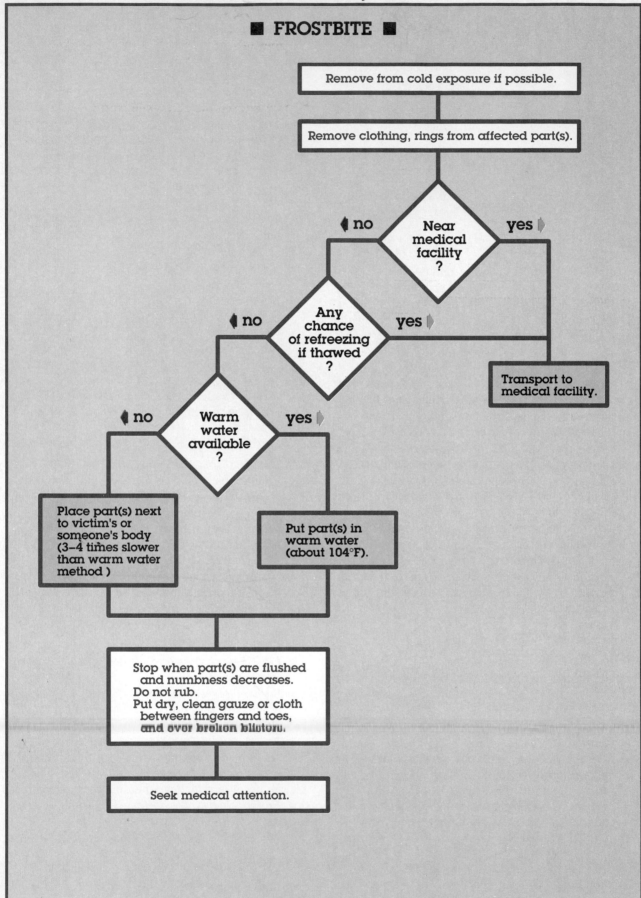

Remove from cold exposure if possible.

Remove clothing, rings from affected part(s).

Near medical facility?
- no
- yes → Transport to medical facility.

Any chance of refreezing if thawed?
- no
- yes → Transport to medical facility.

Warm water available?
- no → Place part(s) next to victim's or someone's body (3–4 times slower than warm water method)
- yes → Put part(s) in warm water (about 104°F).

Stop when part(s) are flushed and numbness decreases.
Do not rub.
Put dry, clean gauze or cloth between fingers and toes, and over broken blisters.

Seek medical attention.

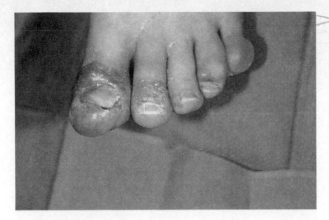

2nd degree frostbite

frostbitten parts seldom takes place outside of a medical facility because such facilities are usually nearby. However, if in a remote situation, the *wet, rapid rewarming method* may be used and is preferred to slow rewarming since the latter is associated with greater tissue damage.

Rapid Rewarming

- Do *not* attempt rewarming if a medical facility is nearby or if there is any chance that the part may refreeze.
- Remove any clothing or constricting items that could impair blood circulation (e.g., rings).
- Put the frostbitten part(s) in warm (not hot) water. Measure the water temperature with a thermometer. The water temperature should be 102–106°F. If you do not have a thermometer, test the water by pouring some water over the inside of your arm. Maintain the water temperature by adding warm water as needed.
- Warming usually takes 20 to 40 minutes and should be continued until the tissues are soft and pliable.
- For ear or facial injuries, apply warm moist cloths and change them frequently.
- To help control pain during the rewarming process, aspirin or acetaminophen may be given.

Post-Care

- Treat victim as a "stretcher" case.
- Maintain total body warmth.
- Protect injured part(s) from direct contact with clothing, bedding, etc.
- Leave any blisters intact.
- Place dry, sterile gauze between toes and fingers to absorb moisture and avoid having them stick together.
- Slightly elevate the affected part to reduce pain and swelling.
- Keep both the victim and affected part as warm as possible without overheating.

Cautions

- Do *not* allow the victim to walk on frostbitten toes or feet, especially after rewarming.
- Do *not* use water hotter than 106°F since burns can result.
- Do *not* break any blisters that may have formed.
- Do *not* rub the part, even with snow.
- Do *not* rewarm the part with a heating pad, hot-water bottle, sunlamp, stove, radiator, exhaust pipe, or over a fire since this produces excessive temperatures and cannot be controlled, thus resulting in burns.
- Do *not* allow the victim to drink alcoholic beverages because they dilate blood vessels and cause a loss of body heat.
- Do *not* allow the victim to smoke since smoking constricts blood vessels, thus impairing circulation.
- Do *not* allow the thawed part to refreeze since ice crystals formed will be larger and more damaging.
- Unless circumstances justify its use (i.e., lack of water or fuel to warm water), do *not* use the "dry, rapid rewarming" technique (putting victim's hands in armpits) since it takes three to four times longer than the wet method to thaw frozen tissue and slow rewarming results in greater tissue damage than rapid rewarming.

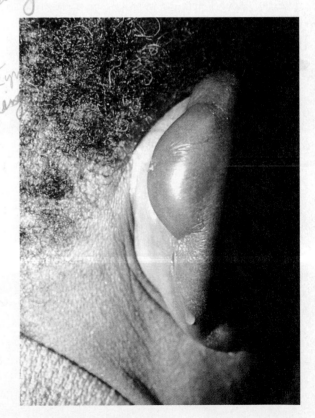

Frostbitten ear 8 hours old

Hypothermia*

Hypothermia results from a cooling of the body's core temperature. Hypothermia can occur at temperatures above freezing as well as below it. The victim may suffer frostbite as well, if the body loses more heat than it produces. If the body temperature falls to 80°F, most people die. Hypothermia does not result from outdoor exposure alone. It is also caused by cool indoor temperatures.

Types of Exposure

1. *Acute exposure* occurs when the victim loses body heat very rapidly, usually in water immersion. Acute exposure is considered to be six hours or less in duration.

2. *Subacute exposure* occurs when exposure is six to 24 hours, and can be either a land based or water immersion experience.

3. *Chronic exposure* involves long-term cooling. It generally occurs on land when exposure exceeds 24 hours.

Types of Hypothermia

A victim's core body temperature determines the type of hypothermia. To take the temperature, you need a low-reading thermometer, not the standard rectal thermometer, which is calibrated from 94 to 108°F. The recommended type is a rectal thermometer capable of reading temperatures between 84 to 108°F. These thermometers are hard to find.

1. *Mild* (above 90°F). Shivering, slurred speech, memory lapses, and fumbling hands. Victims frequently stumble and stagger. They are usually conscious and can talk. While many people suffer cold hands and feet, victims of mild hypothermia experience cold abdomens and backs.

*Source: Based on National Ski Patrol protocols; adapted with permission.

How Cold Is It?

In addition to coldness, two other factors account for body heat loss: moisture and wind. Moisture—whether from rain, snow, or perspiration—speeds the conduction of heat away from the body.

Wind causes sizable amounts of body heat loss. If the thermometer reads 20°F and the wind speed is 20 mph, the exposure is comparable to −10°F. This is called the wind-chill factor. A rough measure of wind speed is: If you feel the wind on your face, the speed is about 10 mph; if small branches move or dust or snow is raised,

20 mph; if large branches are moving, 30 mph; and if a whole tree bends, about 40 mph.

Determine the wind-chill factor by:

1. Estimating the wind speed by checking for the signs described above.

2. Looking at a thermometer reading (in Fahrenheit degrees) outdoors.

3. Determining the wind-chill factor by matching the estimated wind speed with the actual thermometer reading in the "Wind-Chill Factor" table.

Wind-Chill Factor

Estimated Wind Speed (in MPH)	Actual Thermometer Reading (°F)											
	50	40	30	20	10	0	−10	−20	−30	−40	−50	−60
	Equivalent Temperature (°F)											
calm	50	40	30	20	10	0	−10	−20	−30	−40	−50	−60
5	40	37	27	16	6	−5	−15	−26	−36	−47	−57	−68
10	40	28	16	4	−9	−24	−33	−46	−58	−70	−83	−95
15	36	22	9	−5	−18	−32	−45	−58	−72	−85	−99	−112
20	32	18	4	−10	−25	−39	−53	−67	−82	−96	−110	−124
25	30	16	0	−15	−29	−44	−59	−74	−88	−104	−118	−133
30	25	13	−2	−18	−33	−48	−63	−79	−94	−109	−125	−140
35	27	11	−4	−20	−35	−51	−67	−82	−98	−113	−129	−145
40	26	10	−6	−21	−37	−53	−69	−85	−100	−116	−132	−148
(Wind speeds greater than 40 mph have little additional effect.)	Little danger (for properly clothed person). Maximum danger of false sense of security.			Increasing danger. (Flesh may freeze within 1 minute.)			Great danger. (Flesh may freeze within 30 seconds.)					

■ HYPOTHERMIA ■

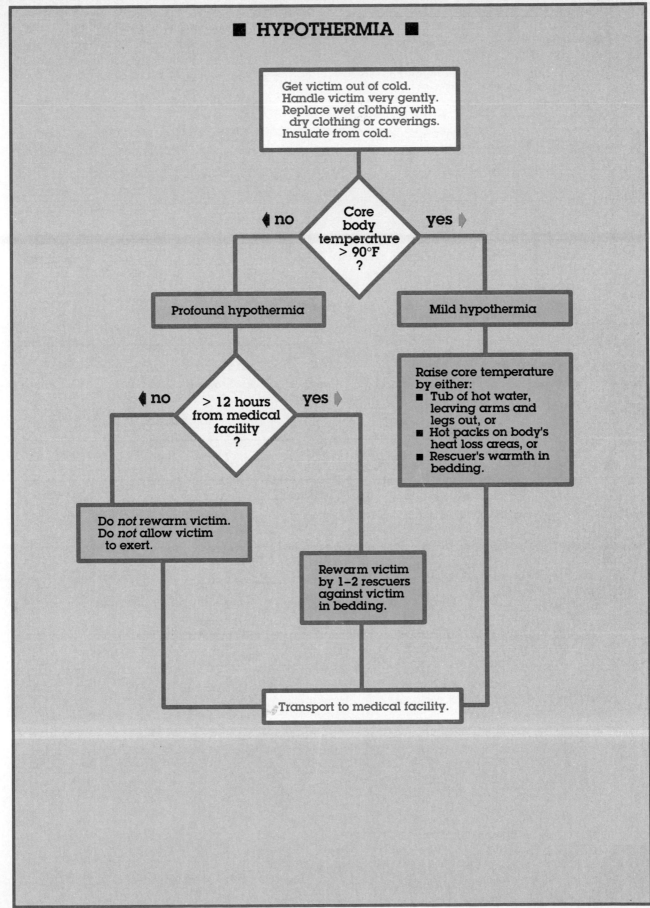

Get victim out of cold.
Handle victim very gently.
Replace wet clothing with
dry clothing or coverings.
Insulate from cold.

Core body temperature > 90°F ?

no → Profound hypothermia

yes → Mild hypothermia

> 12 hours from medical facility ?

no → Do *not* rewarm victim. Do *not* allow victim to exert.

yes → Rewarm victim by 1–2 rescuers against victim in bedding.

Raise core temperature by either:
■ Tub of hot water, leaving arms and legs out, or
■ Hot packs on body's heat loss areas, or
■ Rescuer's warmth in bedding.

Transport to medical facility.

2. *Profound* (below 90°F). Shivering has stopped. Muscles may become stiff and rigid, similar to rigor mortis. The victim's skin has a blue appearance and doesn't respond to pain; pulse and respirations slow down, and pupils dilate. The victim appears to be dead. Fifty to 80 percent of all profound hypothermic victims die.

First Aid

1. General Suggestions
   Stop further heat loss by doing the following:
   a. Get the victim out of the cold environment.
   b. Have a source of heat (e.g., stove, fire).
   c. Add insulation beneath and around the victim. Cover the victim's head since

If a Blizzard Traps You While You Are Driving

- Don't panic.

- Stay in your vehicle. Do not attempt to walk out of a blizzard. Disorientation comes quickly in blowing and drifting snow. Being lost in open country during a blizzard is almost certain death. You are more likely to be found, and more likely to be sheltered, in your car.

- Avoid overexertion and exposure. Exertion from attempting to push your car, shovel heavy drifts, and perform other difficult chores during the strong winds, blinding snow, and bitter cold of a blizzard may cause a heart attack—even for persons in apparently good physical condition.

- Keep fresh air in your car. Freezing, wet snow and wind-driven snow can completely seal the passenger compartment, causing suffocation.

- Beware the gentle killers: carbon monoxide and oxygen starvation. Run the motor and heater sparingly, and only with the downwind window open for ventilation.

- Keep watch. Do not permit all occupants of the car to sleep at one time.

- Exercise by clasping hands and moving arms and legs vigorously from time to time, and do not stay in one position for long.

- Turn on your car's dome light at night, to make the vehicle visible to work crews.

Source: National Oceanic and Atmospheric Administration

Winter Wardrobe

	Advantages	Disadvantages	Wear In
WOOL	Stretches without damage; insulates well even when wet	Heavy weight; absorbs moisture; may irritate skin	Layer 1, 2 or 3
COTTON	Comfortable and lightweight	Absorbs moisture	Layer 1 (for inactive people) or 2
SILK	Extremely lightweight and durable; very good insulator; washes well.	More expensive; does not transfer moisture quickly	Layer 1
POLY-PROPYLENE	Lightweight; transfers moisture quickly and dries quickly	Does not insulate well; low melting point; surface may pill up	Layer 1 or 2 (for active people)
DOWN	Durable, lightweight; most effective insulator by weight	Expensive; loses insulative quality when wet; difficult to dry	Layer 2 or 3 (especially in dry, extreme cold)
NYLON	Lightweight; wind- and water-resistant; durable	May not allow perspiration to evaporate; low melting point; flammable	Layer 3
SYNTHETIC POLYESTER INSULATION	Does not absorb moisture, therefore insulates even when wet	Heavier than down; does not compress as well	Layer 2 or 3 (especially in wet weather)

Source: National Safety Council, Family Safety & Health.

50 percent of the body's heat loss is
through the head.

    d. Replace wet clothing with dry clothing.

    e. Handle the victim gently.

    f. Treat any injuries.

2. Mild Hypothermia (core temperature above 90 °F)

Raise core temperature by one of the following
means available:

    a. Use a tub of hot water (no greater than
106°F) or electric blanket. *Leave victim's
arms and legs out.*

    b. Place hot packs against the body's areas of
high heat loss (e.g., head, neck, chest, and
groin). Do not burn the victim.

    c. Have a rescuer lie trunk to trunk with the
victim in a sleeping bag.

3. Profound Hypothermia (core temperature below
90 °F)

    a. Do *not* rewarm the victim if he or she can
be transported within 12 hours. Keep the
victim from getting colder.

    b. Do *not* jostle or jolt the victim during trans-
portation.

    c. *Avoid* CPR unless the victim has no pulse.
Start CPR immediately in near-drowning
cases. Pulses are difficult to detect so take a
full minute to check them. CPR could actually induce cardiac arrest. Once CPR is
begun, it should be continued until arrival
at a medical facility. Hypothermic victims
have survived after long-term CPR (unlike
those with cardiac arrest from other
causes).

Warm drinks have no warming effect and contain little energy. Warm drinks send a message to
the brain to send more blood to the skin. Dilation
of the skin's blood vessels produces a warm feeling
and some heat loss since the capillaries are dilated.

Avoid cardiac arrest by observing the following
guidelines:

- *Never* allow the victim to physically exert him-
self (i.e., no walking, climbing, etc.).
- Make *no* attempt to rapidly rewarm a profound
hypothermic victim outside of a medical facility. Most circumstances require no rewarming
attempts at all.
- Handle a profound hypothermic victim as carefully and gently as though every arm and leg
were broken.

Cautions

- Do *not* put an unconscious victim in a bathtub.
- Do *not* give the unconscious victim anything to
drink.
- Do *not* give the victim alcohol.

- Do *not* attempt to rewarm the body by rubbing the arms and legs.
- Do *not* allow the victim to move about, walk,
or struggle.
- Do *not* wrap a victim in a blanket without
another source of heat unless it is to protect
the victim against further heat loss since such
victims cannot generate sufficient heat to rewarm themselves, and blankets insulate them
from the warm environment.
- Do *not* stop resuscitative attempts until the victim has been rewarmed and preferably evalu-
ated at a medical facility.
- Do *not* rewarm the victim outside of a medical
facility if he or she can be transported within
12 hours. Victims can be hypothermic for long
periods of time and still recover.
- Do *not* give CPR unless the victim is pulseless.
Use CPR in cases of drowning. Monitor pulse
for a full minute.
- Do *not* rewarm extremities and body core
(chest, abdomen) at the same time.

Heat-Related Emergencies

There are two types of major heat illness—heat stroke
and heat exhaustion, and two types of minor heat
illness—heat cramps and heat syncope.

Heat Stroke (sunstroke)

Heat stroke is the most dangerous heat-related emergency. The death rate from this condition approaches
50 percent, even with appropriate medical care. Untreated victims always die. Heat stroke happens when
the body is subjected to more heat than it can handle.

TABLE 9-1 Heat Index

Relative Humidity	Air Temperature										
	70	75	80	85	90	95	100	105	110	115	120
	Apparent Temperature*										
0%	64	69	73	78	83	87	91	95	99	103	107
10%	65	70	75	80	85	90	95	100	105	111	116
20%	66	72	77	82	87	93	99	105	112	120	130
30%	67	73	78	84	90	96	104	113	123	135	148
40%	68	74	79	86	93	101	110	123	137	151	
50%	69	75	81	88	96	107	120	135	150		
60%	70	76	82	90	100	114	132	149			
70%	70	77	85	93	106	124	144				
80%	71	78	86	97	113	136					
90%	71	79	88	102	122						
100%	72	80	91	108							

*Degrees Fahrenheit.

Above 130°F = heat stroke imminent

105°–130°F = heat exhaustion and heat cramps likely and heat stroke with long exposure and activity

90°–105°F = heat exhaustion and heat cramps with long exposure and activity

80°–90°F = fatigue during exposure and activity

Source: National Weather Service

Types of Heat Stroke

- **Classic.** This type affects the elderly, chronically ill, obese, alcoholic, diabetic, and those with circulatory problems. It results from a combination of a hot environment and body mechanisms incapable of handling heat exposure.
- **Exertional.** This type affects a healthy individual when strenuously working or playing in a warm environment.

Signs and Symptoms

- The skin is always hot, with high body temperature above 104°F, and is usually flushed, although it may appear ashen in more severe cases.
- Mental status can be altered. It first appears as confusion, lethargy, and agitation, and may progress to seizures and coma or unconsciousness.
- Breathing and pulse are rapid.
- Skin may be dry or wet. Dry skin has been cited as the main sign of heat stroke. However, normal or even extreme sweating may be seen in some victims. Victims with dry skin have had their sweat glands fail. Exertional heat stroke victims may have sweat on their skin since they are progressing from heat exhaustion into heat stroke.

First Aid

Heat stroke is a true emergency! Heat stroke victims must be treated rapidly. Every minute of delay increases the likelihood of serious complications or death.

- Monitor the ABCs and treat accordingly.
- Move the victim to a cool place. Remove heavy clothing; light clothing can be left in place.
- Immediately cool the victim by any available means.

   Place ice packs at areas with abundant blood supply (e.g., neck, armpits, and groin). If

Highest Body Temperature

Sustained body temperatures of much over 109°F are normally incompatible with life, although recoveries after readings of 111°F have been noted. Marathon runners in hot weather attain 105.8°F.

Willie Jones, 52 years old, was admitted to Grady Memorial Hospital, Atlanta, Georgia, on July 10, 1980, with heat stroke on a day when the temperature reached 90°F with 44% humidity. His temperature was found to be 115.7°F.

—Guinness Book of World Records

ice is not available, an effective method is to wrap the victim in wet towels or sheets, and fan him or her. Keep the cloths wet with cool water. Continue cooling the victim until his or her temperature drops to 102°F. Stop at this point to prevent seizures and hypothermia.

- Keep the victim's head and shoulders slightly elevated.
- Seek medical attention immediately! All heat stroke victims need hospitalization. During transport, continue cooling.
- Care for seizures if they occur.
- Do *not* use aspirin or acetaminophen (antipyretics). The hypothalamic setpoint during heat stroke is at normal despite the elevated body temperature. Thus, these medications, which reduce fever by resetting this setpoint, have no effect.

Heat Exhaustion

Heat exhaustion results from either excessive perspiration or the inadequate replacement of water lost by sweating. It is less critical than heat stroke, but it requires prompt attention because it can progress to heat stroke if left untreated.

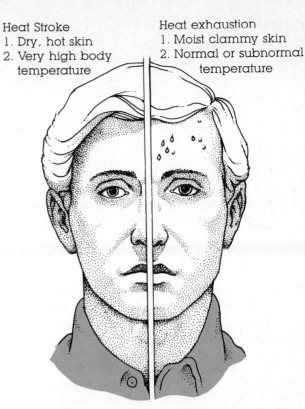

Heat Stroke
1. Dry, hot skin
2. Very high body temperature

Heat exhaustion
1. Moist clammy skin
2. Normal or subnormal temperature

Signs and symptoms of heat stroke and heat exhaustion

TABLE 9–2 Heat-related Emergencies			
Indicators	Heat Cramps (least serious)	Heat Exhaustion (serious)	Heat Stroke (most serious)
Muscle cramps	Yes	No	No
Skin	Normal, moist-warm	Cold, clammy	Hot, dry
Temperature	Normal	Normal or slightly elevated	>105° F.
Loss of consciousness	Seldom	Sometimes	Usually
Perspiration	Heavy	Heavy	Little or none
First aid	Move to cool place.	Move to cool place.	Move to cool place.
	Rest affected muscle.	Elevate legs.	Elevate head and shoulders.
	Give a lot of cold water.	Cool victim.	Immediately cool victim.
	Do *not* massage.	If no improvement in 30 minutes, seek medical attention.	Immediately transport to medical facility.
			Monitor ABCs.
			Heat stroke is life-threatening!

Signs and Symptoms

- Heavy sweating
- Weakness
- Fast pulse
- Normal body temperature
- Headache and dizziness
- Nausea and vomiting

First Aid

- Move the victim to a cool place.
- Keep victim lying down with straight legs elevated 8–12 inches.
- Cool the victim by applying cold packs or wet towels or cloths. Fan the victim.
- Give the victim cold water if he or she is fully conscious.
- If no improvement is noted within 30 minutes, seek medical attention.

Heat Cramps

Heat cramps are painful muscle spasms in the arms or legs. They may occur when an excessive amount of body fluid is lost through sweating. Controversy exists regarding what type of liquid to drink—plain water, a commercial sports drink, or a saltwater solution. The body loses more water than electrolytes (sodium, potassium, etc.) during exercise. Experts generally agree that the primary need for those sweating in hot environments is to replace the water lost from heavy sweating, rather than the electrolytes. No proof exists that muscle cramping results from a shortage of electrolytes.

Routine use of salt tablets to prevent heat cramps is no longer recommended since they can induce high blood pressure and hinder adjustment to heat.

Signs and Symptoms

- Severe cramping, usually affecting arms or legs
- Abdominal cramping

First Aid

- Move the victim to a cool place.
- Rest the cramping muscle.
- Give victim a lot of cold water.
- Do *not* massage since it rarely provides relief and may even worsen the pain.

Hot Weather Precautions

These simple preventive measures can reduce heat stress:

1. Keep cool as possible.
   - Avoid direct sunlight.
   - Stay in the coolest available location (usually indoors)
   - Use air-conditioning, if available.
   - Use electric fans to promote cooling.
   - Place wet towels or ice bags on the body or dampen clothing.
   - Take cool baths or showers.

2. Wear lightweight, loose-fitting clothing.

3. Avoid strenuous physical activity, particularly in the sun and during the hottest part of the day.

4. Increase intake of fluids, such as water and fruit or vegetable juices. Thirst is not always a good indicator of adequacy of fluid intake. Some studies indicate that fluid intake in hot weather should be 1 1/2 times the amount that quenches thirst. Persons who are overweight or large in build or who are engaged in strenuous activities, such as sports, may require more than a gallon of fluid intake daily in very hot weather. Persons for whom salt or fluid is restricted should consult their physicians for instructions on appropriate fluid and salt intake.

5. Do not take salt tablets unless so instructed by a physician.

6. Avoid alcoholic beverages (beer, wine, and liquor).

7. Stay in daily contact with other people.

—*Morbidity and Mortality Weekly Report*

Heat Syncope

This condition resembles fainting and is usually self-correcting. Victims who are not nauseated can drink water. First aid consists of having the victim lie down in a cool place.

■ HEAT-RELATED EMERGENCIES ■

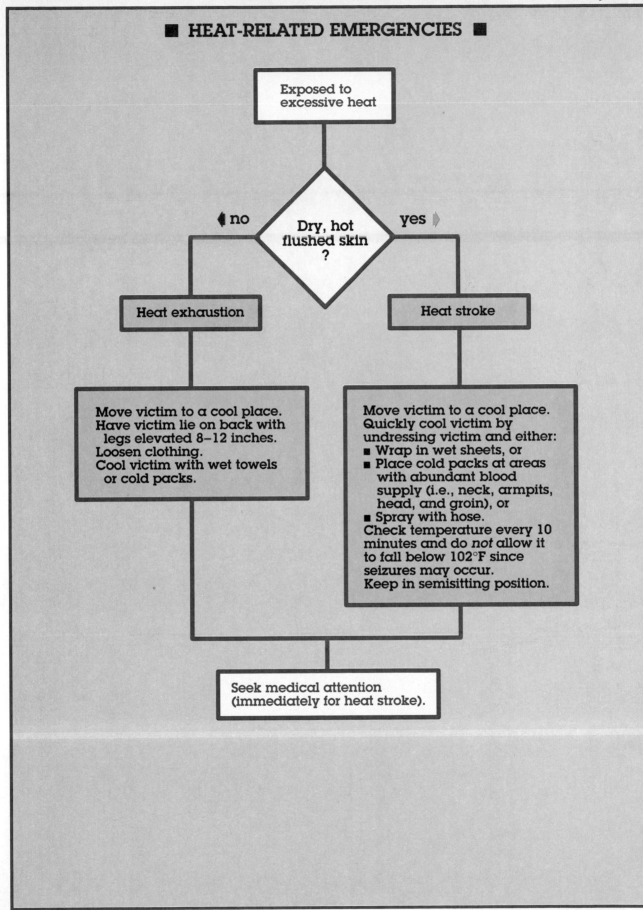

Exposed to excessive heat

Dry, hot flushed skin ?

no — Heat exhaustion

yes — Heat stroke

Heat exhaustion
Move victim to a cool place.
Have victim lie on back with legs elevated 8–12 inches.
Loosen clothing.
Cool victim with wet towels or cold packs.

Heat stroke
Move victim to a cool place.
Quickly cool victim by undressing victim and either:
■ Wrap in wet sheets, or
■ Place cold packs at areas with abundant blood supply (i.e., neck, armpits, head, and groin), or
■ Spray with hose.
Check temperature every 10 minutes and do *not* allow it to fall below 102°F since seizures may occur.
Keep in semisitting position.

Seek medical attention (immediately for heat stroke).

10

Bone, Joint, and Muscle Injuries*

■ Fractures ■ Dislocations ■ Spinal Injuries ■
■ Ankle Injuries ■ Muscle Injuries ■

Fractures

The terms **fracture** and **broken bone** have the same meaning—break or crack in a bone. Fractures are classified as being **open** (when the skin is broken and bleeds externally) or **closed** (when the skin has not been broken).

Fracture Classification

- ***Open (compound) fracture.*** The overlaying skin has been damaged or broken. The wound can be produced either by the bone protruding through the skin or by a direct blow cutting the skin at the time of the fracture. The bone may not always be seen in the wound. Any broken bone which is covered by damaged skin is classified as an open fracture.
- ***Closed (simple) fracture.*** The skin has not been broken and no wound exists anywhere near the fracture site. Open fractures are more serious than closed fractures because of greater blood loss and greater chance of infection.

Signs and Symptoms

- ***Swelling.*** Caused by bleeding; it occurs rapidly after a fracture.

*Source: Based upon American Academy of Orthopaedic Surgeons protocols.

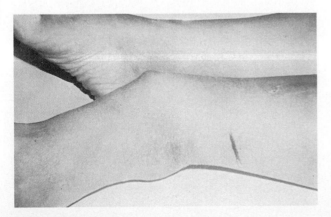

Closed leg fracture

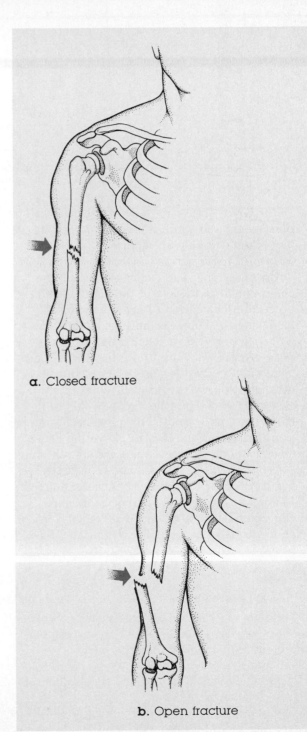

a. Closed fracture

b. Open fracture

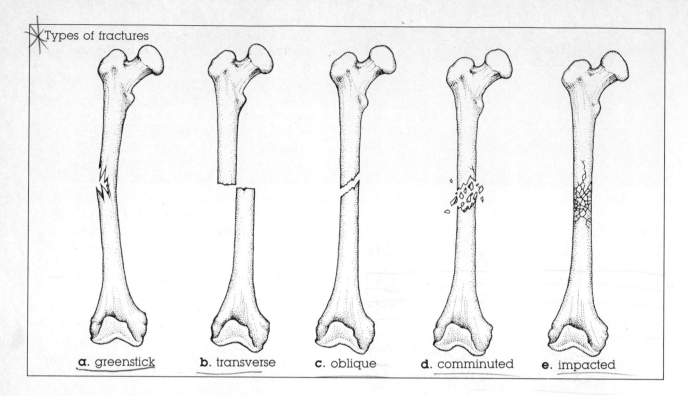

Types of fractures

a. greenstick   **b.** transverse   **c.** oblique   **d.** comminuted   **e.** impacted

- **Deformity.** This is not always obvious. Compare the injured with the uninjured opposite part when checking for deformity. _ask if it was always that way._
- **Pain and tenderness.** Commonly found only at the injury site. The victim will usually be able to point to the site of the pain. A useful procedure for detecting fractures is to gently feel along the bones; complaints about pain or tenderness serve as a reliable sign of a fracture.
- **Loss of use.** Inability to use the injured part. "Guarding" occurs because when motion produces pain, the victim will refuse to use it. However, sometimes the victim is able to move the limb with little or no pain.
- **Grating sensation.** Do *not* move the injured limb as an attempt to see if a grating sensation (called **crepitus**) can be felt and even sometimes heard when the broken bone ends rub together.
- **History of the injury.** Suspect a fracture whenever severe accidents (e.g., motor-vehicle accidents, falls) happen. The victim may have heard or felt the bone snap.

ABCH

First Aid

The first aid procedures listed here are basic guidelines.

- Treat any life-threatening emergencies. Broken bones (except spinal or pelvic breaks) seldom present an immediate threat to life.
- Treat the victim for shock.
- Determine what happened and the location of pain, numbness, tingling.
- Gently remove clothing surrounding the injured area. Do *not* move the injured area un-less necessary. Cut clothing at the seams if necessary. Check for swelling, deformity, tenderness, guarding, and open wounds.
- Control bleeding and cover all wounds before splinting. In open fractures, do *not* attempt to push bone ends back beneath the skin surface. Simply cover them with a sterile dressing.
- Check for a pulse, sensations, and capillary refill. Compare area with an uninjured part.

A quick nerve and circulatory exam is very important. Fractures can injure nerves. Check for nerve damage by checking for sensations and asking the victim to flex the hand or foot, depending upon the fracture location.

A quick circulatory exam is important because prolonged loss of blood to an extremity rapidly results in irreversible damage. Check the radial pulse at the wrist and the dorsalis

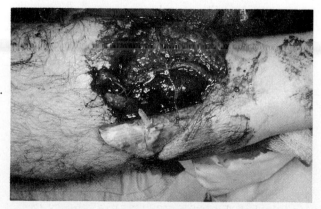

Open tibia, fibula fracture

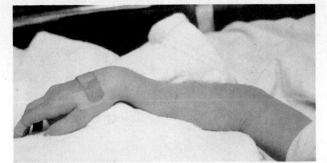

Forearm fracture

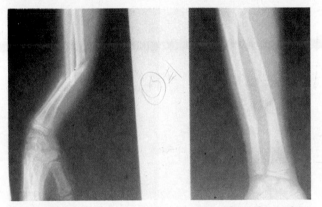

X-rays of victim with forearm fracture. One shows before setting; the other is after.

pedis pulse in the foot. About one person in five has no detectable dorsalis pedis pulse, so if it is absent, check for a posterior tibial pulse. (The dorsalis pedis pulse is located on top of the foot, whereas the posterior tibial pulse can be found behind the inside ankle bone.) If you can not detect a pulse, obtain medical assistance immediately. Capillary refilling can also be used as a check for circulation. Perform this test by pressing on the tip of a nail to cause the nailbed to turn white. Then, release the pressure. Normally the pink color returns by the time it takes to say "capillary refill." If it does not return during this time, suspect a circulation problem. Do *not* wait to see whether circulation will return before getting help.

If the victim's hand or foot is cold, pale, and pulseless, and medical care is more than 15 minutes away, many experts recommend realigning the limb with gentle manual traction. This involves pulling *gently* in line with the normal bone position. If there is great pain or resistance to this gentle traction, splint the fracture as it is.

- All fractures should be splinted before the victim is moved unless the victim's life is endangered. When splinting possible fractures, immobilize the joints above and below the fracture site. Splinting helps prevent further injury to soft tissues, blood vessels, or nerves from sharp

[handwritten margin note: check distal pulse of the injury]

bone fragments and relieves pain by stopping motion at the fracture site. Keep the fingers and toes exposed in order to check circulation even though they may be included within a splint.

- Several commonly available materials can form splints. An arm sling and swathe, a pillow, cardboard, boards, newspapers, blankets—even tying the injured part to an uninjured part—all serve well as splints. Padded splints prevent pressure to nerves and skin.

- Severely deformed fractures should be realigned before splinting if a pulse is absent. This helps preserve or restore circulation. This involves gently pulling in line with the normal bone position. Explain to the victim that straightening the fracture may cause momentary pain, but that it will stop once the fracture is straightened and splinted. If the victim shows increased pain or resistance, splint the extremity in the deformed position. Do *not* straighten dislocations or any fractures involving the spine, shoulder, elbow, wrist, or knee. *[handwritten: Don't Do!]*

- Never reduce open fractures. Cover the wound with a sterile dressing. Then apply the appropriate splint.

- If the victim has a possible spinal injury as well as an extremity injury, the spinal injury takes precedence. Splinting the spine is always a problem. Immobilize the spine with rolled blankets or similar objects placed on either side of the neck and torso. In most cases it is best to wait until an ambulance arrives with trained personnel and proper equipment to handle spinal injuries. Tell the victim not to move.

- Position the injured part slightly above the heart's level to help control swelling and pain. Cold packs help control swelling and pain but avoid overuse because of frostbite.

- Most fractures do not require rapid transportation. An exception involves the arm or leg without a pulse, which means insufficient blood is being provided for the affected arm or leg. This necessitates seeking immediate medical attention.

- If in doubt, splint and treat as if there were a fracture. *[handwritten: 20 to 30 min Ice]*

- Analgesics can help reduce the pain associated with an injury. Do *not* give aspirin or acetaminophen if the victim cannot tolerate it. Cold packs can also help reduce pain.

Dislocations

Dislocations occur in a joint when it is pushed beyond its normal range of motion.

[handwritten bottom margin: numbness — immediate in nerve damage]

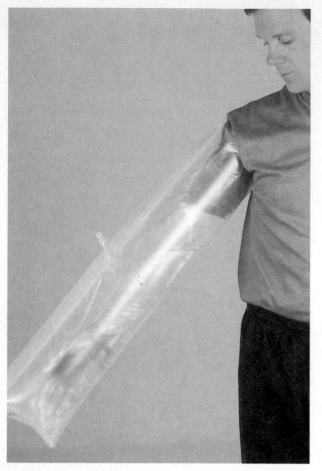

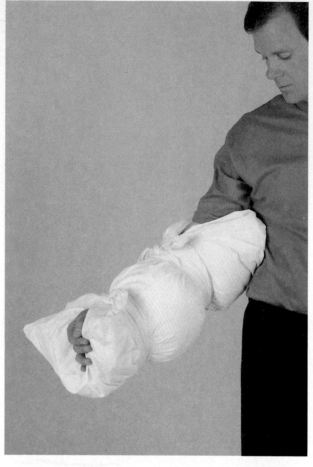

Types of splints: Commercial (air splint)   Improvised (pillow)

Signs and Symptoms

- Deformity of a joint
- Severe pain in a joint
- Swelling around the joint
- Discoloration around the joint
- Inability to move the injured area
- Appearance differing from comparable uninjured joint

First Aid

- Check the pulse, sensation, and capillary refill of the injured extremity (compare with uninjured part).
- Splint as if a fracture.
- Do *not* replace the joint since nerve and blood vessel damage could happen.

Types of Splints

Any device used to immobilize a fracture or dislocation is a splint. Splint by using:

- ***Improvised splint.*** Use pillow, folded newspaper, magazine, cardboard, wooden board, or any other object that can provide stability.

- ***Victim's body.*** Tie injured part to uninjured part (e.g., injured finger to adjacent finger; legs tied together; injured arm tied to chest).
- ***Commercial splint.*** Use wire splints, air splints.

Spinal Injuries

The spine is a column of vertebrae stacked one on the next from the skull's base to the tail bone. Each vertebra has a hollow center through which the spinal cord passes. The spinal cord consists of long tracts of nerves that join the brain with all body organs and parts.

If a broken vertebra pinches spinal nerves, paralysis can result. All unconscious victims should be treated as though they had spinal injuries. All conscious victims sustaining injuries from falls, diving accidents, or auto accidents should be carefully checked for spine injuries before moving them.

A mistake in handling a spinal injured victim could mean a lifetime in a wheelchair or bed for the victim. Suspect a spinal injury in all severe accidents.

■ FRACTURES ■

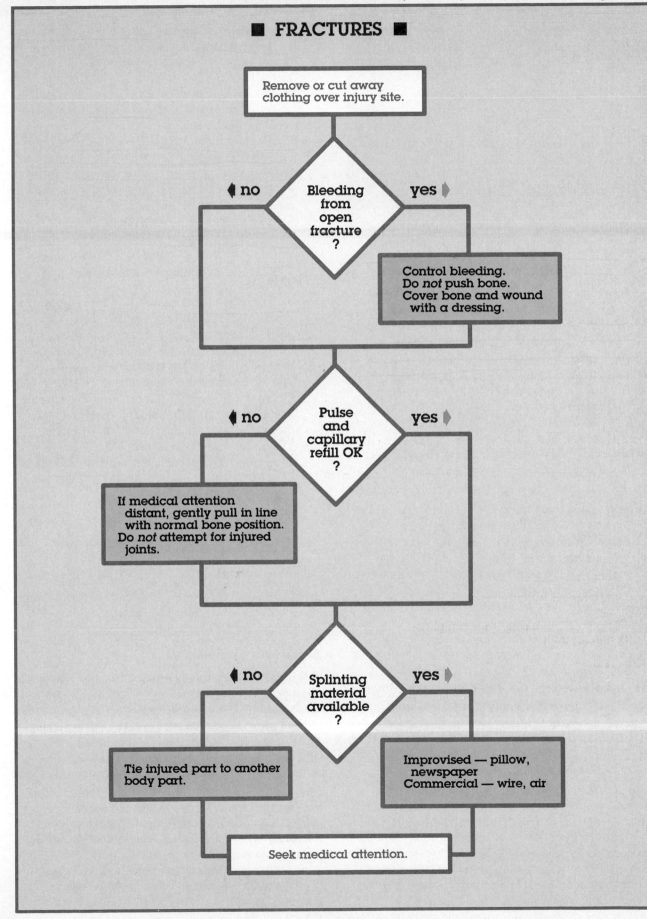

Remove or cut away clothing over injury site.

Bleeding from open fracture ?

no

yes

Control bleeding.
Do *not* push bone.
Cover bone and wound with a dressing.

Pulse and capillary refill OK ?

no

yes

If medical attention distant, gently pull in line with normal bone position. Do *not* attempt for injured joints.

Splinting material available ?

no

yes

Tie injured part to another body part.

Improvised — pillow, newspaper
Commercial — wire, air

Seek medical attention.

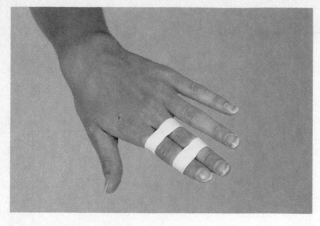

Using victim's body as a splint

Signs and Symptoms

- Head injuries serve as a clue since the head may have been snapped suddenly in one or more directions, endangering the spine. About 15 to 20 percent of head injured victims also have neck and spinal cord injuries.
- Painful movement of arms and/or legs
- Numbness, tingling, weakness, or burning sensation in arms or legs
- Loss of bowel or bladder control
- Paralysis to arms and/or legs
- Deformity; odd-looking angle of the victim's head and neck

Ask the conscious victim the following questions:

- **Is there pain?** Neck injuries (cervical) radiate pain to the arms; upper back injuries (thoracic) radiate pain around the ribs and into the chest; lower back injuries (lumbar) usually radiate pain down the legs. Often the victim describes the pain as "electric."
- **Can you move your feet?** Ask the victim to move his or her foot against your hand. If the victim cannot perform this movement or if the movement is extremely weak against your hand, the victim may have injured the spinal cord.
- **Can you move your fingers?** Moving the fingers is a sign that nerve pathways are intact. Ask the victim to grip your hand. A strong grip indicates that a spinal cord injury is unlikely.

For an unconscious victim:

- Look for cuts, bruises, and deformities.
- Test responses by pinching the victim's hands (either palm or back) and foot (sole or top of the bare foot). No reaction could mean spinal cord damage.
- Ask others about what happened. If not sure about a possible spinal injury, assume that the victim has one until proven otherwise.

First Aid

- Check and monitor the airway, breathing, and circulation, and treat accordingly. Do *not* use the head tilt because it would move the neck. Instead, jut the jaw forward by placing the fingers on the corners of the jaw and pushing forward (known as the "jaw thrust"). Keep the head and neck still.
- First aiders should normally wait for the Emergency Medical Service (EMS) to transport the victim because of their training and equipment. Victims with suspected spine injuries will require cervical collars and immobilization on a spine board. It is better to do nothing than to mishandle these victims. Splinting requires at least two trained people. Do *not* attempt to splint a victim by yourself.
- Stabilize the victim against any movement. Do *not* move the neck to reposition it except when danger is present (e.g., smoking or burning car or burning building). Bring help to the victim, *not* the victim to the help.
- The victim must be immobilized. Tell the victim not to move, if he or she is conscious. Place objects on either side of the head to prevent it from rolling from side to side.
- Victims in water with potential neck or back injury must be floated gently to shore. Before removal from the water, the victim must be secured to a backboard.

Ankle Injuries

The ankle frequently gets injured and it should *not* be handled casually. Careless treatment can have consequences that include a lifelong disability. In some cases, the damage requires surgical correction.

Signs and Symptoms

It is difficult to tell the difference between a severely sprained and a fractured ankle. Treat the injury as a fracture until you can get the advice of a physician. Identification cannot be made on the basis of appearance or the amount of pain.

The following suggestions may help you determine whether the injury is a sprained or a fractured ankle:

1. Ask the victim, "Did you try it?" Putting some weight on the ankle may hurt a little, but if the victim is able to do that, most likely the ankle is sprained. If it is broken, the victim will not even want to try putting any weight on it. If the victim can tolerate pain more than most and he or she feels something grinding or gravelly, suspect a fracture.

■ SPRAINS, STRAINS, CONTUSIONS, DISLOCATIONS ■

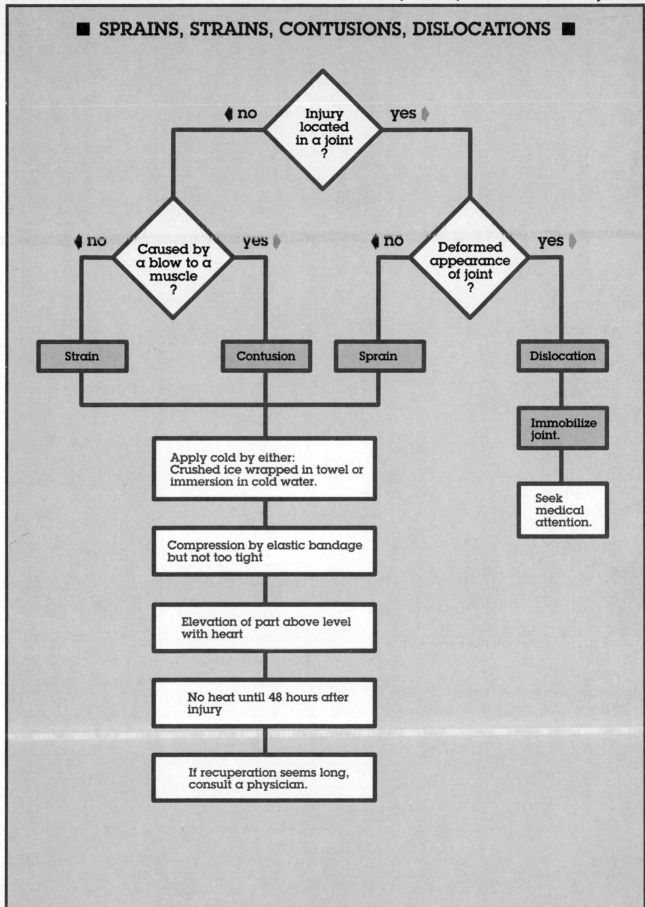

■ SPINAL INJURIES ■

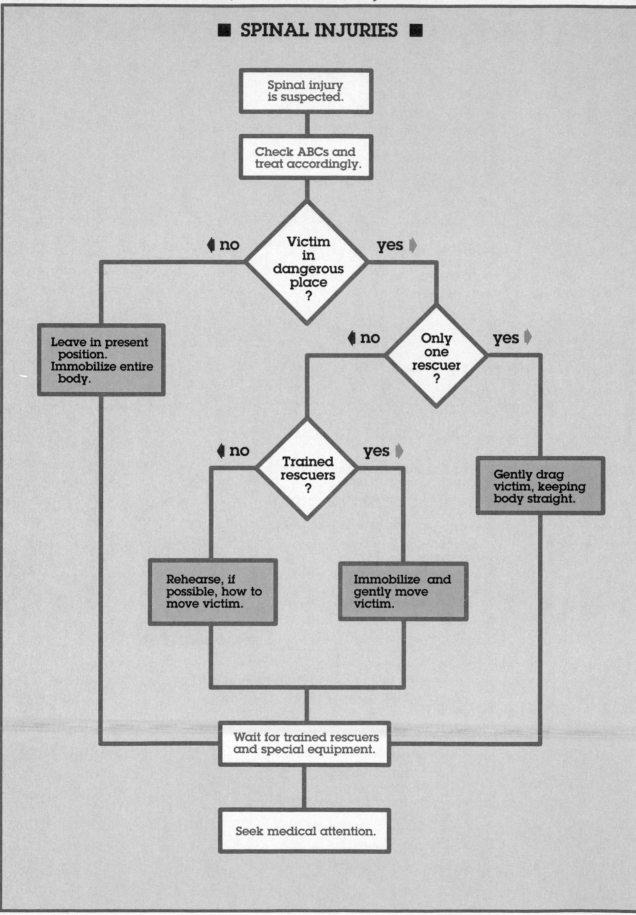

Spinal injury is suspected.

Check ABCs and treat accordingly.

Victim in dangerous place?

no → Leave in present position. Immobilize entire body.

yes → Only one rescuer?

yes → Gently drag victim, keeping body straight.

no → Trained rescuers?

no → Rehearse, if possible, how to move victim.

yes → Immobilize and gently move victim.

Wait for trained rescuers and special equipment.

Seek medical attention.

CONSCIOUS VICTIM—UPPER EXTREMITY CHECKS

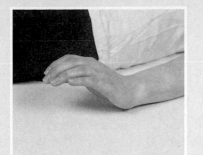 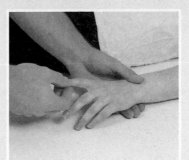 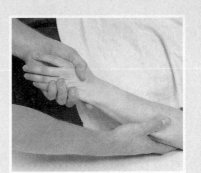

1. Victim wiggles fingers.

2. Rescuer touches fingers.

3. Victim squeezes rescuer's hand.

CONSCIOUS VICTIM—LOWER EXTREMITY CHECKS

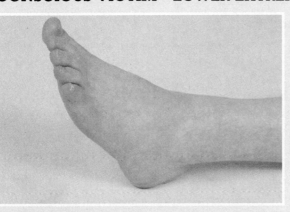

1.

1. Victim wiggles toes.

2. Rescuer touches toes.

3. Victim pushes foot against rescuer's hand.

Victim's failure to perform may mean spinal cord injury!

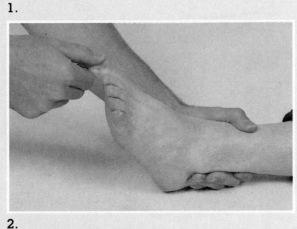

2.

UNCONSCIOUS VICTIM

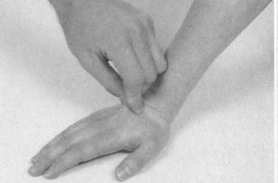

1. Pinch hand.

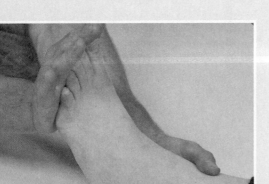

3.

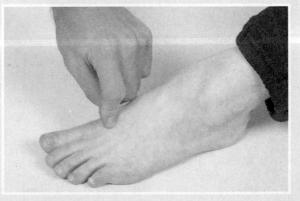

2. Pinch foot.

■ ANKLE INJURIES ■

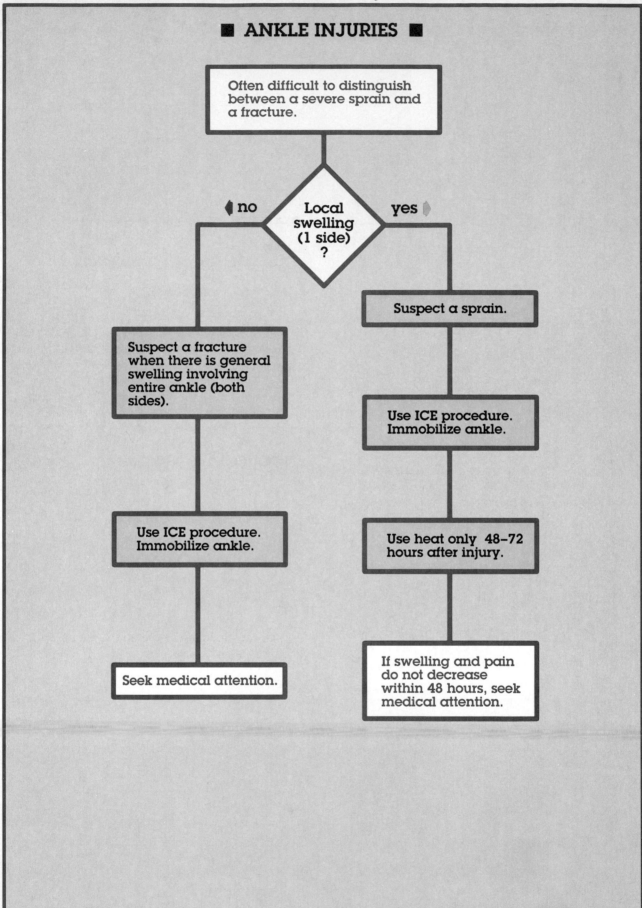

Often difficult to distinguish between a severe sprain and a fracture.

Local swelling (1 side) ?

← no   yes →

no:

Suspect a fracture when there is general swelling involving entire ankle (both sides).

Use ICE procedure. Immobilize ankle.

Seek medical attention.

yes:

Suspect a sprain.

Use ICE procedure. Immobilize ankle.

Use heat only 48–72 hours after injury.

If swelling and pain do not decrease within 48 hours, seek medical attention.

2. If the victim hops on his or her good foot to get off a playing field, court, or some other place, and the injured ankle can not tolerate the jarring, suspect a fracture and obtain medical attention.

3. Some experts say that a feeling of nausea right after an ankle injury indicates a fracture rather than a sprain.

4. It has been observed that ankle sprains tend to swell only on one side of the foot while swelling on both sides of the foot accompanies fractures.

The above tests are not 100% accurate but do serve as useful guidelines.

First Aid

Remember the mnemonic **ICE: I**ce, **C**ompression, **E**levation as a guide to sprained ankle injuries.

- **I** stands for the application of cold, which causes constriction of the blood vessels. This decreases the amount of bleeding, swelling, and pain.

  Cold is available from ice, commercially prepared ice packs, frozen food cans, drinking fountains, etc. The earlier that cold is applied, the better. Try using crushed ice rather than ice cubes since crushed ice contours to the shape of the ankle better.

  Do *not* place ice directly on the skin except in periodic ice massages because it can cause frostbite. Place a towel or washcloth between the ice pack and skin.

  Applying cold for short periods of time does not cool deeper tissues—it only lowers skin temperature. The cold application should be continued for at least 20-30 minutes. This should occur about three times during the first 24 hours after the injury. off the areapply

  A common mistake is the early use of heat. Heat causes swelling and pain if applied too early. A minimum of 24 hours and preferably 48–72 hours should pass before applying any heat.

- **C** represents compression. Swelling is like glue and can lock up a joint within hours. It is important to prevent swelling by using cold promptly, and also make the swelling recede as quickly as possible with a compression (elastic) bandage.

  Some experts believe elastic bandages are often applied too tightly. Do *not* apply the bandage too firmly. Toes should be checked periodically for skin discoloration and coldness, indicating that the bandage has been applied too tightly. Comparing the toes of the injured foot with those of the uninjured foot is also suggested. Pain, tingling, loss of sensation, and loss of pulses also indicate impaired circulation. Loosen the elastic bandage if any of these signs or symptoms appear.

  To counteract swelling, take any soft, pliable material (e.g., sock, T-shirt) and either fold or cut it into the shape of a horseshoe. Place this "horseshoe" around the ankle bone knob on the injured side with the curved part down. Then place a figure-of-eight wrap around the ankle covering the "horseshoe" and foot with an elastic bandage. This technique applies compression to the soft tissue areas, not just the ankle bone and tendon.

- **E** stands for elevation. To further reduce swelling and bleeding, tell the victim to elevate the ankle for the first 24 to 48 hours. Some medical experts say, "Keep the foot higher than the knee and the knee higher than the heart." Avoid any weight on the ankle. Some victims should consider crutches.

  Swelling and pain should begin to subside within 48 hours, and the ankle should be nearly normal within 10 days. If the injury is not healing, consult with a physician.

  If a fracture is suspected, immobilize the ankle with a pillow splint and seek medical attention. Controversy exists regarding whether or not to take off a shoe. Those favoring leaving the shoe on believe it acts as a splint and helps in retarding swelling. Others believe taking off the shoe allows a better examination, including checking the foot's pulse and temperature. Moreover, if a shoe or boot is left on, the swelling may reduce circulation in the foot.

Muscle Injuries

Though muscle injuries pose no real emergency, first aiders have ample opportunities to care for them.

Muscle Strains

A muscle strain, also known as muscle pull, occurs when the muscle is stretched beyond its normal range of motion, resulting in a muscle fiber tear.

Signs and Symptoms

- A sharp pain immediately after the injury
- Extreme tenderness when area is felt
- Disfigurement (indentation, cavity, or bump)
- Severe weakness and loss of function of the injured part
- The sound of a snap when the tissue is torn

■ MUSCLE INJURIES ■

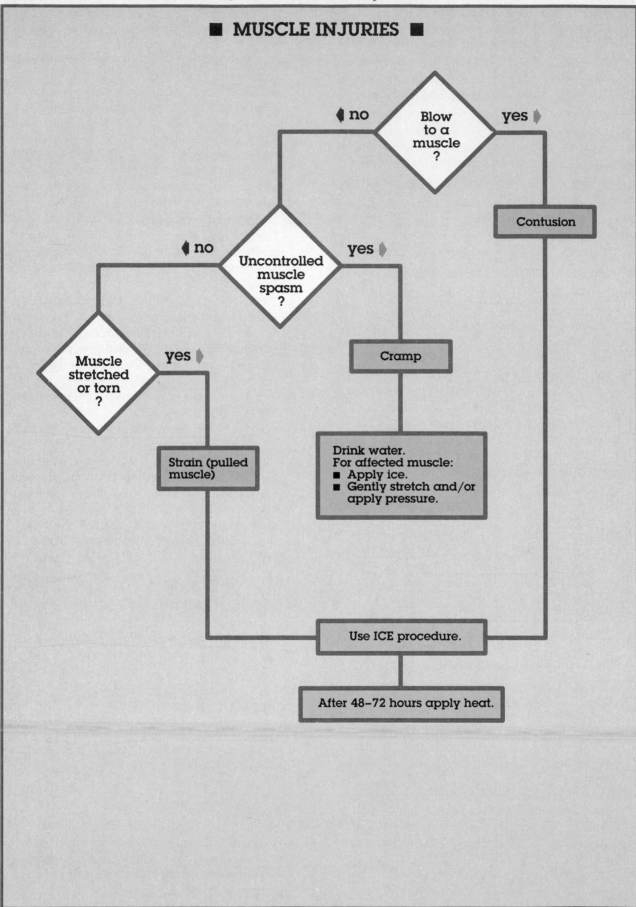

Muscle Contusions

Muscle contusions result from a blow to a muscle. This injury is also known as a bruise.

First Aid for Muscle Strains and Contusions

Even though the ice, compression, and elevation (ICE) procedure is universally used as the first aid for muscle strains and contusions, many first aiders and even hospital emergency department personnel mistakenly treat new muscle injuries with heat packs.

- **_Ice._** Methods of applying cold include using crushed ice as an ice pack or immersion in cold water. The application should continue for 20 to 30 minutes, three to four times during the first day, and if possible, the second day.

  Place towels or elastic bandage between the ice or cold packs and the body to insulate against the full effects of the cold. Frostbite will not occur if cold packs are applied for limited time periods. Constant use of a cold pack is not necessary because of the lasting effect of cold to body tissue.

The use of cold to an injured area reduces the pain, bleeding, and swelling that follow a muscle strain or contusion.

- **_Compression._** A compression (elastic) bandage applied to the injured area serves to limit internal bleeding. Often, the elastic bandage is applied directly to the site, the ice pack is placed over the first layer of elastic bandage wrap, and more compression elastic wrap is put over the ice. The cold with the compression limits internal bleeding common in muscle injuries. The victim should wear the elastic bandage continuously for 18 to 24 hours.

  Elastic bandages may be applied too tightly, thus inhibiting blood circulation. Leave fingers and toes exposed for observing any color and temperature change. Pain, numbness, and tingling also indicate that an elastic bandage is too tight.

- **_Elevation._** Elevating the injured area limits circulation to that area and helps control internal bleeding. The aim of this procedure is to get the injured part up above or even with the heart's level.

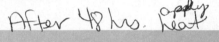

Cryotherapy

Ice is one of the most versatile panaceas available for injuries. The use of ice or other equally cold applications to treat muscle strains, bruises, joint sprains, insect stings, and minor burns is called **cryotherapy**.

Cryotherapy is effective because cold applications reduce tissue temperature. This constricts blood vessels, helps control bleeding, and reduces pain.

Forms of Ice Therapy

- **_Ice massage._** Rubbing ice cubes in a circular motion on the affected area for 7 to 10 minutes on regions with little fat (e.g., elbow, knee, ankle) and about 20 minutes in areas with more fat (e.g., leg muscles) is recommended.

- **_Ice bags._** Apply a bag full of crushed ice or covered ice cubes to the affected area for 10 to 30 minutes. This method penetrates and lasts longer than the ice massage.

- **_Cold water immersion._** An ice slush (ice cubes or crushed ice added to a bucket of water) is useful for injuries to the hand, foot, or elbow. Allow the injured part to soak in the ice slush for 10 to 20 minutes.

- **_Cold packs._** Sealed plastic pouches containing a refreezable gel are available commercially. These can get very cold, so it is important that the cold packs be wrapped in a towel and that they never be applied directly to the skin.

- **_Chemical "snap packs."_** These sealed pouches resemble cold packs but contain two chemical envelopes that, when squeezed, mix the chemicals. A chemical reaction produces a cooling effect. Though they don't cool as well as other methods, snap packs are convenient.

  Precautions include *not* exposing the skin to cold too long which can result in frostbite. Those with any form of cold allergy, Raynaud's phenomenon, or abnormal sensitivity to cold should avoid cryotherapy.

  Other tips when using ice or other forms of cryotherapy include the following:

- Apply ice or cold immediately after an injury.

- Raise the injured area above heart level.

- Apply ice or cold for no more than 30 minutes at a time. Repeat two to four times a day until fully recovered.

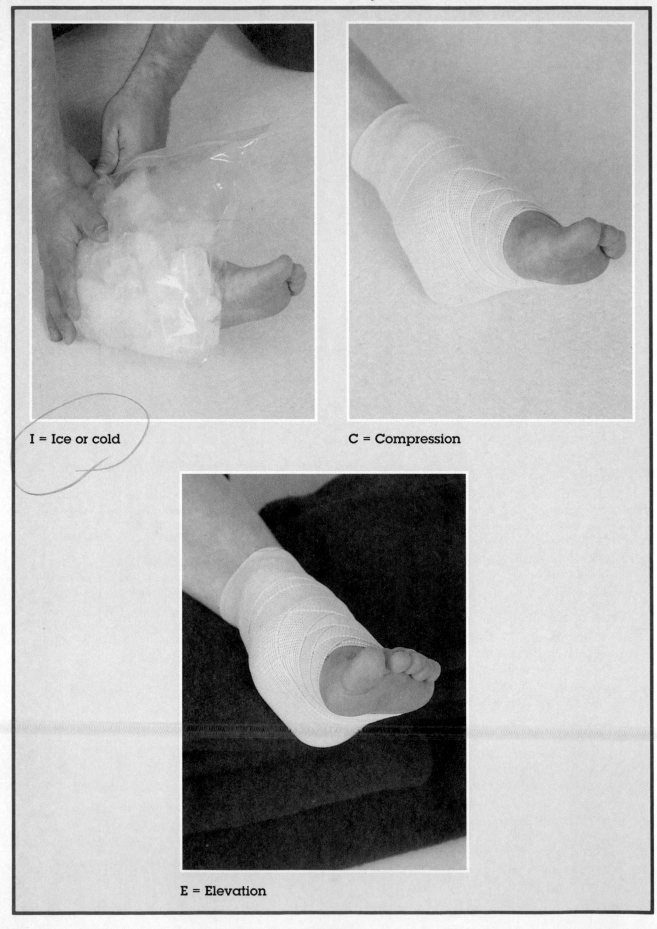

I = Ice or cold

C = Compression

E = Elevation

Muscle Cramps

Muscles can go into an uncontrolled spasm and contraction, resulting in severe pain and a restriction or loss of movement. Some experts believe that diet or fluid loss explains muscle cramping. Nevertheless, many different things can cause muscle cramps; no one knows all the causes.

First Aid

- Attempt to relieve a cramp by gently stretching the affected muscle. Since a muscle cramp is really an uncontrolled spasm or contraction of a muscle, a gradual lengthening of the muscle may help to lengthen those muscle fibers and relieve the cramp.

- Apply ice to the cramped muscle because it causes the muscles to relax. The exception might be during cold weather.
- Relax the affected muscle by applying pressure to it (do *not* massage). ~may have a blood clot there.
- Pinching the upper lip hard (an accupressure technique) has been advocated for reducing calf muscle leg cramping.
- Drinking water is important because fluid deficiency appears to be a main cause. Sport drinks (electrolyte drinks) can work if they do not contain a lot of sugar. Too much sugar slows fluid absorption.
- Do *not* give salt tablets. They can draw fluid out of the circulatory system and into the stomach. They can also irritate the stomach lining.

11
Medical Emergencies

■ Heart Attack ■ Stroke ■ Diabetic Emergencies ■
■ Epilepsy ■ Asthma ■

All because of the blockage area causing the heart not to pump blood properly

Heart Attack*

A heart attack occurs when the blood supply to a part of the heart muscle is severely reduced or stopped because of an obstruction in one of the coronary arteries (these supply the heart with its blood). A buildup of fatty deposits along the coronary artery's inner wall is one reason for blood obstruction. The blood supply can also be reduced when the artery goes into a spasm.

Signs and Symptoms

Heart attacks are difficult to determine. Because medical care at the onset of a heart attack is vital to survival and the quality of recovery, the rule to follow is that if you suspect a heart attack for any reason, seek medical attention at once rather than delaying.

The American Heart Association lists these as possible signs and symptoms of a heart attack:

- Uncomfortable pressure, fullness, squeezing or *or heaviness* pain in the center of the chest lasting two minutes or longer. It may come and go.
- Pain may spread to either shoulder, the neck, the lower jaw, or either arm.
- Any or all of the following: weakness, dizziness, sweating, nausea, or shortness of breath.

Not all of these warning signs occur in every heart attack. Many victims will deny that they might be having a heart attack. If you see some of these signs, however, don't wait to seek medical attention. Time loss can seriously increase the risk of major damage. Get help immediately!

Source: American Heart Association.

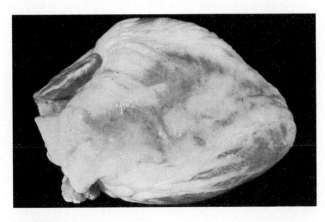

Healthy heart

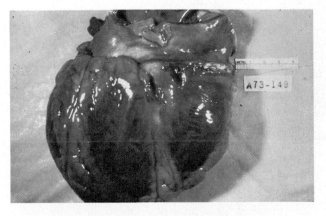

Heart with artery clot after heart attack

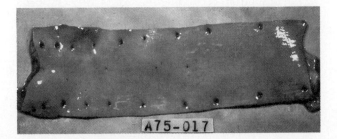

Normal artery (aorta)

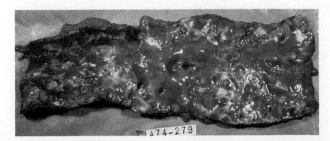

Inside of atherosclerotic artery (aorta)

First Aid

The American Heart Association identifies these proper actions in case of a heart attack:

- Find out which hospitals have 24-hour emergency cardiac care.
- If chest discomfort lasts two minutes or more, call the emergency medical services.
- If you can get to a hospital faster by going yourself and not waiting for an ambulance, drive the victim there.
- If you are with someone experiencing the signs and symptoms of a heart attack—and the warning signs last two minutes or longer—act immediately.
- Expect a denial. It is normal for someone with chest discomfort to deny the possibility of something as serious as a heart attack. But don't take no for an answer. Insist on taking prompt action.
- Call the emergency medical service or get to the nearest hospital emergency room offering 24-hour emergency cardiac care.
- If necessary and if you are properly trained, give CPR.

Knowing these things, you should also:

- Help the victim to the least painful position—usually sitting with legs up and bent at the knees. Loosen clothing around the neck and midriff. Be calm and reassuring.
- Determine if the victim is *known* to have coronary heart disease and is using nitroglycerin. If so, use it. Nitroglycerin in tablets or spray under the tongue or in ointment placed on the skin may relieve chest pain. Nitroglycerin dilates the coronary arteries, which increases blood flow to the heart muscle; and it lowers the blood pressure and dilates the veins, which decreases the work of the heart and the heart muscle's need for oxygen.

  Caution: Since nitroglycerin lowers blood pressure, the victim should be sitting or lying when taking it. Nitroglycerin may normally be repeated for a total of 3 tablets in 10 minutes if the first dose does not relieve the pain. However, a first aider may not know whether the victim has already taken some nitroglycerin. Also, nitroglycerin is prescribed in different strengths so that while 3 tablets of one strength may be a mild dose, 3 tablets of another strength may be a high dose. First aiders should be very cautious when administering nitroglycerin.
- If victim is unconscious, check the ABCs and start CPR if needed.

Handwritten left margin: Dialates the bl. vessels. wks. fast. Relief within 5 min. if its working. repeated every 10 min. Don't exceed 3 times.

Risk Factors of Heart Disease

According to the American Heart Association, several factors contribute to an increased risk of heart attack and stroke. The more risk factors present, the greater the chance a person will develop heart disease.

Risk factors that you cannot change

- Heredity: Tendencies appear in family lines.
- Male sex: Men have a greater risk, yet heart attack is still the leading cause of death among women.
- Age: Most heart attack victims are age 65 or older.

Risk factors that you can change

- Cigarette smoking: Smokers have more than twice as much risk of heart attack as nonsmokers.
- High blood pressure: This adds to the heart's workload. *Controlled diet & medication*
- High blood cholesterol: Too much cholesterol in the blood can cause a buildup on the walls of the arteries. *control cholesterol. Body will produce chole. on its own.*

Other risk factors, which also can be changed

- Diabetes: This condition affects blood's cholesterol and triglyceride levels.
- Obesity: Being overweight influences blood pressure and blood cholesterol, can result in diabetes, and can put an added strain on the heart.
- Physical inactivity: Inactive people have twice as much risk of heart attack as active people.
- Stress: All people feel stress, but react in different ways. Excessive, long-term stress may create problems in some people.

Handwritten: my. Cardio infarction

Stroke*

A stroke is also known as a **cerebrovascular accident (CVA).** A stroke occurs when a blood vessel that is bringing oxygen and nutrients to the brain bursts or becomes clogged by a blood clot, preventing part of the brain from receiving the flow of blood it needs. Stroke is the third largest cause of death in America. It is also a major cause of disability.

Signs and Symptoms

Signs and symptoms of a stroke depend on the area of the brain involved:

- Sudden weakness or numbness of the face, arm and leg on one side of the body

Source: American Heart Association.

Handwritten bottom: If several bl. vessels are involved will cause unconsciousness.

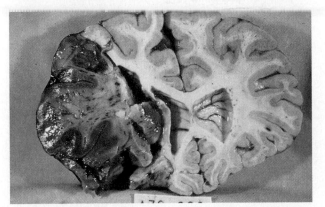

Stroke resulting from a severe hemorrhage

[handwritten: Where it happens will depend]
[handwritten: On what goes out in the brain.]

- Loss of speech, or trouble talking or understanding speech
- Dimness or loss of vision, particularly in only one eye; unequal pupils
- Unexplained dizziness, unsteadiness or sudden falls
- Sudden severe headache
- Loss of bladder and/or bowel control

About 10 percent of strokes are preceded by "little strokes" (**transient ischemic attacks,** or TIAs). *[handwritten: Comes + goes. They get better]* TIAs are extremely important warning signs for stroke. TIA symptoms are very similar to those of a full-fledged stroke. Do *not* ignore TIAs; get medical attention immediately. *[handwritten: If the Diastole in the resting stages isn't low (BP) they may have a CVA.]*

First Aid

- Check and monitor the victim's breathing and pulse. Provide rescue breathing and/or cardiopulmonary resuscitation (CPR) if needed.
- If the victim is semiconscious or unconscious, place him or her on one side, preferably with the paralyzed side down. This position frees the victim's useful extremities. Cushion the paralyzed side. Positioning on the side permits secretions and vomit to drain into the cheek or out the mouth rather than the throat. *[handwritten: elevate head]*
- Keep the victim in a semiprone position, preferably with the upper body and head

slightly elevated to allow for less blood pressure on the brain.
- Remove dentures and any mucus and food from the mouth in a swabbing motion with a piece of cloth wrapped around a finger.
- Do *not* give any liquids—the throat may be paralyzed, which restricts swallowing.
- If an eye has been affected, consider protecting the eye by closing the lid and taping the eyelid down to prevent drying, which can result in vision loss.
- Provide calm reassurance to the victim. *[handwritten: In a medical facility]*

Diabetic Emergencies*

Diabetes is the inability of the body to appropriately metabolize carbohydrates. The pancreas fails to produce enough of a hormone called insulin. The function of insulin is to take sugar from the blood and carry it into the cells to be used. When excess sugar remains in the blood, the body cells must rely on fat as fuel. Since blood sugar is a major body fuel, when it cannot be used, diabetes develops.

When the blood sugar level becomes too high because of too little insulin in the blood, **diabetic coma,** or **ketoacidosis,** may occur. Meanwhile, the cells, deprived of sugar, begin to use fats for fuel. Use of fat results in the production of acids and ketones as wastes. The ketones give the victims' breath a fruity odor.

The opposite condition, **insulin shock,** can result when a person with diabetes has taken too much insulin or has not eaten. The blood sugar level drops dangerously low, and the victim becomes weak and disoriented, or unconscious.

Both of these conditions can be fatal unless something is done to reverse them. **See page 192 for a description of symptoms and first aid for diabetic emergencies.**

Epilepsy**

Types of Seizures

[handwritten: A seizure is an interruption of the nerves sheaths.]

Epileptic seizures may be convulsive or nonconvulsive in nature, depending on where in the brain the malfunction takes place and on how much of the total brain area is involved.

Convulsive seizures are the ones that most people generally think of when they hear the word "epilepsy." In this type of seizure the person undergoes convulsions that usually last from two to five minutes, with complete loss of consciousness and muscle spasm.

Source: American Diabetes Association; reprinted with permission.
**Source: Epilepsy Foundation of America; reprinted with permission.*

[handwritten right margin: Glucose needs insulin to get into the cells. Ketone bodies - are an acid that is left over from fats not used @ 250mg glucose.]

[handwritten bottom: Chronic condition for life]

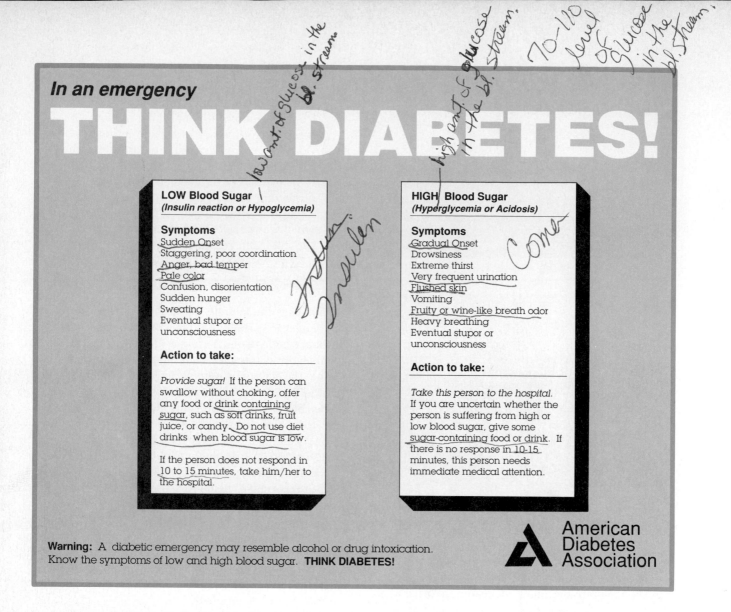

In an emergency

THINK DIABETES!

[handwritten: low amt of glucose in the bl. stream]
[handwritten: high amt of glucose in the bl. stream]
[handwritten: 70-120 level of glucose in the bl. stream]

LOW Blood Sugar
(Insulin reaction or Hypoglycemia)

Symptoms
Sudden Onset
Staggering, poor coordination
Anger, bad temper
Pale color
Confusion, disorientation
Sudden hunger
Sweating
Eventual stupor or
unconsciousness

[handwritten: too little Insulin]

Action to take:

Provide sugar! If the person can
swallow without choking, offer
any food or drink containing
sugar, such as soft drinks, fruit
juice, or candy. Do not use diet
drinks when blood sugar is low.

If the person does not respond in
10 to 15 minutes, take him/her to
the hospital.

HIGH Blood Sugar
(Hyperglycemia or Acidosis)

Symptoms
Gradual Onset
Drowsiness
Extreme thirst
Very frequent urination
Flushed skin
Vomiting
Fruity or wine-like breath odor
Heavy breathing
Eventual stupor or
unconsciousness

[handwritten: Coma]

Action to take:

Take this person to the hospital.
If you are uncertain whether the
person is suffering from high or
low blood sugar, give some
sugar-containing food or drink. If
there is no response in 10-15
minutes, this person needs
immediate medical attention.

Warning: A diabetic emergency may resemble alcohol or drug intoxication.
Know the symptoms of low and high blood sugar. **THINK DIABETES!**

American
Diabetes
Association

Nonconvulsive seizures may take the form of a blank stare lasting only a few seconds, an involuntary movement of an arm or leg, or a period of automatic movement in which awareness of one's surroundings is blurred or completely absent.

Since these seizure types are so different, they require different kinds of action from a first aider, and some require no action at all. Table 11.2 describes seizures in detail and how to handle each type.

First Aid

An uncomplicated convulsive seizure due to epilepsy is not a medical emergency, even though it looks like one. After a few minutes it stops naturally, without ill effects. The average victim is able to resume normal activity after a rest period and may need little or no assistance in getting home.

However, several medical conditions other than epilepsy can cause seizures. These require immediate medical attention and include:

encephalitis   pregnancy

meningitis   hypoglycemia
heat stroke   high fever
poisoning   head injury

The following guidelines are designed to help people with epilepsy avoid unnecessary and expensive trips to the emergency room and to help you decide whether or not to call an ambulance when someone has a convulsive seizure. Do *not* call an ambulance if:

1. Medical identity jewelry or card identifies the person as epileptic, *and*

2. The seizure ends in less than *ten minutes, and*

3. Consciousness returns without further incident, *and*

4. There are no signs of injury, physical distress, or pregnancy.

Call an ambulance if:

1. The seizure has happened in water.

2. There is no medical identity jewelry or card and no way of knowing whether the seizure is caused by epilepsy, *and*

TABLE 11-2 Seizure: Recognition and First Aid

Seizure Type	What It Looks Like	What it is Not	What To Do	What Not To Do
Generalized Tonic-Clonic (Also called grand mal)	Sudden cry, fall, rigidity, followed by muscle jerks, shallow breathing or temporarily suspended breathing, bluish skin, possible loss of bladder or bowel control, usually lasts a couple of minutes. Normal breathing then starts again. There may be some confusion and/or fatigue, followed by return to full consciousness.	Heart attack *[handwritten: From tightening & relax of the muscles.]* Stroke	Look for medical identification. Protect from nearby hazards. Loosen tie or shirt collars. Protect head from injury. Turn on side to keep airway clear. Reassure when consciousness returns. If single seizure lasted less than 5 minutes, ask if hospital evaluation wanted. If multiple seizures, or if one seizure lasts longer than 5 minutes, call an ambulance. If person is pregnant, injured or diabetic, call for aid at once.	Don't put any hard implement in the mouth. Don't try to hold tongue. It can't be swallowed. Don't try to give liquids during or just after seizure. Don't use artificial respiration unless breathing is absent after muscle jerks subside, or unless water has been inhaled. Don't restrain.
Absence (Also called petit mal)	A blank stare, lasting only a few seconds, most common in children. May be accompanied by rapid blinking, some chewing movements of the mouth. Child is unaware of what's going on during the seizure, but quickly returns to full awareness once it has stopped. May result in learning difficulties if not recognized and treated.	Daydreaming / Lack of attention / Deliberate ignoring of adult instructions	No first aid necessary, but if this is the first observation of the seizure(s), medical evaluation should be recommended.	*[handwritten: Status epilepticus if it lasts more than 10 min.]*
Simple Partial	Jerking may begin in one area of the body, arm, leg, or face. Can't be stopped, but patient stays awake and aware. Jerking may proceed from one area of the body to another, and sometimes spreads to become a convulsive seizure. Partial sensory seizures may not be obvious to an onlooker. Patient experiences a distorted environment. May see or hear things that aren't there, may feel unexplained fear, sadness, anger, or joy. May have nausea, experience odd smells, and have a generally "funny" feeling in the stomach.	Acting out, bizarre behavior / Hysteria / Mental Illness / Psychosomatic illness / Parapsychological or mystical experience	No first aid necessary unless seizure becomes convulsive, then first aid as above. No action needed other than reassurance and emotional support. Medical evaluation should be recommended.	
Complex Partial (Also called psychomotor or temporal lobe)	Usually starts with blank stare, followed by chewing, followed by random activity. Person appears unaware of surroundings, may seem dazed and mumble. Unresponsive. Actions clumsy, not directed. May pick at clothing, pick up objects, try to take clothes off. May run, appear to be afraid. May struggle or flail at restraint. Once pattern established, same set of actions usually occur with each seizure. Lasts a few	Drunkenness / Intoxication on drugs / Mental Illness / Disorderly conduct	Speak calmly and reassuringly to patient and others. Guide gently away from obvious hazards. Stay with person until completely aware of environment. Offer to help getting home.	Don't grab hold unless sudden danger (such as a cliff edge or an approaching car) threatens. Don't try to restrain. Don't shout. Don't expect verbal instructions to be obeyed.

193

TABLE 11-2 Seizure: Recognition and First Aid (continued)

Seizure Type	What It Looks Like	What it is Not	What To Do	What Not To Do
Complex Partial Cont.	minutes, but post-seizure confusion can last substantially longer. No memory of what happened during seizure period.			
Atonic Seizures (Also called drop attacks)	A child or adult suddenly collapses and falls. After 10 seconds to a minute he recovers, regains consciousness, and can stand and walk again.	Clumsiness Normal childhood "stage" In a child, lack of good walking skills In an adult, drunkenness, accute illness	No first aid needed (unless he hurt himself as he fell), but the child should be given a thorough medical evaluation.	
Myoclonic Seizures	Sudden brief, massive muscle jerks that may involve the whole body or parts of body. May cause person to spill what they were holding or fall off a chair.	Clumsiness Poor coordination	No first aid needed, but should be given a thorough medical evaluation.	
Infantile Spasms	These are clusters of quick, sudden movements that start between 3 months and two years. If a child is sitting up, the head will fall forward, and the arms will flex forward. If lying down, the knees will be drawn up, with arms and head flexed forward as if the baby is reaching for support.	Normal movements of the baby Colic	No first aid, but doctor should be consulted.	

Source: © Epilepsy Foundation of America; reprinted with permission.

3. The seizure continues for more than *five* minutes. Setting a five-minute limit on a seizure of unknown origin before calling for emergency assistance (as opposed to ten minutes if medical identification is worn) is a precaution based on the possibility that a serious condition other than epilepsy may be causing the convulsion.

If an ambulance arrives after the person has regained consciousness, you should ask the person whether the seizure was associated with epilepsy and whether emergency room care is wanted. The same questions should be asked of a person without medical identification whose seizure lasts less than five minutes and for whom an ambulance has not yet been called.

Asthma

Asthma results from a narrowing of the airway bronchial tubes, causing breathing difficulty, especially while exhaling. Wheezing is a whistling, high-pitched sound produced by air forced through a constricted airway. Not all wheezes involve asthma.

The sight of a person suffering an acute asthmatic attack is most distressing and, to first aiders inexperienced with this form of illness, very frightening. At some time in their lives, 5 to 10 percent of the population are believed to be affected by asthma. It is a common cause of emergency department visits. It kills 5,000 of its victims annually.

All asthmatics have hyperirritable airways, making the bronchial tree sensitive and overreactive to substances and conditions that do not normally bother other people.

Signs and Symptoms

- Breathing difficulty while exhaling
- Wheezing or whistling sound
- Tense, frightened, nervous behavior
- Bluish skin color in severe attacks due to lack of oxygen
- Preference for sitting up (since it is easier to breathe).

First Aid

In most cases, the first aider can do little other than recognize asthma and, if needed, obtain medical assistance. Provide the following for the victim:

- Comfort and reassure victim since emotional stress can make the condition worse.
- Many asthmatics carry tablets or <u>inhalers that relax bronchial spasms.</u> Help them in using these medicines.
- Help the victim into a comfortable breathing position that he or she chooses. <u>The best position is usually sitting upright.</u>
- Place the victim in a room that is as free as possible of common offenders (e.g., dust, feathers, animals). It should also be free of odors (e.g., tobacco smoke, paint).
- <u>Keep conversations with asthmatics brief since they are struggling to breathe.</u>

- <u>Increase the drinking of water if possible.</u>
- Seek medical attention, for:

  1. Severe, prolonged asthma attacks

  2. Reactions happening after an insect sting or contact with another source that produces an allergic reaction, which could progress to anaphylactic shock

  3. Failure to improve with medication

  4. Breathing that can barely be heard

  5. Increasing bluish skin color

  6. Pulse rate of more than 120 beats per minute

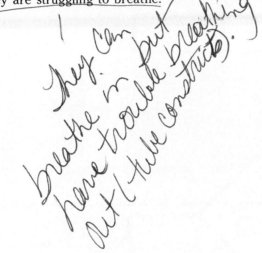

They can. but have trouble breathing in. breathe in. have trouble breathing out (tube constricts).

Hyperventilation—
too much breathing
from: stress

breathe again after 5 min.

S/S: Dizzy
light headed
tingling in head
start to faint
if continues goes to Resp. alcolosis

F.A.
1) Decrease resp. by calming down
2) 1 deep breathe + let it out slowly.

mimic Heart attack

195

■ HEART ATTACK ■

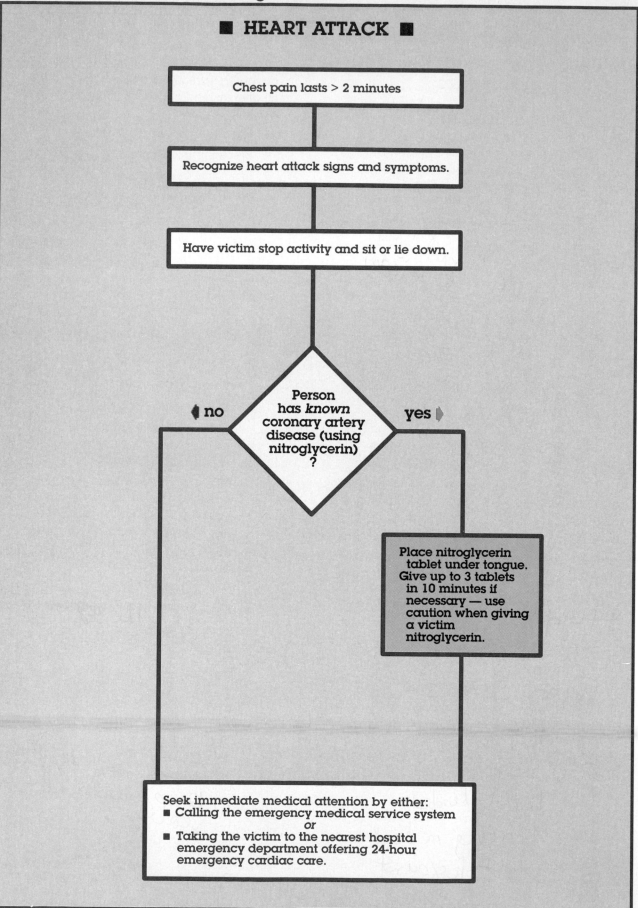

Chest pain lasts > 2 minutes

Recognize heart attack signs and symptoms.

Have victim stop activity and sit or lie down.

Person has *known* coronary artery disease (using nitroglycerin)?

◀ no   yes ▶

Place nitroglycerin tablet under tongue. Give up to 3 tablets in 10 minutes if necessary — use caution when giving a victim nitroglycerin.

Seek immediate medical attention by either:
■ Calling the emergency medical service system
  or
■ Taking the victim to the nearest hospital emergency department offering 24-hour emergency cardiac care.

■ STROKE ■

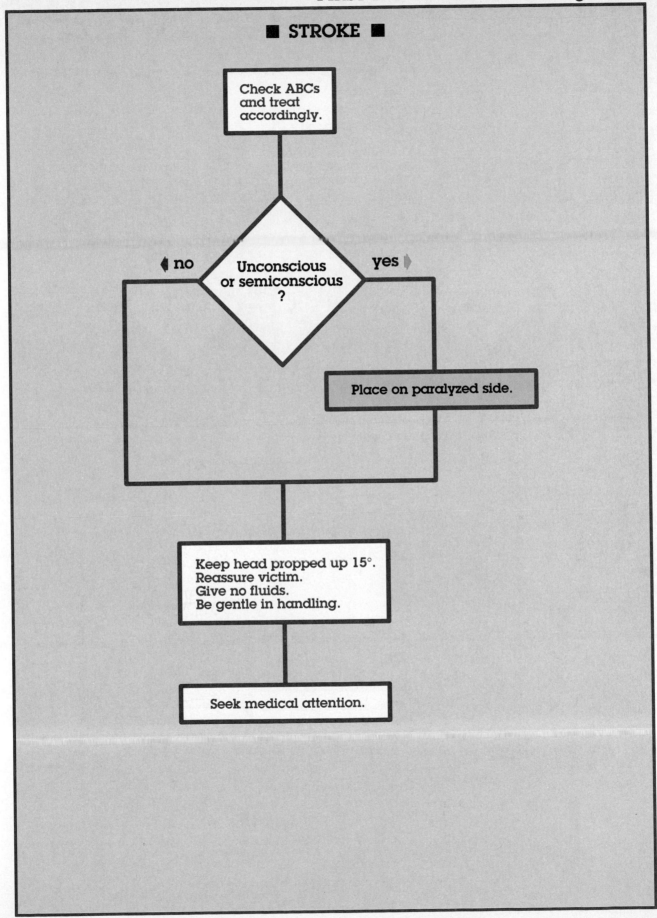

Check ABCs and treat accordingly.

Unconscious or semiconscious?

no

yes

Place on paralyzed side.

Keep head propped up 15°.
Reassure victim.
Give no fluids.
Be gentle in handling.

Seek medical attention.

■ DIABETIC EMERGENCIES ■

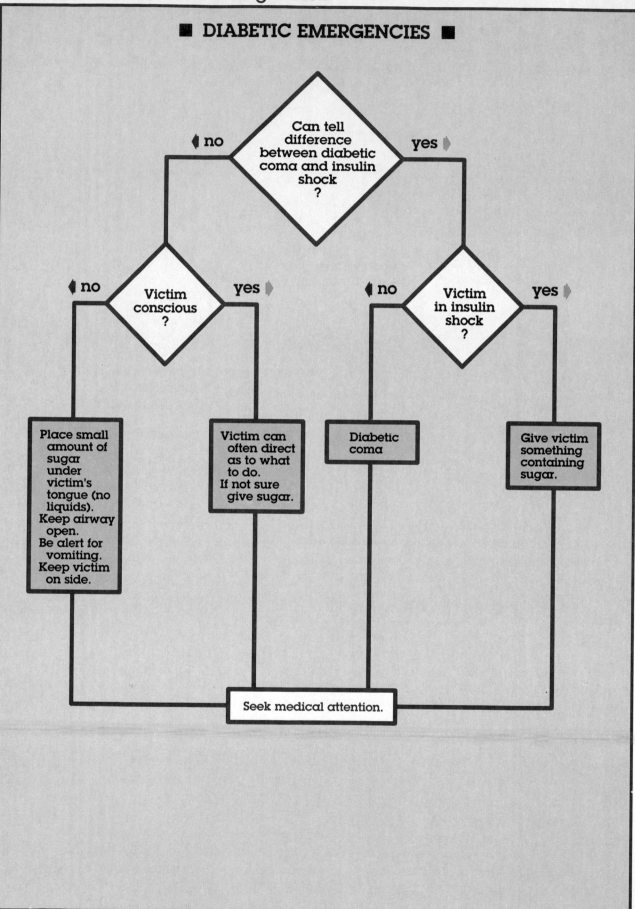

no ◀ **Can tell difference between diabetic coma and insulin shock ?** ▶ yes

no ◀ **Victim conscious ?** ▶ yes

no ◀ **Victim in insulin shock ?** ▶ yes

Place small amount of sugar under victim's tongue (no liquids). Keep airway open. Be alert for vomiting. Keep victim on side.

Victim can often direct as to what to do. If not sure give sugar.

Diabetic coma

Give victim something containing sugar.

Seek medical attention.

■ SEIZURES ■

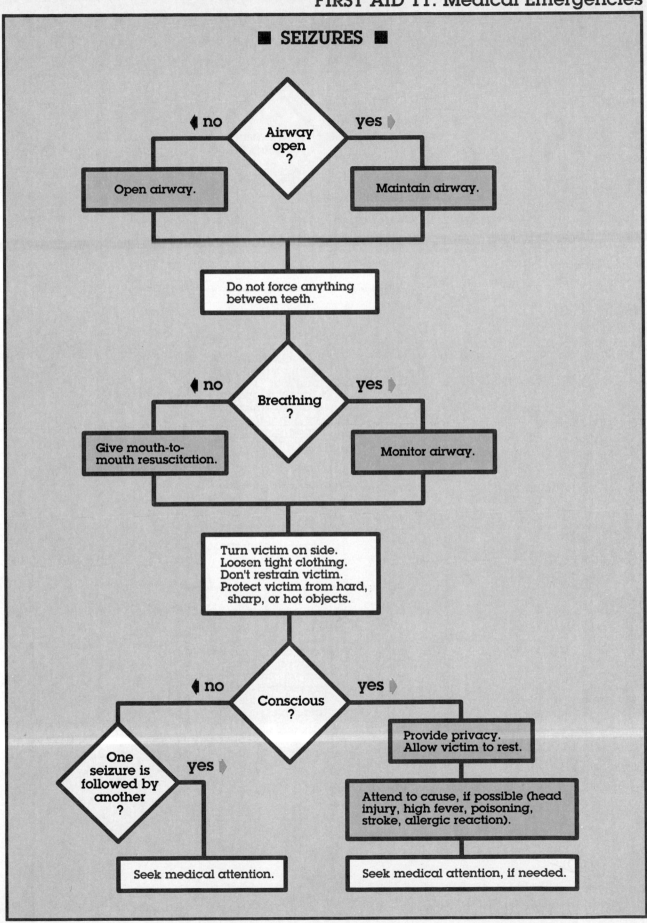

Airway open?
- no → Open airway.
- yes → Maintain airway.

Do not force anything between teeth.

Breathing?
- no → Give mouth-to-mouth resuscitation.
- yes → Monitor airway.

Turn victim on side.
Loosen tight clothing.
Don't restrain victim.
Protect victim from hard, sharp, or hot objects.

Conscious?
- no → One seizure is followed by another?
  - yes → Seek medical attention.
- yes → Provide privacy. Allow victim to rest.
  - Attend to cause, if possible (head injury, high fever, poisoning, stroke, allergic reaction).
  - Seek medical attention, if needed.

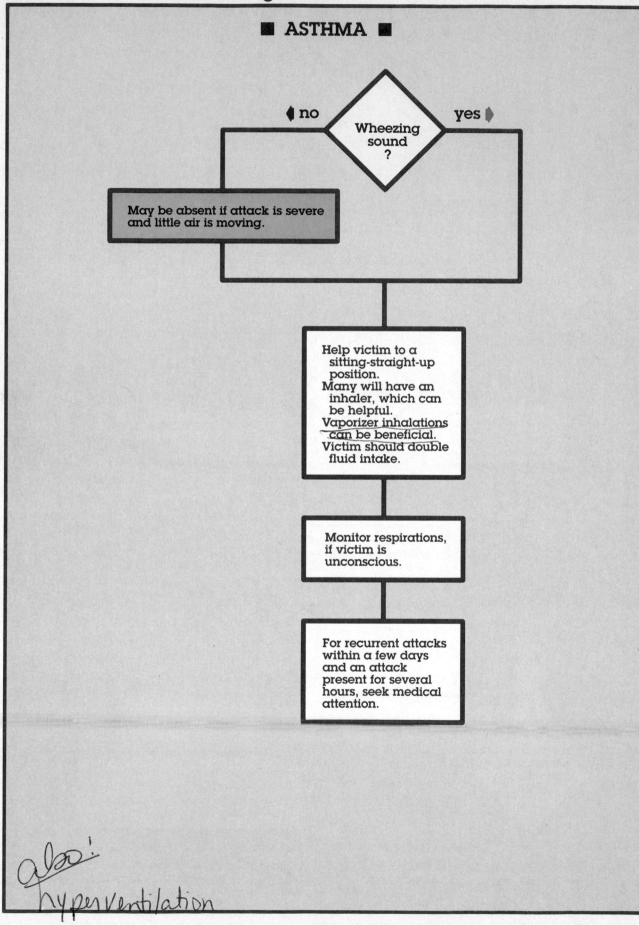

■ ASTHMA ■

Wheezing sound ?

← no   yes ►

May be absent if attack is severe and little air is moving.

Help victim to a sitting-straight-up position.
Many will have an inhaler, which can be helpful.
Vaporizer inhalations can be beneficial.
Victim should double fluid intake.

Monitor respirations, if victim is unconscious.

For recurrent attacks within a few days and an attack present for several hours, seek medical attention.

hyperventilation

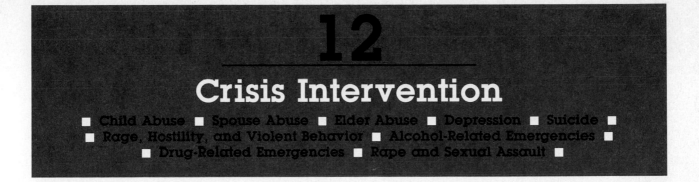

12

Crisis Intervention

■ Child Abuse ■ Spouse Abuse ■ Elder Abuse ■ Depression ■ Suicide ■
■ Rage, Hostility, and Violent Behavior ■ Alcohol-Related Emergencies ■
■ Drug-Related Emergencies ■ Rape and Sexual Assault ■

A first aider dealing with a crisis usually provides emotional support as well as first aid for any physical injury. A few principles hold true for most crisis situations, regardless of type. The first and perhaps main principle is to talk with the person in a warm, caring, empathetic manner. Get on the victim's eye level and establish eye contact. Use a calm, steady voice to provide honest reassurance.

Child Abuse

Child abuse is a general term encompassing physical abuse, psychological or emotional abuse, sexual abuse, and neglect. Because there is no standard definition of child abuse, each state has created its own legal definition. An estimated two million cases of child abuse and neglect are reported yearly.

The terms **abused** or **battered** are applied to children who are deliberately injured by an adult, usually a parent. However, the abuser may be an older brother or sister, a baby sitter, or an acquaintance of a parent, especially if the parent is single. Child abuse is a major problem and occurs in all socioeconomic groups. An estimated 10 percent of all children seen in emergency rooms are victims of child abuse. Child abuse can cause serious mental distress and physical injury—sometimes death.

Types of Child Abuse and Neglect

Child abuse is usually divided into four major types: physical abuse, neglect, sexual abuse, and emotional maltreatment. Each has recognizable characteristics, and all may be encountered by a first aider. Physical and behavioral indicators are found in Table 12.1. The list is not intended to be exhaustive; many more indicators exist than can be included. In addition, the presence of a single indicator does not necessarily prove that child abuse or neglect has occurred. However, the repeated occurrence of an indicator, the presence of several indicators in combination, or the appearance of serious injury should alert the first aider to the possibility of child abuse or neglect.

One or more of the following signs indicate that the child may have been abused:

- Multiple extremity fractures
- Multiple bruises and abrasions, especially on the trunk and buttocks
- Both old and new bruises (Remember that bruises change color as time passes.)
- Burns, especially cigarette burns or scalds
- Multiple soft-tissue injuries and injuries about the mouth (for example, black eyes, split lips, missing teeth)
- Evidence of poor nourishment or poor care in general
- History of one or more suspicious accidents
- Apathetic attitude; absence of crying, despite injuries
- An injury that occurred several days before medical attention was sought

Some cases of child abuse are obvious, and some are not. If the evidence leads you to suspect that the child has suffered abuse, do the following:

- Examine the child for abrasions, bruises, lacerations, and evidence of internal injury.
- Look for signs of head injury, closely looking at the ears and nose for blood and cerebrospinal fluid, and at the eyes for unequal pupils.
- Conduct the assessment as you would with any injured victim. Keep any suspicions quiet, but make careful notes of the assessment and your observations at the scene (the condition of the home or of any objects that might have been used against the child, such as belts or straps). Later, report your findings to the proper authority, but never openly accuse the parents of abuse.

The sexually molested child is a special case and must be handled with tact and composure. The child may be frightened and upset; the parents, very anxious. Keep in mind that a parent or close relative may have been the molester.

TABLE 12-1 Physical and Behavioral Indicators of Child Abuse and Neglect

Type of Child Abuse/Neglect	Physical Indicators	Behavioral Indicators

PHYSICAL ABUSE	Unexplained bruises and welts:
	  on face, lips, mouth
	  on torso, back, buttocks, thighs
	  in various stages of healing
	  clustered, forming regular patterns
	  reflecting shape of articles used to inflict (electric cord, belt buckle)
	  on several different surface areas
	  regularly appearing after absence, weekend, or vacation
	  especially about the trunk and buttocks
	  be particularly suspicious if there are old bruises in addition to fresh ones
	
	Unexplained burns:
	  cigar, cigarette burns, especially on soles, palms, back or buttocks
	  immersion burns (socklike, glove-like doughnut shaped on buttocks or genitalia)
	  patterned like electric burner, iron, etc.
	  rope burns on arms, legs, neck or torso
	
	Unexplained fractures:
	(particularly if multiple)
	  to skull, nose, facial structure
	  in various stages of healing
	  multiple or spiral fractures
	
	Unexplained lacerations or abrasions:
	  to mouth, lips, gums, eyes
	  to external genitalia
		Wary of adult contacts
		Apprehensive when other children cry
		Behavioral extremes:
		  aggressiveness or withdrawal
		Frightened of parents
		Afraid to go home
		Reports injury by parents
		Acts apathetic and *does not cry* despite his injuries
		Has been seen by emergency personnel recently for related complaints
		Was injured several days before you were called

PHYSICAL NEGLECT	Consistent hunger, poor hygiene, inappropriate dress Consistent lack of supervision, especially in dangerous activities or for long periods Unattended physical problems or medical needs Abandonment	Begs, steals food Extended stays at school (early arrival and late departure) Constant fatigue, listlessness, or falling asleep in class Alcohol or drug abuse Delinquency (e.g., thefts) States there is no caretaker
SEXUAL ABUSE	Difficulty in walking or sitting Torn, stained, or bloody underclothing Pain or itching in genital area Bruises or bleeding in external genitalia, vaginal, or anal areas Venereal disease, especially in pre-teens Pregnancy	Unwillingness to change for gym or participate in physical education class Withdrawal, fantasizing, or infantile behavior Bizarre, sophisticated, or unusual sexual behavior or knowledge Poor peer relationships Delinquency or truancy Reports sexual assault by caretaker

Type of Child Abuse/Neglect	Physical Indicators	Behavioral Indicators

EMOTIONAL MALTREATMENT	Speech disorders
	Lags in physical development
	Failure-to-thrive
		Habit disorders (sucking, biting, rocking, etc.)
		Conduct disorders (antisocial, destructive, etc.)
		Neurotic traits (sleep disorders, inhibition of play)
		Psychoneurotic reactions (hysteria, obsession, compulsion, phobias, hypochondria)
		Behavior extremes:
		    compliant, passive-aggressive, demanding
		Overly adaptive behavior:
		    inappropriately adult
		    inappropriately infantile
		Developmental lags (mental, emotional)
		Attempted suicide

Source: National Center on Child Abuse and Neglect

Spouse Abuse

The most common feature of domestic violence among adults is that it is perpetrated by men against women (95 percent of serious partner assaults). Although women may hit men during conflicts, there is no evidence of a "battered man" syndrome comparable to the syndrome among women. Nationally, about one million women use emergency medical services each year for treatment of injuries related to battering. Between two and four million women are physically battered each year by husbands, former husbands, boyfriends, or lovers. About half of these women are single, separated or divorced. Between 20 and 30 percent of all women in this country have been beaten by a partner at least once. Studies show that women in this country are more at risk for assault, rape, and murder by a male partner than by a stranger.

Abuse may be the single most common source of serious injury to women, accounting for almost three times as many medical visits as traffic injuries. Studies indicate that about 20 percent of women using emergency rooms are battered.

In addition, battered women comprise a significant percentage of rape victims, suicide attempts, psychiatric patients, mothers of abused children, substance abusers, and women who miscarry and abort. Clearly, this makes battering a major health concern.

Physical violence may include slapping, punching, kicking, choking, and attacks with weapons. Women also report being shot, stabbed, and bludgeoned. Injuries tend to be on the head, neck, chest, breast, abdomen, and perineum rather than the extremities. Rape and traumatic injuries during pregnancy also indicate abuse.

First aid includes calling the police and the emergency medical services system. First aid for injuries should also be given.

Elder Abuse

Between 1 and 10 percent of the nation's elderly have been abused, according to various studies. The House Select Committee on Aging estimates that each year more than one million of older Americans are physically, financially, and emotionally abused by their relatives.

The types of physical abuse vary from passive neglect to active assault. Some physically abused elderly report having had something thrown at them; some are pushed, grabbed, or shoved; some are slapped, bitten, or kicked.

Depression

Depression can lead to suicide (50 percent of all suicides involve depression). Depressed persons can be recognized by their sad appearance, crying spells, and listless or apathetic behavior. They feel worthless, guilty, and extremely pessimistic. Asserting that no one understands or cares about them and their problems cannot be solved, they often express the desire to be

TABLE 12-2 Psychological First Aid for Emergency Reactions

Reaction	Symptoms	Do	Don't
Normal	Trembling Muscular tension Perspiration Nausea Mild diarrhea Urinary frequency Pounding heart Rapid breathing Anxiety	Give reassurance. Provide group iden- tification. Motivate. Talk with victim. Observe to see that individual is gain- ing composure, not losing it.	Don't show resentment. Don't overdo sympathy.
Individual Panic (flight reaction)	Unreasoning attempt to flee Loss of judgment Uncontrolled weeping Wild running about	Try kindly firmness at first. Give something warm to eat or drink. Get help to isolate if necessary. Be empathetic. Encourage victim to talk. Be aware of your own limitations.	Don't use brutal re- straint. Don't strike. Don't douse with water. Don't give sedatives.
Depression (underactive reactions)	Stands or sits without moving or talking Vacant expression Lack of emotional display	Make contact gently. Secure rapport. Get victim to tell you what happened. Be empathetic. Recognize feelings of resentment in vic- tim and yourself. Give simple, routine task. Give warm food, drink.	Don't tell victim to "snap out of it." Don't overdo pity. Don't give sedatives. Don't act resentful.
Overactive	Argumentative Talks rapidly Jokes inappropriately Makes endless sug- gestions Jumps from one ac- tivity to another	Let victim talk about it. Find victim jobs which require physical effort. Give warm food, drink. Supervision necessary. Be aware of own feelings.	Don't suggest that victim is acting abnormally. Don't give sedatives. Don't argue with victim.
Physical (conversion reaction)	Severe nausea and vomiting Can't use some part of the body	Show interest in victim. Find small job for vic- tim to make him or her forget. Make comfortable. Get medical help if possible. Be aware of own feelings.	Don't tell victim that there's nothing wrong with him/her. Don't blame. Don't ridicule. Don't ignore disability openly.

Source: Modified from M 51-400-603-1, Department of Nonresident Instruction, Medical Field Service School, Brooke Army Medical Center, Fort Sam Houston, Texas.

left alone. Their speech may be as if they have hardly enough energy to talk. Sleeping difficulties may accompany the depressed.

Some depressed persons, however, do not feel like talking. In such cases, you might say, "You look very sad," which often allows persons to talk about their depressed feelings. Such persons may burst into tears. Do *not* discourage their crying. Maintain a sympathetic silence and let them "cry themselves out."

Depressed persons need sympathetic attention and reassurance. They need to know that the first aider is concerned about them. It is usually best if these persons are interviewed in private, as the presence of several people may make depressed persons uncomfortable. These persons should be told that though many people have periods of unhappiness, they can be helped to feel better. At this point, you can mention community resources where such help can be found.

Suicide

Suicide is defined as any willful act designed to end one's own life. Each year, the suicide deaths of 25,000 to 30,000 Americans are recorded. Suicide in the United States is increasingly a problem of adolescents and the very old.

The male rate for suicides is more than three times that for females. It is most common in men who are single, widowed, or divorced. Slightly more than half of all suicides—both men and women—use firearms. The next most common method is hanging. Poisoning by solids or liquids is the most common method used by women attempting but not completing suicide. Jumping from high places, carbon monoxide poisoning by auto exhaust, drowning, and cutting oneself with a sharp instrument are less common methods.

The frequency of suicide peaks during spring months, rises again in the fall, and is lowest in December. Suicide rates are lowest in the Northeast and highest in the West. This may reflect the greater availability of firearms in the western states.

Suicide attempts are eight times more common than completed suicides. In addition, it is known that while males complete suicide three times more often than females, females are reported to attempt suicide three times more often than males. It is not known whether males are more reluctant to seek help and are therefore less likely to report their attempts. And it is not known whether the lower rate of suicide among females results from their choice of less lethal methods despite an equal desire to die.

Despite its role as a major cause of death, suicide is a rare event. Except in the case of suicide clusters (groups of deaths closely related in time and place, involving at least three completed suicides), no community is likely to experience many suicides.

Suicide is often attempted by depressed persons and alcoholics. At least 60 percent of all suicide victims previously attempted suicide, and 75 percent gave clear warning that they intended to kill themselves. Typically, a suicide attempt will occur when an individual's close emotional attachments are in danger or when he or she loses a significant family member or friend. Suicidal people often feel unable to manage their lives. Frequently, they lack self-esteem.

Every suicidal act or gesture should be taken seriously, and the person should be referred to a professional counselor. Always contact the police about an attempted suicide.

Many suicides will make last-minute attempts to communicate their intentions. When an individual phones to threaten suicide, someone should stay on the line with that person until the emergency medical service system reaches the scene.

If faced with an attempted or threatened suicide situation, discreetly remove any dangerous articles. Talk quietly with the person. Encourage him or her to discuss the situation. Find out the following: Has there been a previous suicide attempt? Have any concrete plans concerning the method of suicide been made? Has any family member ever committed suicide?

Persons who have made previous attempts, who have detailed suicide plans, or whose close relatives have attempted suicide are most likely to attempt to kill themselves. These persons must be reassured and taken to medical help, usually at a hospital. They must *not* be left alone under any circumstances.

When persons attempt suicide, their first aid care has priority. Drug overdoses must be managed. Persons with slashed wrists must have their bleeding controlled. Even under these circumstances, you should try to talk with the person, if he or she is conscious, and encourage him or her to speak about the situation. When dealing with drug overdoses, collect any medication containers, pills, or other drugs found on the scene and bring the items to the hospital emergency department with the victim.

Rage, Hostility, and Violent Behavior

The angry, violent person is ready to fight with anyone who approaches and may be difficult to control. Remember that anger may be a response to illness and that aggressive behavior may be the person's way of coping with feelings of helplessness. Avoid responding with anger. Many angry or violent persons can be calmed by a trained person who appears confident that the person will behave well. Encourage them to speak directly about the cause of their anger. A statement such as "I'm not sure I understand why you are angry"

These Statements are Not True

FABLE: People who talk about suicide do not commit suicide.

FABLE: Suicide happens without warning.

FABLE: Suicidal people are fully intent on dying.

FABLE: Once a person is suicidal, he is suicidal forever.

FABLE: Improvement following a suicidal crisis means that the suicidal risk is over.

FABLE: Suicide strikes more often among the rich—or, conversely, it occurs more frequently among the poor.

FABLE: Suicide is inherited or "runs in a family" (i.e., is genetically determined.)

FABLE: All suicidal individuals are mentally ill, and suicide is always the act of a psychotic person.

These Statements Are True

FACT: Of every ten people who kill themselves, eight have given definite warnings of their suicidal intentions. Suicide threats and attempts *must* be taken seriously.

FACT: Studies reveal that the suicidal person gives many clues and warnings regarding his suicidal intentions. Alertness to these cries for help may prevent suicidal behavior.

FACT: Most suicidal people are undecided about living or dying, and they gamble with death, leaving it to others to save them. Almost no one commits suicide without letting others know how he or she is feeling. Often this cry for help is given in code. These distress signals can be used to save lives.

FACT: Fortunately, individuals who wish to kill themselves are suicidal only for a limited period of time. If they are saved from self-destruction, they can go on to lead useful lives.

FACT: Most suicides occur within three months after the beginning of improvement, when the individual has the energy to put his morbid thoughts and feelings into effect. Relatives and physicians should be especially vigilant during this period.

FACT: Suicide is neither the rich man's disease nor the poor man's curse. Suicide is very democratic and is represented proportionately among all levels of society.

FACT: Suicide does *not* run in families. It is an individual matter, and can be prevented.

FACT: Studies of hundreds of genuine suicide notes indicate that although the suicidal person is extremely unhappy, he is not necessarily mentally ill. His overpowering unhappiness may result from a temporary emotional upset, a long and painful illness, or a complete loss of hope. It is circular reasoning to say that suicide is an insane act, and therefore all suicidal people are psychotic.

Source: U.S. Department of Health and Human Resources

often brings results. Reassure them that you are there to help them.

A person who is violent and out of control presents a special problem. Notify the police if you are unable to communicate with persons who are dangerous to themselves or others. Only law enforcement officers have the legal right to subdue a violent person against his or her will.

Alcohol-Related Emergencies

Alcohol is a depressant, not a stimulant. Many people think alcohol is a stimulant because its first effect is to reduce tension and give a mild feeling of euphoria or exhilaration.

Alcohol affects a person's judgment, vision, reaction time, and coordination. In very large quantities, it can cause death by paralyzing the respiratory center of the brain.

Alcohol often causes disturbed behavior. In most states, an individual is considered to be legally intoxicated when he or she has consumed enough alcohol to raise the blood alcohol level above 0.10 percent (some states use the 0.08 percent level). Signs of alcohol intoxication include odor of alcohol on the breath, poor impulse control, drowsiness, lack of coordination, slurred speech, nausea and vomiting, flushed face, and sometimes combativeness. If individuals are not combative, they should simply be allowed to sleep until the alcohol wears off. If they are combative, seek medical assistance for them. Remember, however, that the person who appears intoxicated may be suffering from the effects of a more serious medical problem.

Drug-Related Emergencies

Drugs are classified according to their effects on the user:

1. **Uppers** are stimulants of the central nervous system. They include amphetamines, cocaine, caffeine, antiasthmatic drugs, and vasoconstrictor drugs.

2. **Downers** are depressants of the central nervous system. They include barbiturates, tranquilizers, marijuana, narcotics, and anticonvulsants.

3. **Hallucinogens** alter and frequently enhance the processing of sensory and emotional information in brain centers. They include LSD, mescaline, psilocybin, and peyote. Marijuana also has some hallucinogenic properties.

Amphetamines and cocaine. These provide relief from fatigue and a feeling of well-being. Blood pressure, breathing, and general body activity are increased. Some users take a "speed run" of repeated high doses. Results are hyperactivity, restlessness, and belligerence. Such persons need to be protected from hurting themselves and others. Acute cases need medical attention.

Hallucinogens. These produce changes in mood and sensory awareness—a person may "hear" colors and "see" sounds. They can cause hallucinations and bizarre behavior that can make users dangerous to themselves and others. Acute cases need medical attention. Users should be protected from hurting themselves.

Marijuana. Marijuana provides a feeling of relaxation and euphoria. Users report distortions of time and space. In some persons, use can result in a reaction similar to a bad LSD trip.

Barbiturates. These drugs result in relaxation, drowsiness, and sleep. Overdoses can produce respiratory depression, coma, and death. Withdrawal can cause anxiety, tremors, nausea, fever, delirium, convulsions, and ultimately death.

Tranquilizers. They are used to calm anxiety. High doses produce the same effects as barbiturates. Withdrawal may cause the addict problems similar to those occurring from withdrawal from barbiturates.

Inhaled substances. Inhaling glue or other solvents (gasoline, lighter fluid, nail polish, etc.) produces effects similar to those of ingesting alcohol. The person can die through suffocation. In addition, some inhalants can cause death by changing the rhythm of the heartbeat.

Opiates (narcotics). They are used medicinally to relieve pain and anxiety. Overdoses can result in deep sleep (coma), respiratory depression, and death. The pupils of opiate users are described as "pin-point" in size. Withdrawal symptoms include intense agitation, abdominal discomfort, dilated pupils, increased breathing and body temperatures, and a strong craving for a "fix."

In cases involving drug abuse, first aid should include:

- Maintaining an open airway and checking for breathing and pulse
- Treating for shock
- Providing first aid for injuries (e.g., bleeding).
- Handling vomiting (Make no attempt to induce vomiting unless instructed by poison control center personnel or other medical authorities. Telephone them for instructions.
- Positioning unconscious and semiconscious victim on one side
- Being calm and reassuring
- Collecting all materials (e.g., empty bottles, packages, and vomitus) at the scene to assist medical personnel in identifying when and how much of the drug was taken

- Seeking medical attention for the victim
- Leaving police work to the police
- Avoiding the risk of personal injury (Let law enforcement officers handle dangerous situations.)

Rape and Sexual Assault

The definitions of rape and sexual assault vary widely. Rape is generally defined as forcible intercourse without the consent of one participant. Categories of rape include the following:

- *Acquaintance rape* involves individuals who knew each other prior to the rape, including relatives, neighbors, or friends.
- *Date rape* takes place within a relationship but without the consent of the woman and when harm or the threat of harm is used by the man.
- *Marital rape* occurs when the victim and offender are spouses.
- *Stranger rape* occurs when victim and offender have no relation to each other.

The FBI considers rape the second most serious crime, following murder. One estimate says only one in five rapes is reported while another says that it is only one in twenty. The victim herself may hesitate to report rape for various reasons, such as shame, guilt, fear of retaliation, or disbelief from law enforcement officials. She may even question herself as to whether a "real" rape occurred.

Rape is a traumatic crisis that disrupts the physical, psychological, social, and sexual aspects of the victim's life. The most common injuries are bruises, black eyes, and cuts.

The first aider must use tact and sensitivity with the victim. The victim may find it extremely difficult to discuss what happened and may feel fear or hostility toward a male first aider. Every effort should be made to understand the person's feelings and to respond with kindness and reassurance. The emotional trauma of rape is usually more prolonged and severe than the physical trauma. The attitude shown toward the victim during her care can have a serious influence, for good or ill, on her future psychological and physical recovery. Convince the victim to seek counseling through community resources (e.g., a rape crisis center), and to report the crime to the police. Ask the victim not to change her clothes or bathe since doing so can alter legal evidence. For the same reason, suggest that the woman not urinate, douche, defecate, or wash before being examined by a physician. Care for any injuries incurred during the attack.

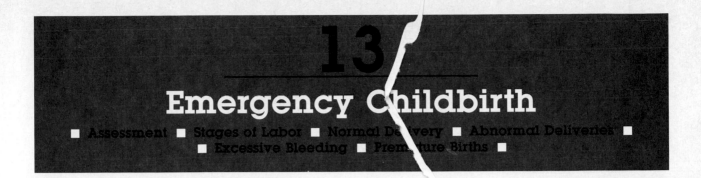

Most births in developed countries occur in hospitals. Often forgotten, however, is the fact that throughout history, most people were born outside of a medical facility. Today, a first aider rarely sees a pregnant woman so far along into the birth process that there is not time to get her to a hospital. However, it sometimes happens, and when it does the first aider should be prepared to help the mother deliver her child.

The first aider should receive the baby, tie and cut the cord, receive the placenta (afterbirth), and provide proper care for the mother and baby following delivery.

Assessment

When confronted with a woman in labor, first aiders will need to determine whether there is time to transport the woman to the hospital. To make this decision, the first aider should get answers to the following questions:

1. **Has the woman had a baby before?** Labor during a first pregnancy usually lasts about 16 hours. The time in labor is considerably shorter for each subsequent baby. For a first baby there may be more time for transport to a hospital.

2. **How often are the contractions?** Contractions more than five minutes apart are a good indication that there will be enough time to get the woman to a nearby hospital. Contractions less than two minutes apart, especially in a woman who has had more than one pregnancy, indicate an imminent delivery. The first aider can time the frequency and length of the contractions.

3. **Has the amniotic sac (the "bag of waters") ruptured and, if so, when?** If the sac ruptures more than 18 hours before birth occurs, the likelihood of infection is increased, and medical advice should be sought.

Only if the preceding answers seem to indicate an imminent birth should a first aider examine the mother for **crowning.** This is looking to see if there is bulging at the vaginal opening or if part of the baby is visible. Crowning indicates that the baby is about to be born, and that there will not be time to go to the hospital before delivery. This procedure may be embarrassing to the mother, father, and bystanders, and it is therefore important that the first aider fully explain what is being done and why. Make every effort to protect the mother from embarrassment during such an examination by removing only enough clothing to expose the vaginal area. Consider transporting the woman to a hospital if she is not straining or crowning and this is her first pregnancy.

If there is enough time to transport the woman to the hospital, she should be placed on her left side to counteract or prevent a possible drop in blood pressure caused by pressure on the inferior vena cava (large vein found between the spine and the abdominal organs), which reduces venous blood return to the heart. Any underclothing that may obstruct delivery should be removed. The first aider should:

- *Never* allow the mother to go to the toilet, if delivery seems imminent.
- *Never* attempt to delay or restrain delivery in any way (e.g., holding the woman's legs together).

If the woman is straining, crowning, and has had prior pregnancies, and if there is not enough time to get to the hospital, the first aider must prepare to assist in the delivery. If the mother-to-be is in a crowded or public place, the first aider should try to find a private, clean area. The woman may find it reassuring to have a companion, such as her husband, friend, or relative present.

Stages of Labor

Labor, which is the process of childbirth, consists of contractions of the walls of the uterus (womb). These contractions force the expulsion of the baby into the outside world. Labor is divided into three stages. The *first stage* usually lasts several hours (possibly 18 hours or more for a first baby), from the first contraction to full dilation of the cervix. The small opening at the lower end of the uterus (the cervix) gradually stretches until it is large enough to let the baby pass through. The contractions usually begin as an acutely aching sensation in the small of the back; in a short time, they turn into cramplike pains recurring regularly in the lower abdomen. At first, these contractions are from 10 to 15 minutes apart, are not very severe, and last but a few moments. Gradually, the intervals between contractions grow shorter and they increase in intensity. A slight, watery, bloodstained discharge from the vagina may accompany contractions or occur before labor begins.

At the end of the *first stage* of labor, the bag of waters, which encases the baby in the uterus, breaks. A pint or more of watery fluid discharges. Sometimes the bag of waters breaks during the first stage of labor. This should not cause the first aider any concern because it usually does not affect labor. If the bag of waters breaks prematurely and labor does not begin within 12 hours, the danger of infection to mother and baby is potentially great.

The *second stage* lasts about 30 minutes to two hours. It begins when the neck of the cervix is fully open, and it ends with the actual birth of the baby.

During the *third stage*, lasting about 15 minutes or more, the afterbirth (placenta) is expelled.

Normal Delivery

Position the woman on her back and place under her buttocks a folded sheet, blanket, towels, or even newspapers with a sheet over them for a cushion. She then should bend her knees and spread her thighs apart. If in a car, have the mother place one of her legs over the back of the seat and one on the floor of the car.

Other positions for the woman include her sitting up or even squatting, with someone behind supporting her. These optional positions place less tension on the vaginal tissues, reducing the likelihood of a tear. These positions also allow the force of gravity to help. Another common position is to lay her on her left side. This position improves blood return to her heart. Someone should hold the woman's right leg up out of the way. Another position is the kneeling knee-chest position used in less developed countries and in cases of breech presentations. These last two positions provide protection against possible aspiration (inhalation of foreign material) if the mother vomits.

Be prepared for vomiting by having someone with a basin or pail near the woman's head—she could aspirate vomit while lying flat on her back.

Supplies to assist the delivery include:

- Clean sheets, towels, and blankets to cover the mother and baby
- New or clean shoelaces or similar materials to tie the cord (Do *not* use thread, wire, or string, since they might cut through the cord.)
- A plastic bag or towel to wrap the placenta for delivery to a hospital
- Clean, unused vinyl or latex gloves (If not available, wash hands thoroughly, if possible. Vinyl or latex gloves reduce the likelihood of infection.)
- Sanitary napkins or pads
- Sterile scissors
- Newspapers, plastic, or cloth sheet to place under the woman to provide for a clean delivery area
- Rubber bulb syringe for suctioning the baby's mouth and nostrils
- Sterile gauze pads for wiping blood and mucous from baby's mouth and nose

Hands should be washed. If vinyl or latex gloves are available, wear them. Encourage the woman to relax and to take slow, deep breaths through her mouth.

When the baby's head begins to emerge from the birth canal, it should be supported gently to prevent explosive delivery. Do *not* attempt to pull the baby from the mother. If the membranes cover the head after it emerges, tear the sac with your fingers and remove it from the baby's face, permitting the amniotic fluid to escape so the baby can breathe. Be sure the umbilical cord is not wrapped around the infant's neck; if it is, slip it gently over the shoulder or head. If this maneuver fails and the cord is tight around the baby's neck, tie the cord two inches apart and cut it between the ties to release pressure from the infant's neck. Support the head at all times. Avoid touching the mother's anus during the delivery.

After the baby is fully delivered, support him or her along the length of your arm, with one hand supporting the baby's head. The baby's head should be held downward to aid drainage. Do *not* raise the baby above the mother's abdomen (location of the placenta) while the umbilical cord is intact because this will cause the baby's blood to flow back toward the placenta and may put the baby in shock. Do *not* hold the baby below the mother's abdomen (location of placenta) since blood can run into the baby, where the extra blood cells can cause jaundice.

Because they are slippery, babies must be held carefully. Blood and mucus from the nose and mouth should be wiped away with sterile gauze. If a rubber bulb syringe is available, use it to suction the mouth and both nostrils. Use sterile gauze to wipe blood and mucus from around the baby's mouth and nose.

If the baby does not breathe within 30 seconds, give stimulation by gently rubbing the back or slapping the soles of the feet. Do *not* hold the baby up by the feet and slap its bottom. If there is no response, the first aider should start rescue breathing. If the baby still does not breathe, and you cannot feel a pulse at the brachial artery, start cardiopulmonary resuscitation

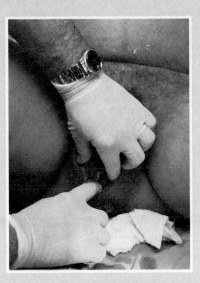

a. Gentle pressure on perineum controls tearing

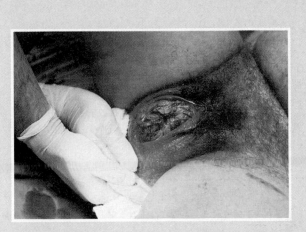

b. Crowning means baby's head is visible

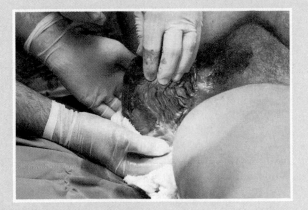

c. Head leaving the vagina

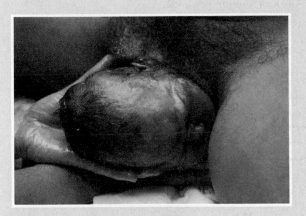

d. Head delivers and turns

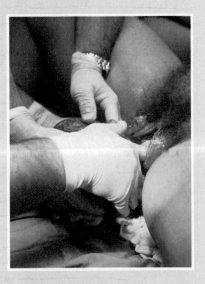

e. Head and shoulders deliver

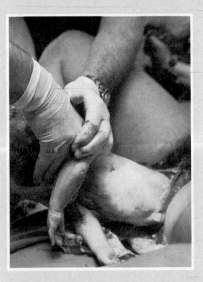

f. Support baby's head and body

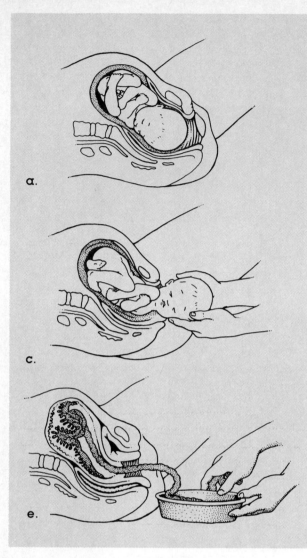

Normal stages of childbirth
a. End of the first stage of labor
b. Head delivers face down
c. Support the head
d. Tie the cord tightly
e. Placenta expelled in five to twenty minutes

and continue it on the way to the hospital. Keep the baby wrapped in a blanket as much as possible.

If, however, the baby has been delivered normally and is breathing well, and the strong pulsations of the cord have stopped, tie the cord (using clean shoelaces or similar material) to protect the mother and baby from bleeding. The cord should be tied about six to eight inches from the baby's navel, with a second tie made two to three inches nearer to the baby. At this point the cord is useless to the baby since oxygen is supplied through breathing rather than from the mother through the cord. The cord should be cut between the two ties and handled gently, because it will tear easily. Examine the end of the cord that is attached to the infant to be certain there is no bleeding. If there is bleeding from the cut end, make another tie on the cord and reexamine it for bleeding. Do *not* untie a cord once it is cut. Do *not* retie a knot. Should bleeding continue, apply another tie as close to the original as possible. Then wrap the baby in a clean blanket to maintain body temperature.

The next stage of delivery involves the delivery of the placenta ("afterbirth"). The placenta usually is delivered within 15 to 20 minutes after the baby's birth. Bleeding can be expected as the placenta separates from the uterine wall. When bleeding occurs, the mother's uterus should be gently massaged. The uterine massage will stimulate the uterus to contract, thus constricting blood vessels within its walls and decreasing bleeding. Allowing the baby to nurse following the delivery of the placenta, stimulates uterine contractions which helps control bleeding.

Never pull on the umbilical cord to deliver the placenta. When the placenta is delivered, wrap it in a towel, plastic bag, or newspaper and take it to the hospital, where it will be examined for completeness. This procedure is necessary because pieces of placenta retained in the uterus cause persistent bleeding and/or infection. Look for lacerations on the skin between the anus and the vagina (called the perineum) and apply pressure to any bleeding tears. Place a sanitary napkin over the vagina, lower the mother's legs, and prepare her for transport to the hospital.

If the placenta is not delivered within 15 to 20 minutes after the baby's delivery, the mother and her baby should be taken to the hospital without delay.

Abnormal Deliveries

Births occurring when the baby's head does not present first are classified as abnormal deliveries. Three abnormal presentations are discussed in this section: breech presentation, prolapsed umbilical cord, and limb presentation. Because these three situations can be life-threatening to the infant, the first aider should become familiar with the special problems of each situation.

Breech Presentation

Breech presentation occurs when the buttocks present first, rather than the head. This is the most common type of abnormal delivery, occurring in 3 to 4 percent of all deliveries. If birth is imminent, the woman should be prepared as discussed earlier, and the buttocks and trunk of the baby should be allowed to deliver. Once the legs are clear, the baby's body should be supported on the first aider's hand and arm, thus allowing the head to deliver. If the head is not delivered within three minutes, act to prevent suffocation of the baby. Suffocation can occur when the baby's face is pressed against the vaginal wall or when the umbilical cord is compressed by the baby's head in the vagina. To establish an airway in the first instance, the first aider should:

- Place a hand in the vagina, positioning the palm toward the baby's face.
- Form a *V* with the fingers on either side of the baby's nose.
- Push the vaginal wall away from the baby's face until the head is delivered.

The first aider should not try to pull the baby out of the vagina. If the head does not deliver within three minutes after an airway has been established, lay the woman on her back with her legs elevated or in the kneeling knee-chest position and get her to the hospital quickly. The baby's airway should be maintained throughout transport.

Prolapsed Umbilical Cord

Prolapsed umbilical cord occurs when the cord comes out of the vagina before the baby. The baby is, therefore, in danger of suffocation. The first aider should:

- Place the mother on her back or on her left side in an exaggerated shock position with her hips elevated on a pillow, and make sure she is kept warm.
- Gently push the baby back up into the vagina several inches.

- Never attempt to push the cord back.
- Take the mother and the baby to the hospital at once, while maintaining pressure on the baby's head. (Pressure should be evenly distributed to avoid injury to the baby's soft skull.)

Breech presentation and prolapsed umbilical cord are the only two cases in which the first aider should place his or her hand in the mother's vagina.

Limb Presentation

The presentation of an arm or leg through the vagina indicates the need for immediate transport to the hospital, the only place where such a delivery should be attempted. Keep the woman on her left side or her back in the delivery position and treat her for shock. Do *not* pull on the baby or attempt to push the limb into the vagina.

Excessive Bleeding

Prebirth

If a woman in labor begins to bleed excessively from her vagina, first aid should include the following:

- Lay the woman on her left side and treat her for shock. Do *not* hold the woman's legs together.
- Place a sanitary napkin or any sterile or clean pad over the opening of the vagina. Do *not* put anything in the vagina.
- Replace but save any blood-soaked pads and all tissues that are passed.
- Arrange for immediate transportation to a hospital.

Postbirth

Normally, the actual blood lost after childbirth amounts to half a pint. It always appears to be much more, especially to a first aider. Control bleeding as follows:

- Do *not* put anything in the vaginal opening.
- Place a sanitary napkin over the vaginal opening.
- Straighten and raise the mother's legs, keeping them together. She does not have to squeeze them.
- Gently massage her lower abdomen. You will feel an object about the size of a grapefruit (the uterus). Rub it gently in a circular motion. This encourages uterine contractions, which reduce bleeding.
- If the mother agrees, have her nurse her baby. This also induces contractions and controls bleeding.

Premature Births

Any baby who weighs less than 5.5 pounds or is born before seven months of pregnancy is defined as premature and needs special care. Premature babies develop problems because they are so small and their organs are immature.

To care for the premature baby, the first aider should:

- Keep the baby warm. Wrap the baby in aluminum foil and blankets to reduce heat loss.
- Keep the baby's nose and mouth clear of fluid with a rubber bulb syringe.

- Prevent bleeding from the umbilical cord, because these infants cannot tolerate the loss of even small amounts of blood.
- Prevent contamination because premature babies are highly susceptible to infection.

Childbirth is an important event. In the majority of births the event is normal and natural. First aiders must be prepared to care for the mother and baby during uncomplicated birth. In addition, they should be competent in handling complications that put mothers and newborns at risk. It is essential that the first aider be calm, deliberate, and gentle.

Babies

Heaviest

The heaviest baby on record of normal parentage was a boy of 22 lb. 8 oz., born to Signora Carmelina Fedele of Aversa, Italy, in September 1955. Tying the record at 22 lb. 8 oz., a boy named Sithandive was delivered by Caesarean section to Mrs. Christina Samane on May 24, 1982, at Sipetu Hospital, Transkie, South Africa. He weighed 77 lb. at 16 months, and 112 lb. at age 5.

Mrs. Anna Bates, *née* Swan, the 7-ft.-5½-in. Canadian giantess, gave birth to a boy weighing 23 lb. 12 oz. (length 30 in.) at her home in Seville, Ohio, on Jan. 19, 1879, but the baby died 11 hours later. Her first child, an 18-lb. girl (length 24 in.), was stillborn when she was delivered in 1872.

On Jan. 9, 1891, Mrs. Florentin Ortega of Buenos Aires, Argentina, produced a stillborn boy weighing 25 lb.

In May 1939, a deformed baby weighing 29 lb. 4 oz. was born in a hospital at Effingham, Ill., but died two hours later from respiratory problems.

Lightest

The lowest birth weight recorded for a surviving infant of which there is definite evidence is 10 oz. in the case of Mrs. Marion Taggart *née* Chapman, born six weeks prematurely, on June 5, 1938, in South Shields, northwest England. She was born unattended (length 12¼ in.) and was nursed by Dr. D. A. Shearer, who fed her hourly for the first 30 hours with brandy, glucose and water through a fountain-pen filler. At three weeks she weighed 1 lb. 13 oz., and by her first birthday her weight had increased to 13 lb. 4 oz. Her weight on her 21st birthday was 106 lb. She died May 31, 1983.

A weight of 8 oz. was reported on March 20, 1938, for a baby born prematurely to Mrs. John Womack, after she had been knocked down by a truck in East St. Louis, Ill. The baby was taken alive to St. Mary's Hospital and died a few hours later. On Feb. 23, 1952, it was reported that a 6 oz. baby only 6⅓ in. in length lived for 12 hours in a hospital in Indianapolis. A twin was stillborn.

—*Guinness Book of World Records*

■ EMERGENCY CHILDBIRTH ■

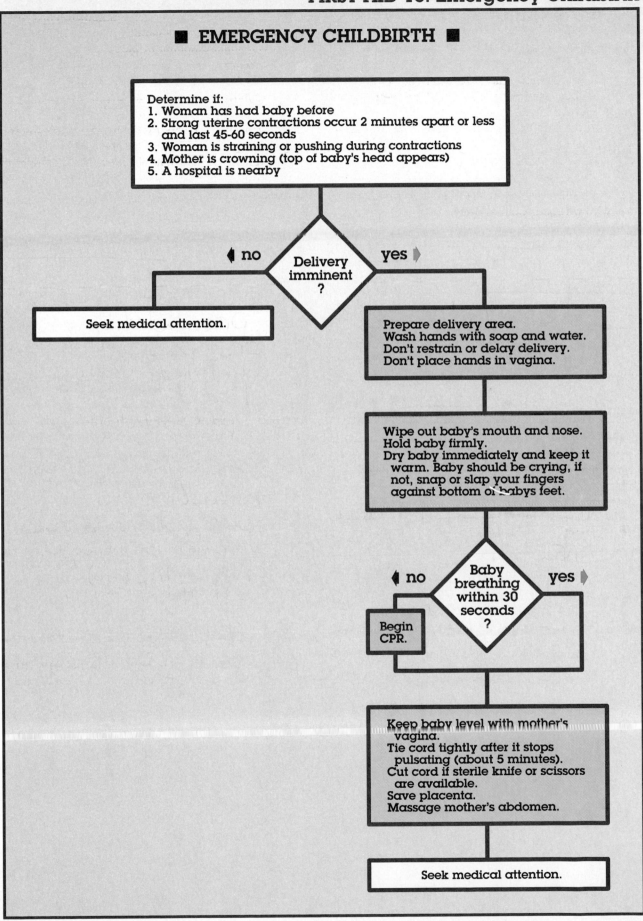

Determine if:
1. Woman has had baby before
2. Strong uterine contractions occur 2 minutes apart or less and last 45-60 seconds
3. Woman is straining or pushing during contractions
4. Mother is crowning (top of baby's head appears)
5. A hospital is nearby

Delivery imminent?

◀ no

yes ▶

Seek medical attention.

Prepare delivery area.
Wash hands with soap and water.
Don't restrain or delay delivery.
Don't place hands in vagina.

Wipe out baby's mouth and nose.
Hold baby firmly.
Dry baby immediately and keep it warm. Baby should be crying, if not, snap or slap your fingers against bottom of babys feet.

Baby breathing within 30 seconds?

◀ no

yes ▶

Begin CPR.

Keep baby level with mother's vagina.
Tie cord tightly after it stops pulsating (about 5 minutes).
Cut cord if sterile knife or scissors are available.
Save placenta.
Massage mother's abdomen.

Seek medical attention.

14

First Aid Skills

■ Bandaging ■ Splinting ■

Dressings control bleeding and prevent contamination. Bandages hold dressings in place. Dressings come in many different forms. Sterile gauzes are most commonly used. When these cannot be found, nonsterile substances such as towels or handkerchiefs can be applied. Many different forms of bandages exist. Roller gauze, triangular, and cravat bandages make up the bandages most often used by first aiders. However, self-adhering and formfitting bandages have become popular especially with emergency medical technicians.

Bandages need not be textbook perfect as long as they hold the dressings in place. Care should be taken, however, so that bandages are not applied too tightly or too loosely. Too tightly applied bandages will restrict blood flow, and too loose bandages fail to hold the dressing in place. When extremities are bandaged,

the fingers and toes should be left exposed so that any color changes in them can be noted. Such changes may indicate impaired circulation. Pain, color change, numbness, and tingling are other signs of a too-tight bandage.

Methods of applying dressings and bandages vary greatly and differ according to the types used and the injured part to which they are applied. Because of the variety of good bandaging techniques, the examples shown on the following pages represent a consensus among first aid experts as to the appropriate methods.

These illustrations show suggested bandaging and splinting skills. This compilation represents the skills needed for first aid situations most likely to be encountered.

TABLE 14-1 Splinting Guide

Injured Part	Suggested splinting materials and methods
Spine	Long backboard, best applied by trained EMS personnel; immobilize and wait
Collarbone	Sling and swathe*
Ribs	Victim holds pillow over injury
Upper arm	Rigid** splint on outside; wrist sling and swathe*
Elbow	**Straight:** rigid** splint on inside of arm **Bent:** rigid** splint on inside or outside of arm; wrist sling
Forearm/Wrist	Rigid** splint; sling and swathe*
Hand	Keep hand in position of function with a wadded cloth in palm; tie hand to rigid** splint; sling and swathe*
Finger(s)	Splint same as hand or tape finger to uninjured finger and apply sling
Pelvis/Hip	Long backboard, best applied by trained EMS personnel
Thigh	Tie legs together or use 6 long boards or traction splint applied by trained EMS personnel
Knee	**Straight:** rigid** splint behind leg **Bent:** rigid** splint on outside of leg
Lower leg	Rigid** splints on sides or tie legs together
Foot/ankle	Pillow splint
Toe	Tape toe to uninjured toe

KEY: **Swathe*** = binder (usually a cravat bandage) tied around body to hold arm against body to decrease movement; used on most upper extremity fractures.

Rigid** = must be long enough to include adjacent joints; examples include padded boards, 40 pages of folded newspapers, or cardboard.

MAKING A CRAVAT

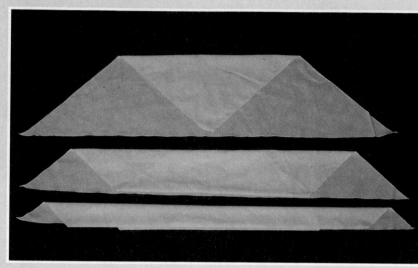

Cravat bandage for head, ears, or eyes

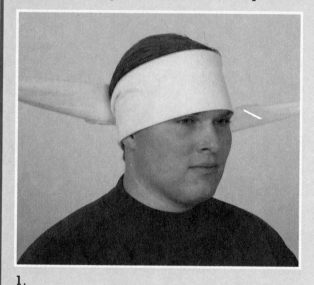

1.

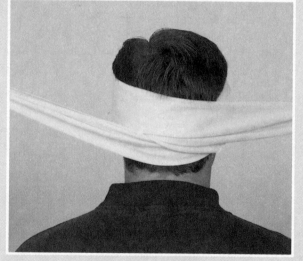

2.

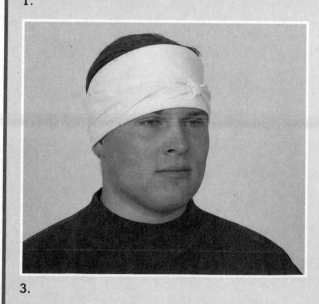

3.

1. Place middle of bandage over the dressing covering the wound.

2. Cross the two ends snugly over each other.

3. Bring the ends back around to where the dressing is and tie the ends in a knot.

SKILL SCAN: Bandaging—Cravat

Cravat bandage for arm or leg

Cravat bandage for elbow or knee

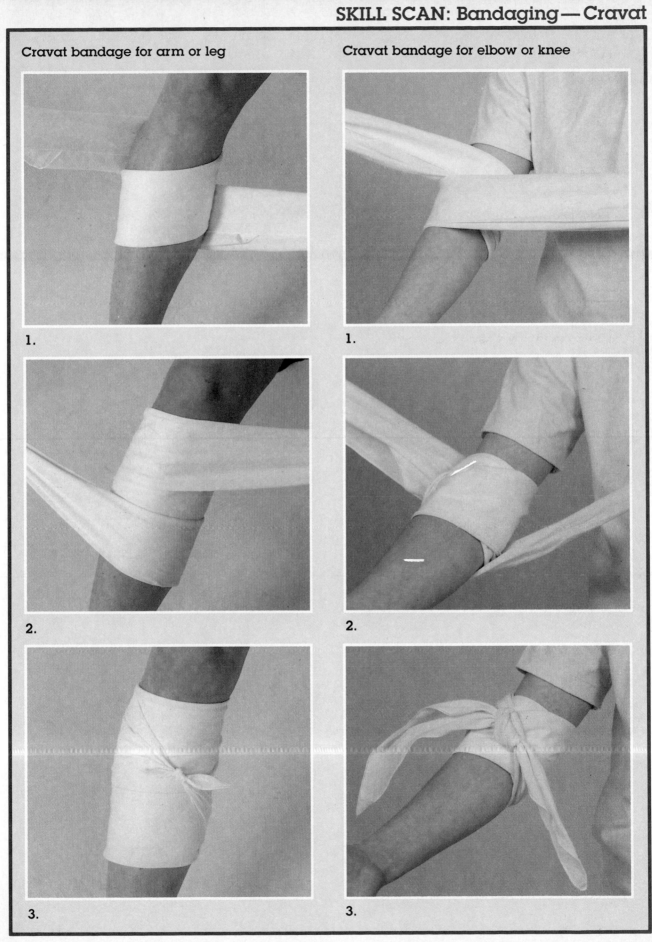

1.

1.

2.

2.

3.

3.

Roller bandage for hand

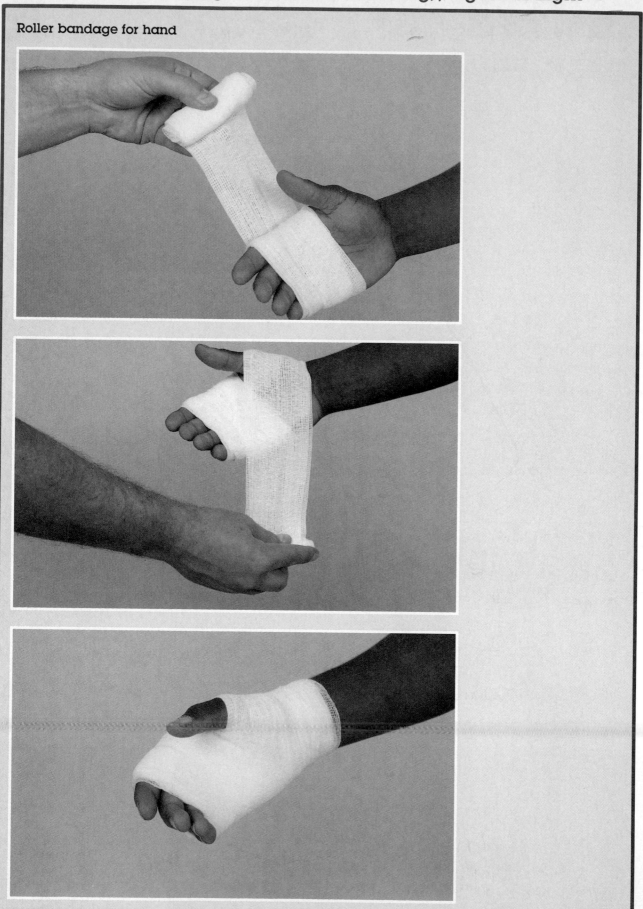

Roller bandage for elbow or knee

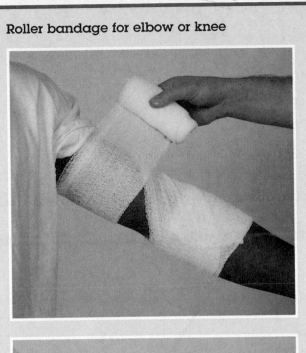

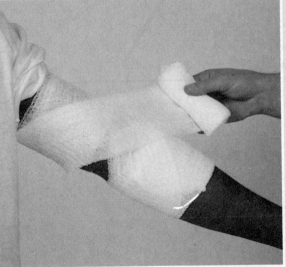

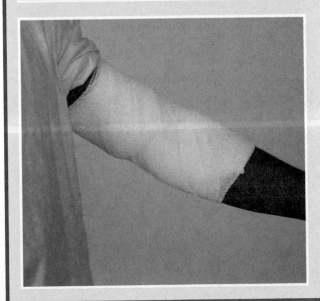

Roller bandage for ankle

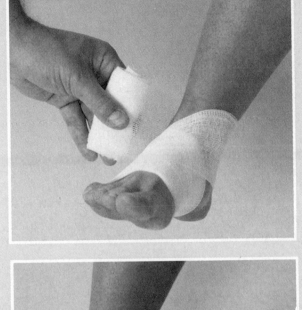

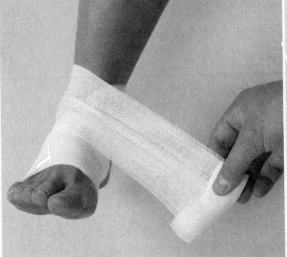

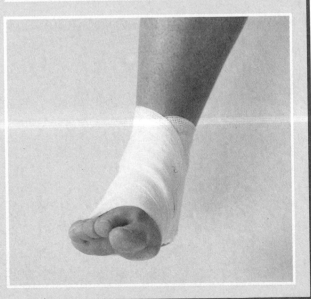

CLAVICLE AND ARM SLING

UPPER ARM (HUMERUS)

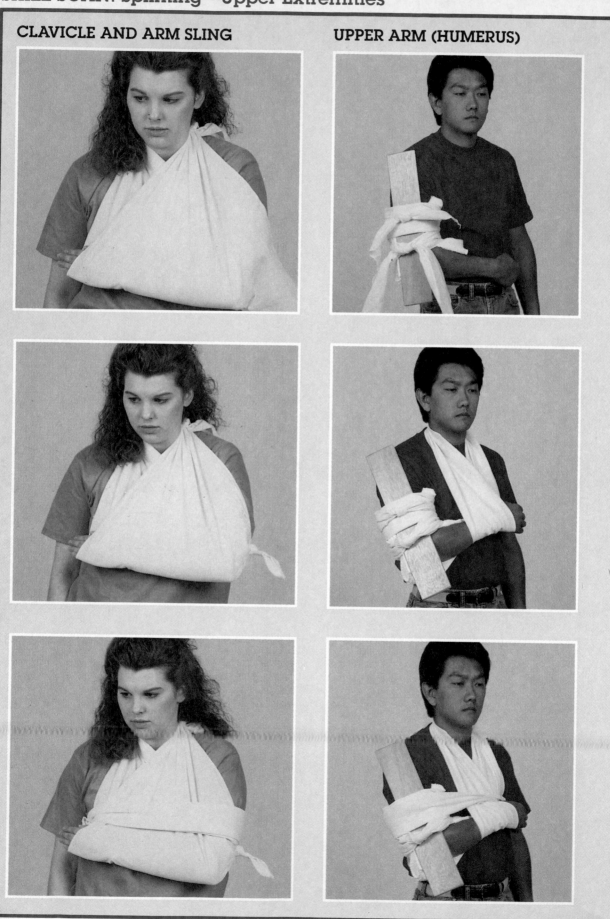

**FOREARM
(RADIUS/ULNA)**

**FINGERS AND HAND
(POSITION OF FUNCTION)**

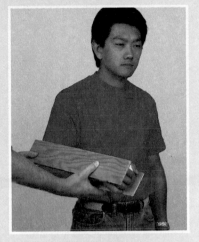

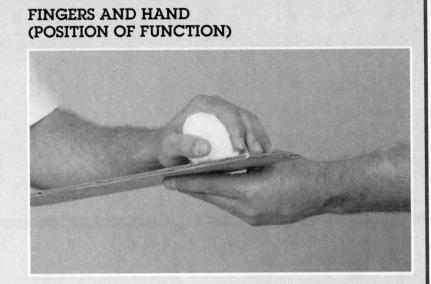

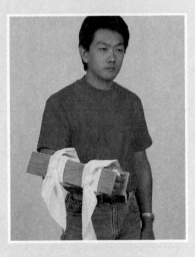

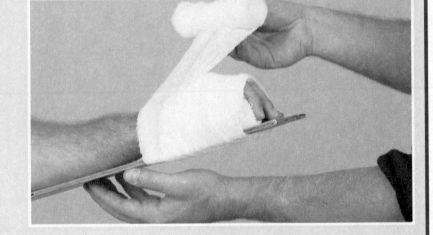

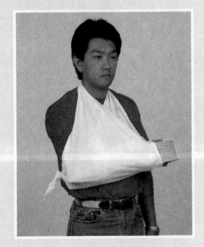

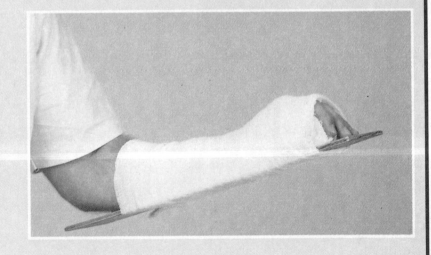

ELBOW IN BENT POSITION   **ELBOW IN STRAIGHT POSITION**

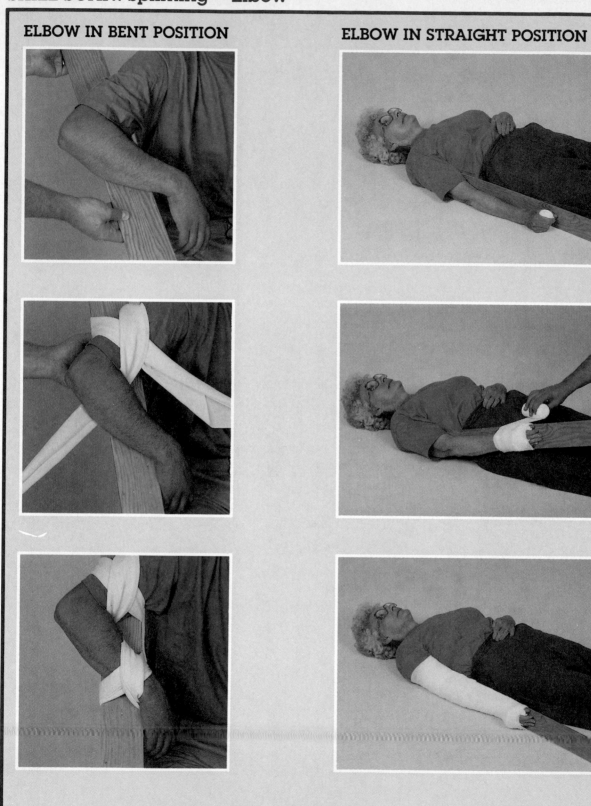

KNEE IN BENT POSITION

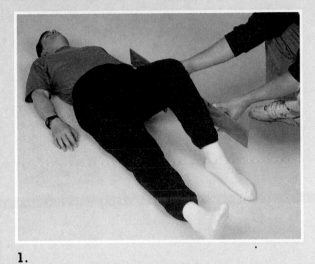

1.

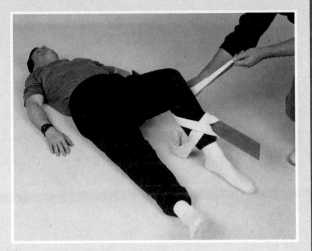

2.

KNEE IN STRAIGHT POSITION

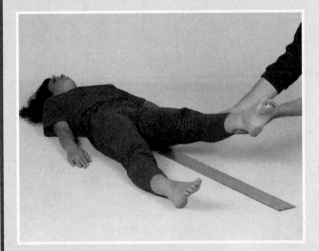

1.

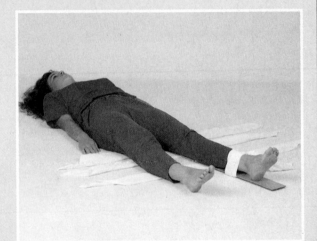

2.

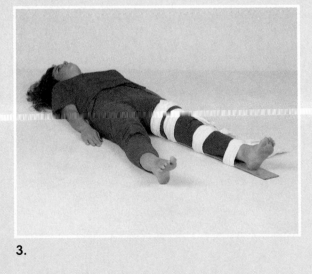

3.

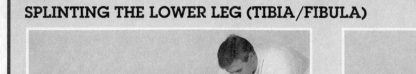
SKILL SCAN: Splinting—Lower Extremities

SPLINTING THE LOWER LEG (TIBIA/FIBULA)

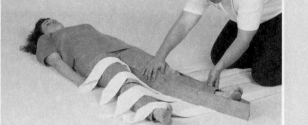

1.

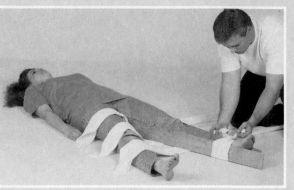

2.

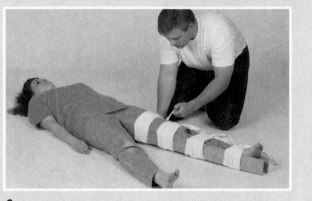

3.

THIGH (FEMUR)

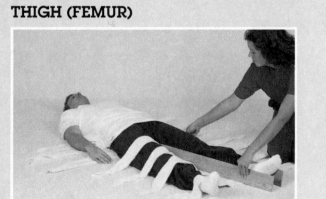

1.

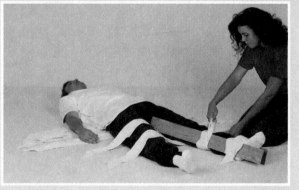

2.

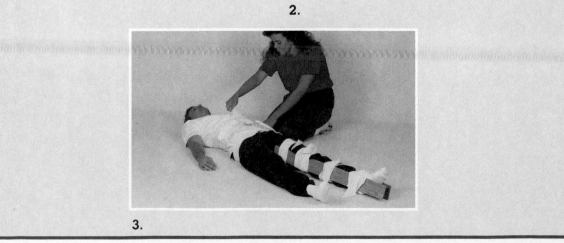

3.

ANKLE/FOOT

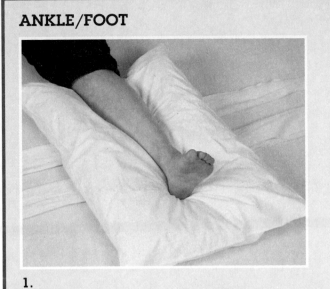

1.

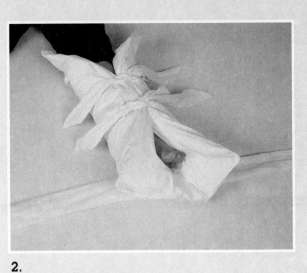

2.

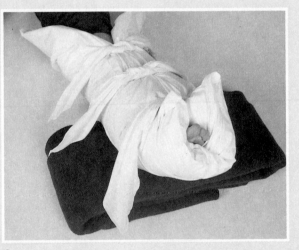

3.

SPLINTING—SELF-SPLINT

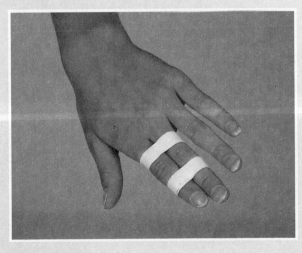

Fingers/toes

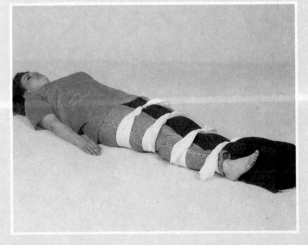

Leg

15

Moving and Rescuing Victims

■ **Emergency Moves** ■ **Nonemergency Moves** ■
■ **Water Rescue** ■

Don't move them unless you have too!

In general, a victim should not be moved until he or she is ready for transportation to a hospital, if required. All necessary first aid should be provided first. A victim should be moved only if there is an immediate danger, that is:

- There is a fire or danger of fire.
- Explosives or other hazardous materials are involved.
- It is impossible to protect the accident scene.
- It is impossible to gain access to other victims in a vehicle who need life-saving care.

Note that a cardiac arrest victim would typically be moved unless he or she were on the ground or floor because cardiopulmonary resuscitation must be performed on a firm surface.

If it is necessary to move a victim, the speed of movement depends on the reason for moving, for example:

- *Emergency move.* If there is a dangerous situation, pull the victim away from the area as quickly as possible.
- *Nonemergency move.* If the victim needs to be moved, give due consideration to injuries before and during movement.

Emergency Moves

The major danger in moving a victim quickly is the possibility of aggravating a spine injury. In an emergency, every effort should be made to pull the victim in the direction of the long axis of the body to provide as much protection to the spine as possible. If victims are on the floor or ground, you can drag them away from the scene by tugging on their clothing in the neck and shoulder area. It may be easier to pull a victim onto a blanket and then drag the blanket away from the scene. Such moves are emergency moves only. They do not adequately protect the spine from further injury.

Nonemergency Moves

Unless of danger or if they're dead to get to a live person.

All injured parts should be immobilized before moving and then protected during the moving. To protect yourself, you should use the following principles in all nonemergency moves:

- Keep in mind physical capabilities and limitations and do not try to handle too heavy a load. When in doubt, seek help.
- Keep yourself balanced when carrying out the move.
- Maintain a firm footing.
- Maintain a constant and firm grip.
- Lift and lower by bending your legs and not your back—keep your back as straight as possible at all times; bend knees and lift with one foot ahead of the other.
- When holding or transporting, keep your back straight and rely on shoulder and leg muscles; tighten muscles of your abdomen and buttocks.
- When performing a task that requires pulling, keep your back straight and pull, using your arms and shoulders.
- Carry out all tasks slowly, smoothly, and in unison with your partner.
- Move your body gradually; avoid twisting and jerking when conducting the various victim-handling tasks.
- When handling a victim, try to keep your arms as close as possible to the body in order to maintain balance.
- Do not keep your muscles contracted for a long period of time.

Transporting an injured victim by stretcher is safer and more comfortable for the victim than by other methods. It is also easier for the rescuers. A common type of stretcher is the army or canvas stretcher. It consists of two poles with canvas attached. Stretchers can be improvised using various materials, for example: a house door removed from its hinges, a ladder, or any two strong poles and material (e.g., blanket, canvas). If strong material is available but there is nothing for poles, you can place the victim in the center

CARRIES

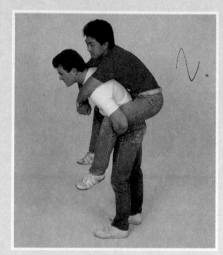

Pack-strap carry

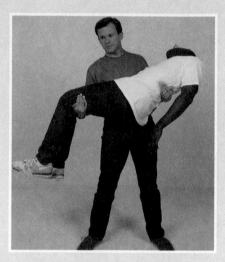

Cradle carry

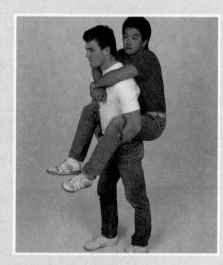

Piggyback carry

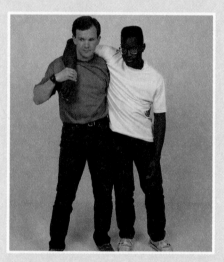

One-person assist

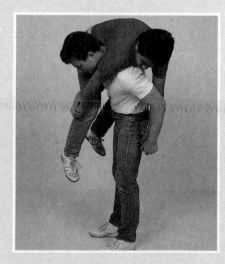

Fireman's carry

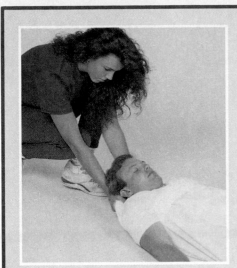

Sling drag

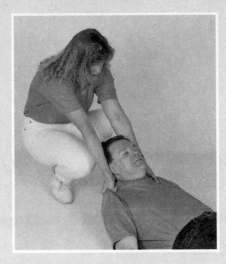

Clothing drag

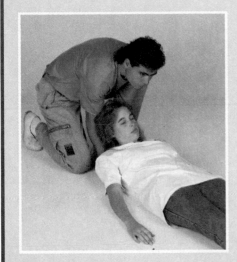

Shoulder drag

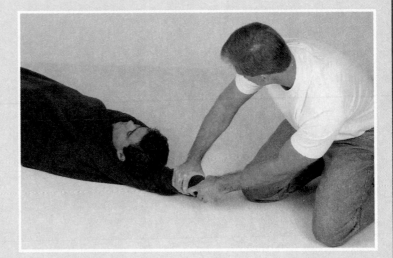

Blanket drag

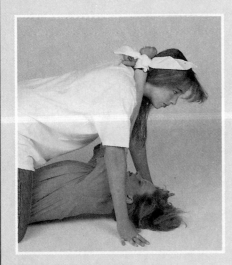

Fireman's drag

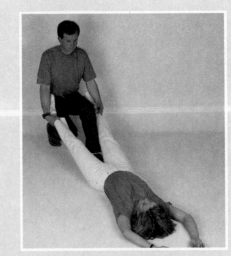

Ankle drag

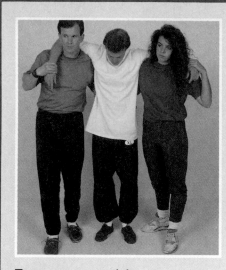

Two-person assist

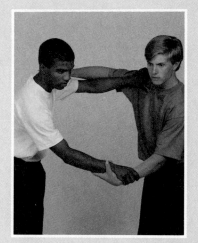

Extremity carry

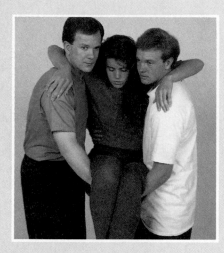

Two-handed seat carry

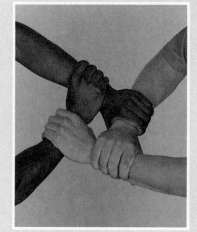

Four-handed grip

Two-handed grip

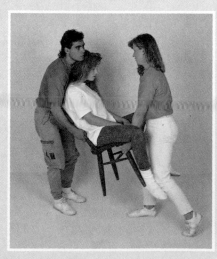

Chair carry

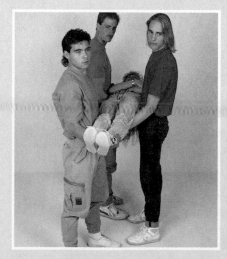

Hammock carry

of the material, tightly roll the sides snug against the victim, and use them for handholds to be carried by four or more people. Test the improvised stretcher before using.

Many improvised stretchers are not rigid enough to be used for victims needing CPR or those with potential spinal injuries. Whenever possible, moving seriously injured or ill victims should be left to trained EMS personnel.

Water Rescue

About 7,000 Americans die each year from drowning, making it the third leading cause of accidental death. Drowning statistics do not reflect the whole problem. An estimated 70,000 people are near-drowning victims each year. Even this figure does not give the entire picture because in many instances the victim recovers and the incident is not reported.

Since drowning situations seem to happen all the time, especially during the summer months, all adults and teenagers should be familiar with the basic rescue techniques available to poor swimmers or nonswimmers.

Types of Drowning

- **Dry drowning** Lungs have no water in them due to a laryngospasm; accounts for estimated 10 percent of drownings.

- **Wet drowning** Water is aspirated (lungs are wet with water); accounts for estimated 80–90 percent of drownings. Freshwater and saltwater have different effects on victim.
- **Hyperventilation drowning** Swimmers hyperventilate before entering the water for a long underwater swim. Hyperventilating lowers their carbon dioxide levels, which decreases the stimulus to breathe.
- **Immersion syndrome** Sudden death following contact with very cold water.
- **Post-immersion syndrome or secondary drowning syndrome** Affects adults following a submersion incident from hours to days after a near-drowning.

Reach-Throw-Row-Go

Reach-throw-row-go identifies the priority list for attempting a rescue.

Reach

The first and simplest rescue technique is the reach. This method is easily mastered, but it requires the ability to judge distance accurately and a lightweight pole, ladder, long stick, or any object that can be extended to the victim.

Once you have your "reacher," secure your footing. Also have a bystander grab your belt or pants for stability. Make sure you are secure before reaching down to assist the victim. Keep talking; this not only calms the victim, it helps you think through each step.

Typical Drowning Situations

Immediate Disappearance Syndrome

- Enters water but does not return to the surface
- Little chance to rescue
- Causes:
    1. Diving from height and striking head
    2. Hyperventilation before underwater swimming
    3. Cold-induced heart attack

Distressed Nonswimmer

- Struggles 20 to 60 seconds before sinking
- Signs of distress: flailing arms, head tilted back, no vocalizing, appears to be playing.

Sudden Disappearance Syndrome

- Fully clothed
- Apparently able to swim but fatigued and/or cold
- Disappears after 5 to 10 minutes on surface (Disappears after clothing loses entrapped air)

Hypothermia-Induced

- Seriously affected after about 15 minutes of cold water exposure
- Rule of 50s: Average unaware, unpracticed, and unprotected 50-year-old man would approach the 50/50 life/death point after 50 minutes of exposure to 50°F water.

Source: Adapted from David S. Smith, Ph.D.

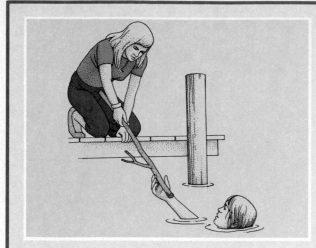

1. Reach the person from shore.

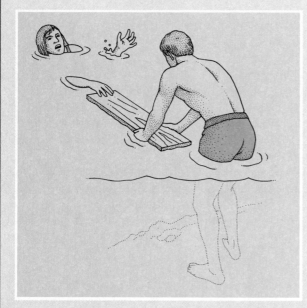

2. If you cannot reach the person from shore, wade closer.

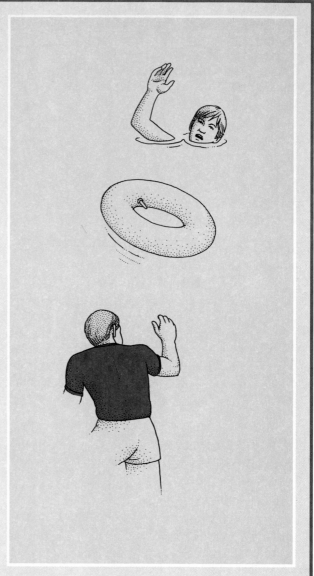

3. If an object that floats is available, throw it to the person.

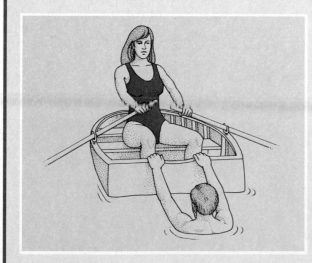

4. Use a boat if one is available.

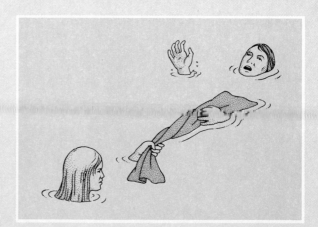

5. If you must swim to the person, use a towel or board for him or her to hold onto. Do not let the person grab you.

Throw

Throwing is another elementary rescue. It provides a maximum range of about fifty feet for the average untrained rescuer. You can throw anything that floats—objects such as empty fuel or paint cans, plastic containers, life jackets or floating cushions, short pieces of wood—whatever is available. If there is rope handy, tie it to the object to be thrown because you can retrieve it in case you miss.

Row

If the victim is beyond reach and you can find a nearby sailboard, boogie board, rowboat, canoe, or an outboard craft that can be started, you may attempt this form of rescue. Using these crafts requires skill only acquired through practice. In a life-or-death situation, however, even the inept use of these craft will be safer and faster than a swimming rescue. There is an element of danger for the rescuer that should be considered.

Craft powered by hand, paddle, or oar may be slower, but they are safer than a motor-driven craft with which you are unfamiliar. Inexperienced hands on a throttle are more dangerous than inexperienced hands on an oar.

If rowing out to a victim, align with an object on the shoreline and in line with the victim. Fix this in your memory. Since you must row facing the opposite direction, you will need to turn your head every five or so strokes to check on the victim and your position.

Upon reaching the victim, never attempt to pull the victim in over the sides of a boat but over the stern or rear end. The former method has been the cause of countless double drownings.

Go

If the previous "reach-throw-row" priorities are impossible to do, you must make an assessment, weighing the potential risk to yourself versus the reward to the victim. Entering even calm water to make a swimming rescue is difficult and hazardous. It takes skill, training, and excellent physical condition. All too frequently a would-be rescuer becomes a victim as well.

After the Rescue

Once the victim is out of the water, protect yourself and the victim against the cold. Get into dry clothing as soon as possible. Be prepared to administer mouth-to-mouth or CPR resuscitation. All rescued victims should be seen by a physician and hospitalized because victims can die of secondary complications a few minutes or up to 96 hours after the incident. Aspiration pneumonia is a late complication of near-drowning episodes, occurring after 48 to 72 hours have elapsed.

Ice Rescue

Attempt to reach the person from shore with a long object (e.g., a branch, a rope, or a board). If there is no equipment, form a human chain reaching from the shore. Lie flat to distribute the weight. Seek medical attention immediately for someone who has fallen through broken ice.

Underwater Duration

In 1986, two-year-old Michelle Funk of Salt Lake City, Utah, made a full recovery after spending 66 minutes underwater. The toddler fell into a swollen creek near her home while playing. When she was eventually discovered, rescue workers found she had no pulse or heartbeat. Her life was saved by the first successful bypass machine to warm blood, which had dropped to 66°F. Doctors at the hospital described the time she had spent underwater as the "longest documented submergence with an intact neurological outcome."

The record for voluntarily staying underwater is 13 minutes 42.5 seconds by Robert Foster, aged 32, of Richmond, California, who stayed under 10 feet of water in a swimming pool in San Rafael, California on March 15, 1959. He hyperventilated with oxygen for 30 minutes before his descent. *It must be stressed that record-breaking of this kind is extremely dangerous.*

—Guinness Book of World Records

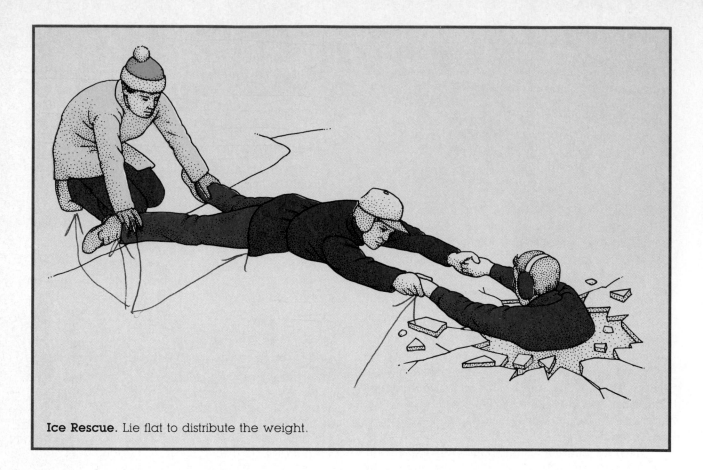

Ice Rescue. Lie flat to distribute the weight.

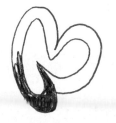

Appendix A
Atlas of the Human Body

1 Skeleton
Front and side view
Skull

2 Spinal Column
Lumbar vertebra
Cervical spine

3 Muscular System
Front and back view

4 Circulatory System
Arteries and major veins
Heart

5 Nervous System
Major nerves
Brain and Spinal Cord

6 Respiratory System

7 Digestive System

8 Endocrine System

9 Urinary System
Kidney (cross section)

10 Reproductive System
Male and Female

11 Skin / Teeth

1 Skeleton

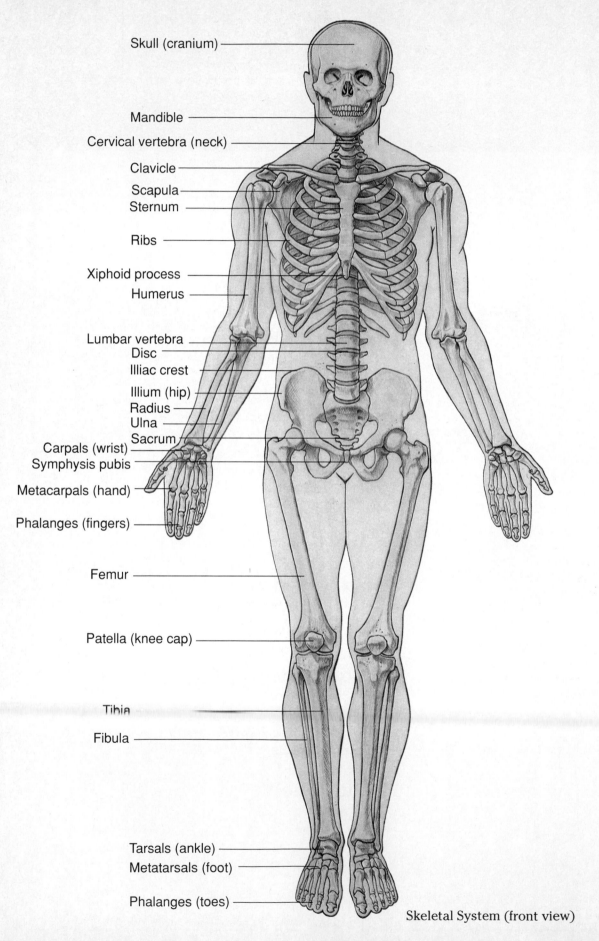

Skull (cranium)

Mandible

Cervical vertebra (neck)

Clavicle

Scapula

Sternum

Ribs

Xiphoid process

Humerus

Lumbar vertebra

Disc

Illiac crest

Illium (hip)

Radius

Ulna

Sacrum

Carpals (wrist)

Symphysis pubis

Metacarpals (hand)

Phalanges (fingers)

Femur

Patella (knee cap)

Tibia

Fibula

Tarsals (ankle)

Metatarsals (foot)

Phalanges (toes)

Skeletal System (front view)

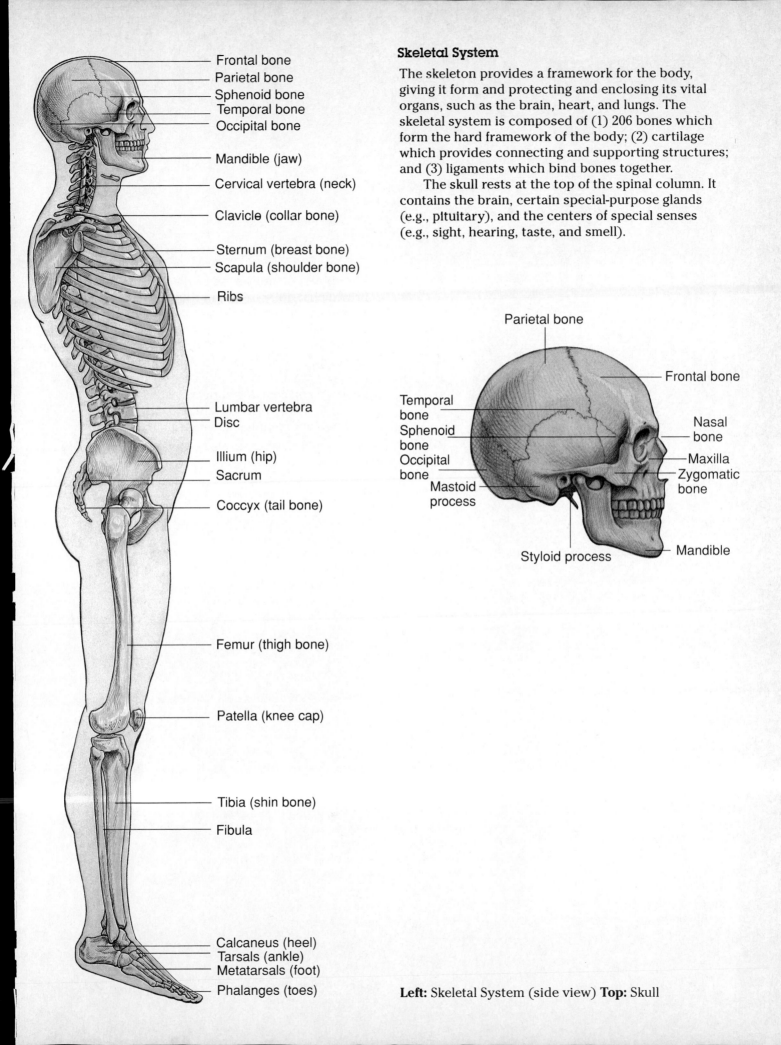

Frontal bone
Parietal bone
Sphenoid bone
Temporal bone
Occipital bone

Mandible (jaw)

Cervical vertebra (neck)

Clavicle (collar bone)

Sternum (breast bone)
Scapula (shoulder bone)

Ribs

Lumbar vertebra
Disc

Illium (hip)
Sacrum

Coccyx (tail bone)

Femur (thigh bone)

Patella (knee cap)

Tibia (shin bone)

Fibula

Calcaneus (heel)
Tarsals (ankle)
Metatarsals (foot)
Phalanges (toes)

Skeletal System

The skeleton provides a framework for the body, giving it form and protecting and enclosing its vital organs, such as the brain, heart, and lungs. The skeletal system is composed of (1) 206 bones which form the hard framework of the body; (2) cartilage which provides connecting and supporting structures; and (3) ligaments which bind bones together.

The skull rests at the top of the spinal column. It contains the brain, certain special-purpose glands (e.g., pituitary), and the centers of special senses (e.g., sight, hearing, taste, and smell).

Parietal bone

Frontal bone

Temporal bone
Sphenoid bone
Occipital bone

Nasal bone

Maxilla
Zygomatic bone

Mastoid process

Styloid process

Mandible

Left: Skeletal System (side view) **Top:** Skull

2 Spinal Column

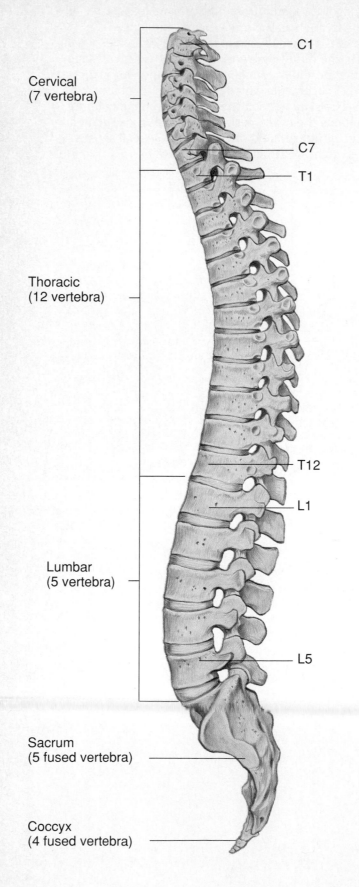

Cervical
(7 vertebra)

C1

C7

T1

Thoracic
(12 vertebra)

T12

L1

Lumbar
(5 vertebra)

L5

Sacrum
(5 fused vertebra)

Coccyx
(4 fused vertebra)

The spinal column serves as the main axis of the body, providing rigidity but permitting some degree of movement. It also serves as a protective case, enclosing the spinal cord and the roots of the spinal nerves. The spinal column includes 33 bones, called vertebra. Lying one on top of the other to form a strong flexible column, the vertebra are bound together by strong ligaments. Between adjacent vertebra are pads of tough elastic cartilage. These intervertebral disks cushion the vertebra and permit some motion in the spine

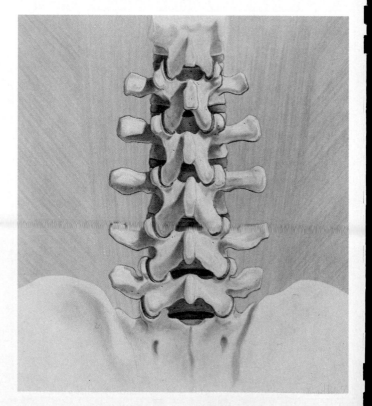

Left: Spinal column (regions) **Above:** Lumbar vertebra (back view)

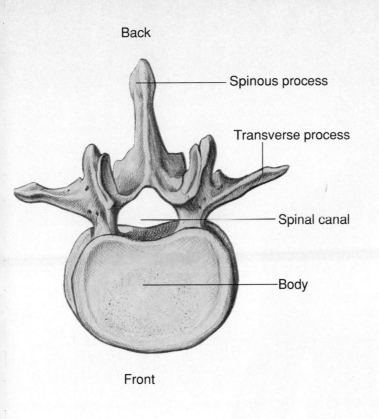

Back

Spinous process

Transverse process

Spinal canal

Body

Front

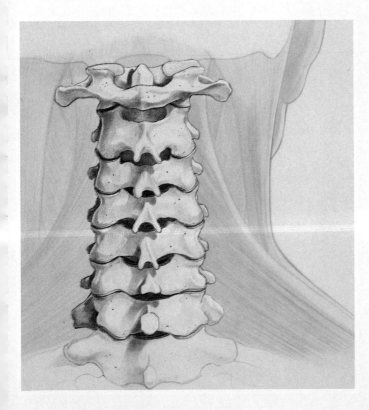

Top: A typical vertebra, second lumbar, (top view)
Bottom: Cervical spine (back view)

3 Muscular System

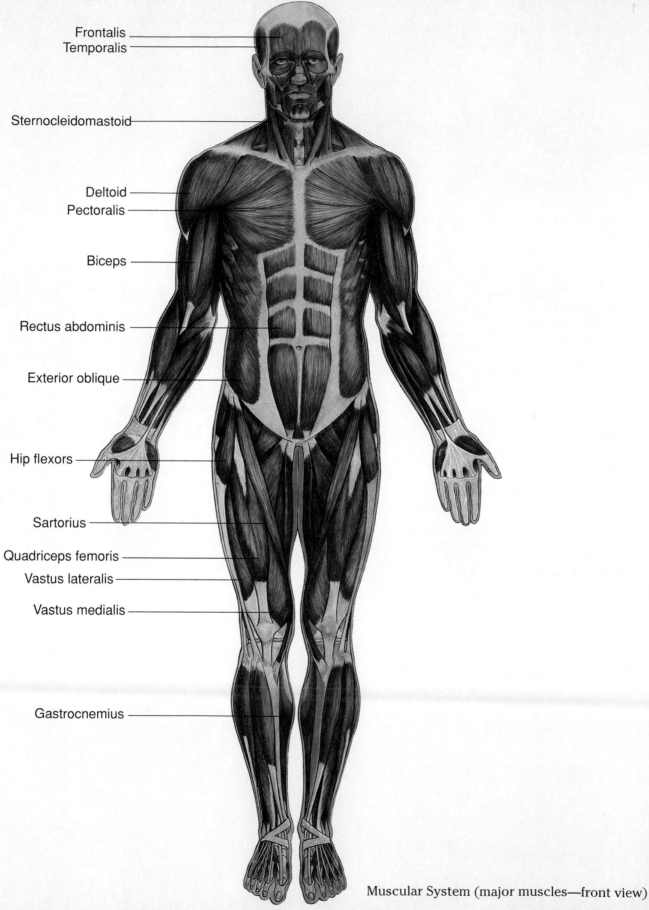

Frontalis
Temporalis
Sternocleidomastoid
Deltoid
Pectoralis
Biceps
Rectus abdominis
Exterior oblique
Hip flexors
Sartorius
Quadriceps femoris
Vastus lateralis
Vastus medialis
Gastrocnemius

Muscular System (major muscles—front view)

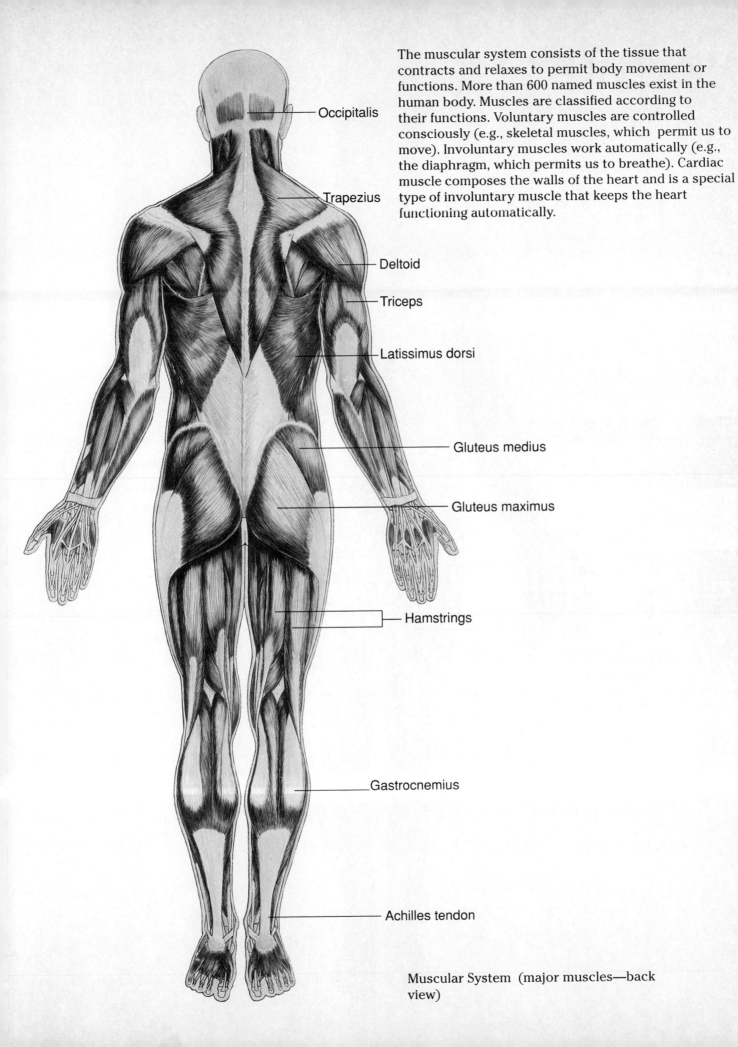

The muscular system consists of the tissue that contracts and relaxes to permit body movement or functions. More than 600 named muscles exist in the human body. Muscles are classified according to their functions. Voluntary muscles are controlled consciously (e.g., skeletal muscles, which permit us to move). Involuntary muscles work automatically (e.g., the diaphragm, which permits us to breathe). Cardiac muscle composes the walls of the heart and is a special type of involuntary muscle that keeps the heart functioning automatically.

Occipitalis

Trapezius

Deltoid

Triceps

Latissimus dorsi

Gluteus medius

Gluteus maximus

Hamstrings

Gastrocnemius

Achilles tendon

Muscular System (major muscles—back view)

4 Circulatory System

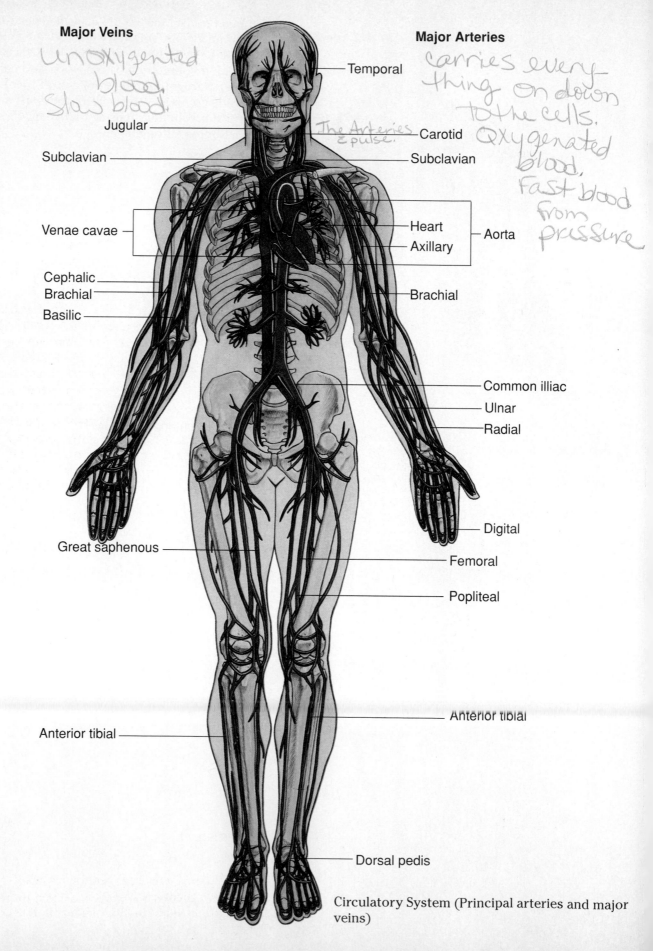

Major Veins

Unoxygenated blood, Slow blood.

- Jugular
- Subclavian
- Venae cavae
- Cephalic
- Brachial
- Basilic
- Great saphenous
- Anterior tibial

Major Arteries

carries everything on down to the cells. Oxygenated blood, Fast blood from pressure

The Arteries & pulse.

- Temporal
- Carotid
- Subclavian
- Heart
- Axillary
- Aorta
- Brachial
- Common illiac
- Ulnar
- Radial
- Digital
- Femoral
- Popliteal
- Anterior tibial
- Dorsal pedis

Circulatory System (Principal arteries and major veins)

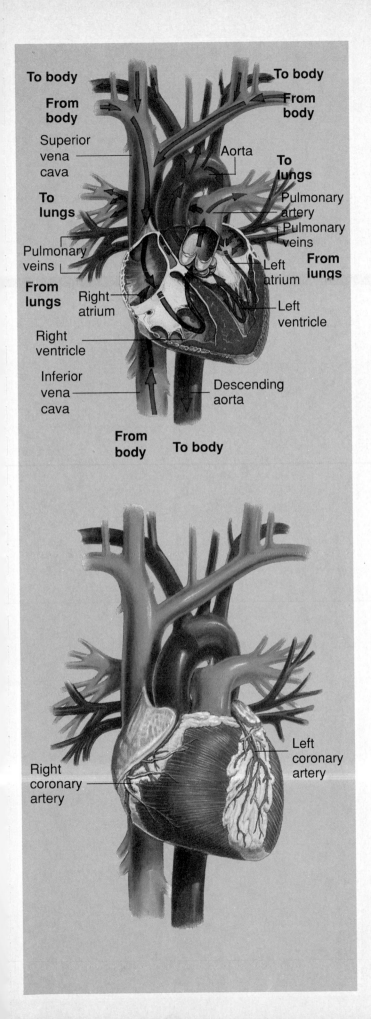

To body

From body

Superior vena cava

To lungs

Aorta

To lungs

Pulmonary artery

Pulmonary veins

Pulmonary veins

From lungs

Left atrium

From lungs

Right atrium

Left ventricle

Right ventricle

Inferior vena cava

Descending aorta

From body

To body

To body

From body

Right coronary artery

Left coronary artery

Circulatory System

The circulatory system consists of the heart, some 60,000 miles of blood vessels of various sizes, about six quarts of blood, and a series of tubes that carry blood throughout the body. The tubes include (1) arteries which carry blood rich in oxygen and other materials **to** other body cells; (2) veins, which carry deoxygenated blood and waste products **from** the body cells; and (3) capillaries through which oxygenated and deoxygenated blood are exchanged with the body cells.

The Heart

The heart is a muscular hollow organ about the size of a clenched fist that pumps blood throughout the body. The heart is located in the chest cavity under the sternum and the lungs. A wall divides the heart into two upper chambers (atriums) and two lower chambers (ventricles).

The heart is a two sided pump. The left side of the heart receives oxygenated blood from the lungs and pumps it out to all body parts through a system of arteries . The right side of the heart receives from the veins blood that has circulated through the body and pumps it to the lungs to be reoxygenated. A system of one-way valves keeps blood moving in the proper direction and prevents backflow of the blood.

Two coronary arteries carry oxygenated blood from the aorta. These form a branching network over the surface of the heart and supply it with the nutrient-rich blood it needs to function. A "heart attack" occurs when a branch of a coronary artery becomes obstructed.

Top: the heart in cross section showing circulation. Arrows indicate direction of blood flow. **Bottom:** exterior view of the heart showing the coronary arteries

5 Nervous System

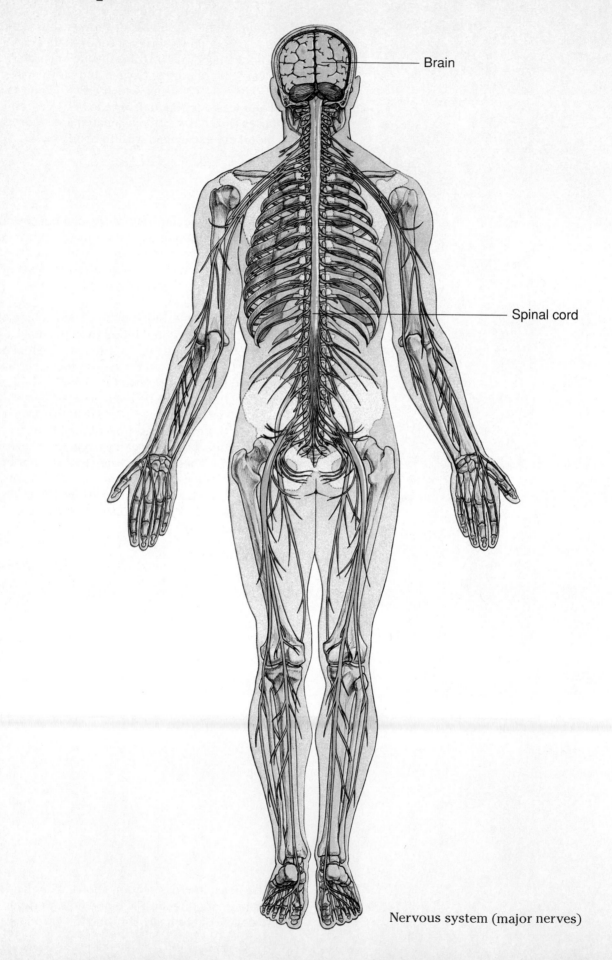

Brain

Spinal cord

Nervous system (major nerves)

Nervous System

The nervous system functions as the body's master control system, continually gathering information about the internal and external environment and relaying appropriate directions to the muscles and glands. The nervous system is divided structurally into two parts: the central nervous system (including the brain and spinal cord) and the peripheral nervous system (containing the sensory and motor nerves).

The nervous system consists of the brain, spinal cord, and nerves that control and permit all body activities and sensations. A muscle will not move if the nerves that serve it are cut.

The Brain

The brain is the controlling organ of the body and the center of consciousness. It occupies the entire space within the cranium. Each type of brain cell has a specific function, and certain parts of the brain perform certain functions.

Spinal Cord

The spinal cord consists of long tracts of nerves that join the brain with all body organs and parts. It is protected by the spinal column.

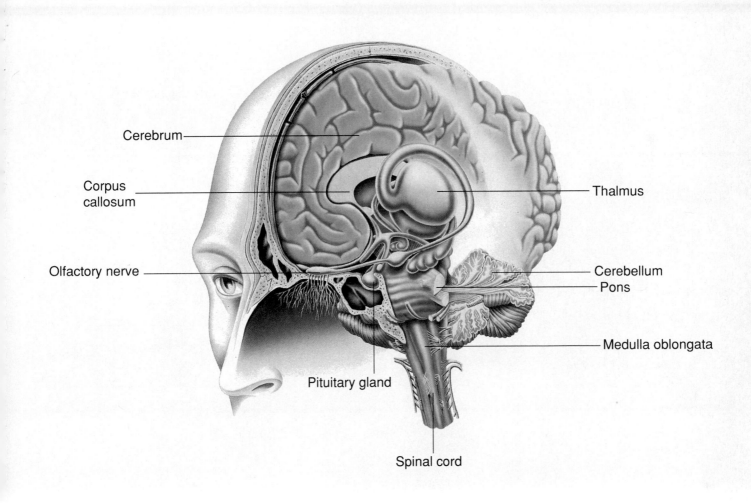

Cerebrum

Corpus callosum

Olfactory nerve

Pituitary gland

Thalmus

Cerebellum
Pons

Medulla oblongata

Spinal cord

6 Respiratory System

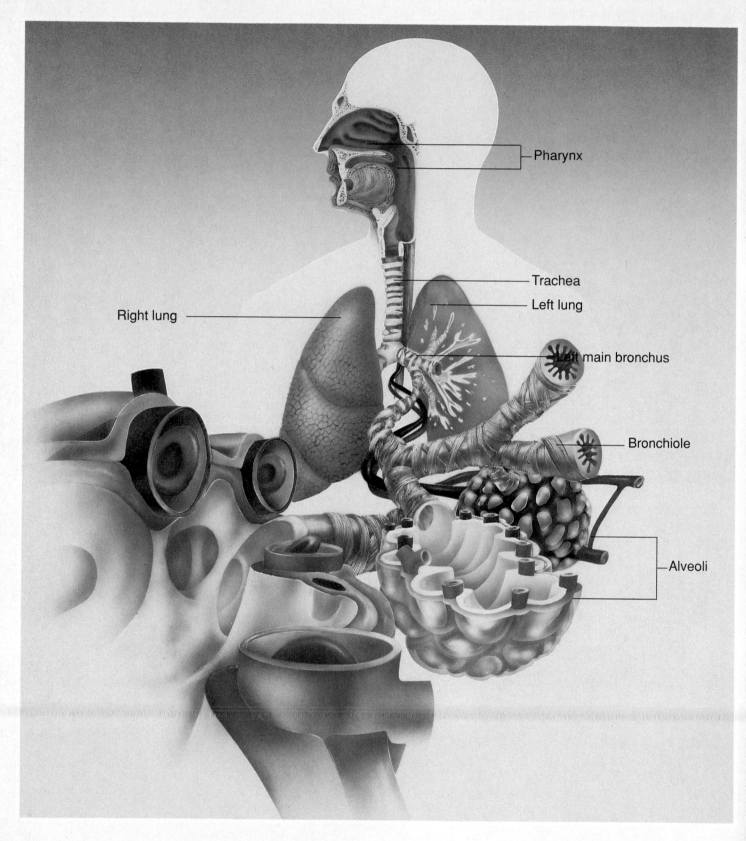

Pharynx

Trachea

Left lung

Right lung

Left main bronchus

Bronchiole

Alveoli

Respiratory System

The respiratory system consists of the organs of the body that enable breathing. It provides for the intake of oxygen needed by the body 5nd the release of carbon dioxide and other substances.

7 Digestive System

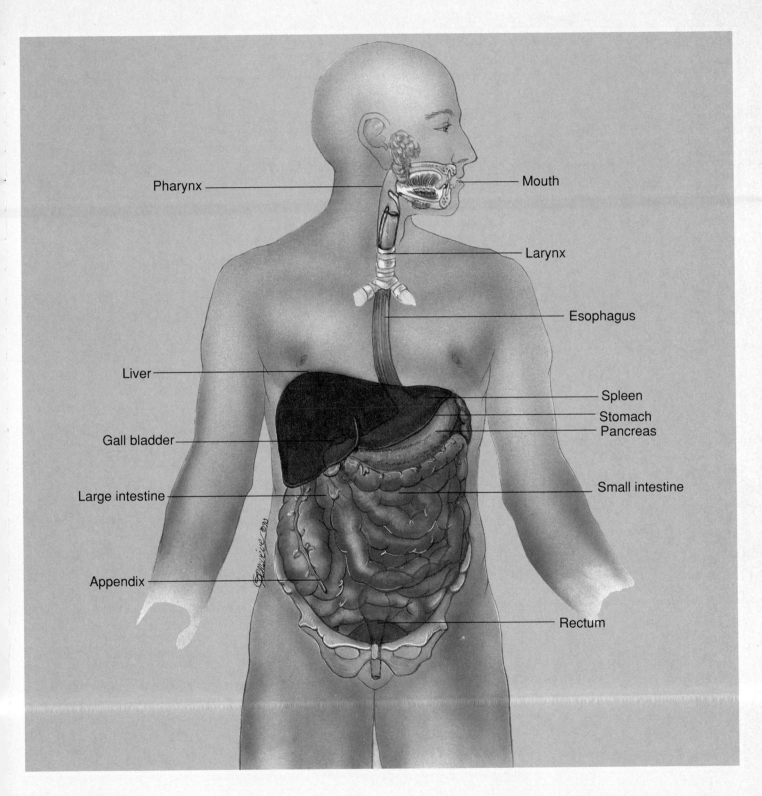

Pharynx

Mouth

Larynx

Esophagus

Liver

Spleen

Stomach

Pancreas

Gall bladder

Large intestine

Small intestine

Appendix

Rectum

Digestive System

The digestive system consists of the organs that enable us to eat, digest, and eliminate foods. It's one long tube (more than 30 feet) that extends from the mouth to the anus. Its various bulges, turns, and regions have special names, such as "stomach." It has muscular mechanisms that propel materials along its course and valves that regulate delivery of partially processed materials at different points in the tube. Here and there, chemicals produced by specialized tissues are introduced through connecting tubes or surfaces. Digestion is a process of continuous chemical simplification of materials that enter via the mouth. Materials are split into smaller and simpler chemical fragments which can then be absorbed through the walls of the tract and thus, finally, into the body.

8 Endocrine System

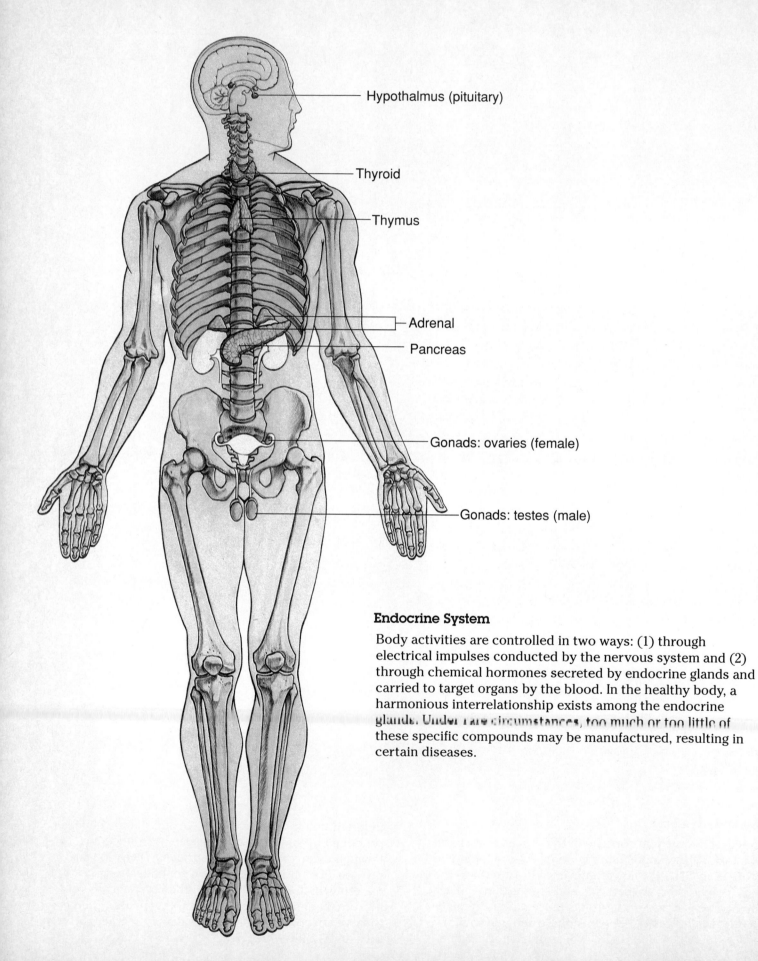

Hypothalmus (pituitary)

Thyroid

Thymus

Adrenal

Pancreas

Gonads: ovaries (female)

Gonads: testes (male)

Endocrine System

Body activities are controlled in two ways: (1) through electrical impulses conducted by the nervous system and (2) through chemical hormones secreted by endocrine glands and carried to target organs by the blood. In the healthy body, a harmonious interrelationship exists among the endocrine glands. Under rare circumstances, too much or too little of these specific compounds may be manufactured, resulting in certain diseases.

9 Urinary System

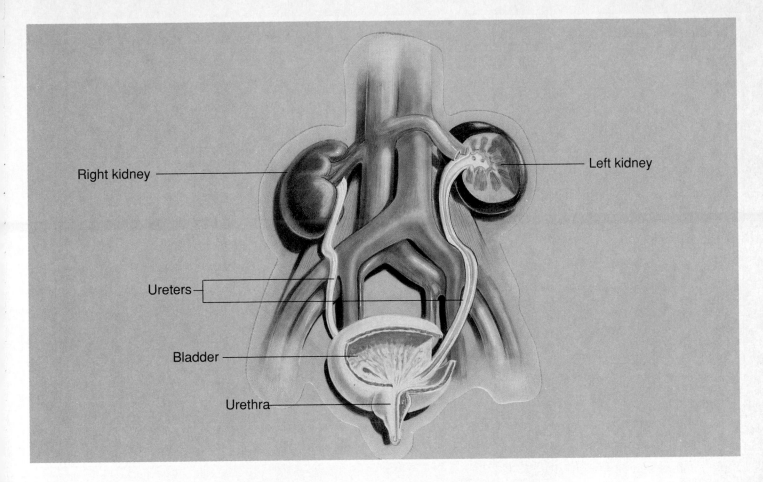

Right kidney

Left kidney

Ureters

Bladder

Urethra

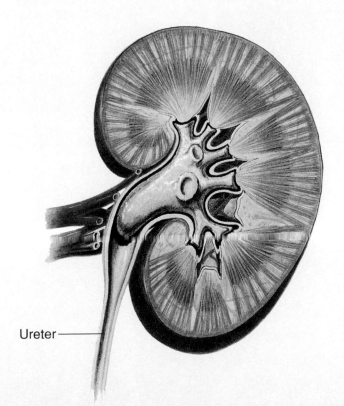

Ureter

Urinary System

The urinary system consists of the organs that enable us to eliminate waste materials filtered from the blood, in the form of urine.

Above: A cross-section of a kidney.

10 Reproductive System

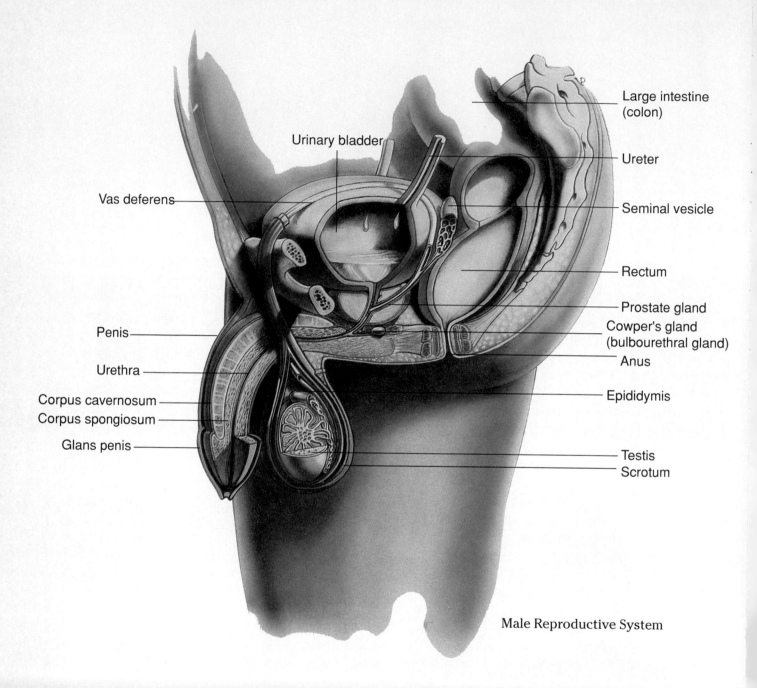

Large intestine (colon)

Urinary bladder

Ureter

Vas deferens

Seminal vesicle

Rectum

Prostate gland

Penis

Cowper's gland (bulbourethral gland)

Anus

Urethra

Corpus cavernosum

Epididymis

Corpus spongiosum

Glans penis

Testis

Scrotum

Male Reproductive System

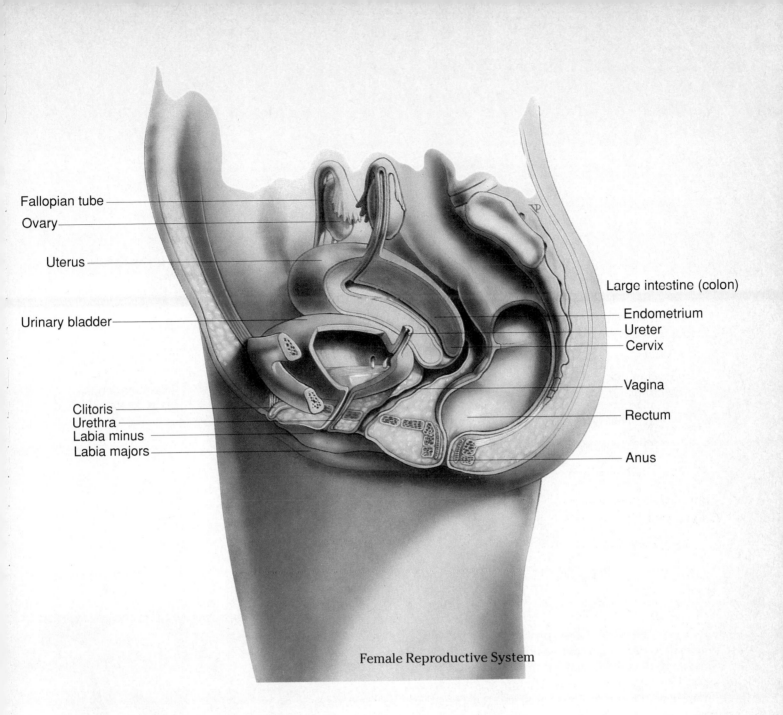

Fallopian tube

Ovary

Uterus

Urinary bladder

Clitoris
Urethra
Labia minus
Labia majors

Large intestine (colon)

Endometrium
Ureter
Cervix

Vagina

Rectum

Anus

Female Reproductive System

Reproductive System

The reproductive system is made up of glands, organs,
and supporting structures involved with human
sexuality and procreation. The male produces
spermotazoa and the hormone testosterone in the
testes. The female produces ova (eggs) and the
hormones estrogen and progesterone in her ovaries. A
single cell called a zygote is formed from the union of
ovum and sperm. The new individual develops and
matures through growth, cell division, and cellular
differentiation (specialized cell formation).

11 Skin / Teeth

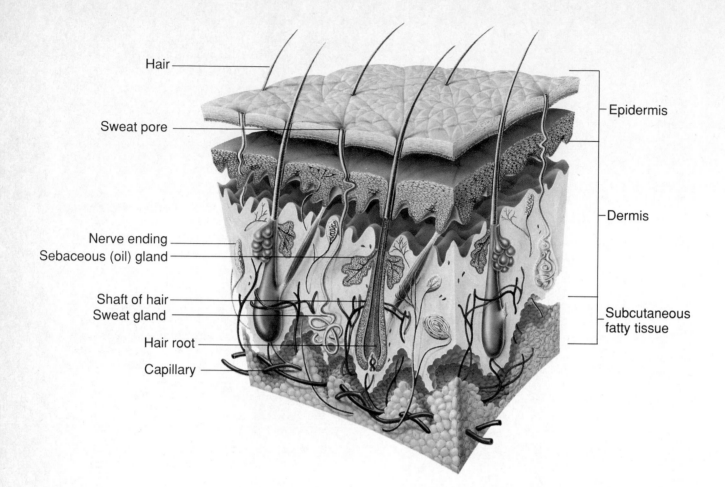

Hair
Sweat pore
Nerve ending
Sebaceous (oil) gland
Shaft of hair
Sweat gland
Hair root
Capillary

Epidermis
Dermis
Subcutaneous fatty tissue

The Skin

The skin covers the whole body, protecting its tissues from injury, dehydration, and invasion by bacteria and other foreign bodies. It consists of the dermis and epidermis. The skin helps to regulate body temperature and eliminate water and various salts, and it acts as the receptor organ for touch, pain, heat, and cold.

Teeth

Teeth break the food eaten into pieces that can be easily swallowed and digested. They help one's personal appearance and are important for proper speech.

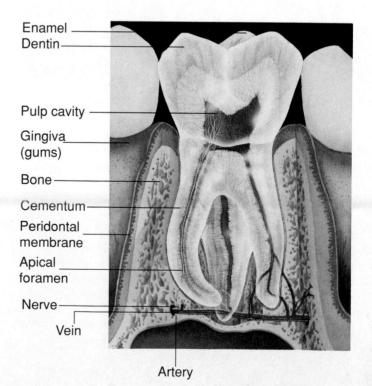

Enamel
Dentin
Pulp cavity
Gingiva (gums)
Bone
Cementum
Peridontal membrane
Apical foramen
Nerve
Vein
Artery

Medicine Chest and First Aid Supplies

Medicine Chest

It is a good idea to have useful medical supplies on hand for emergencies and to treat minor ills, but the family medicine chest does not have to be a minidrugstore. What should be kept in the average household depends on the makeup of the family.

Generally, medicine chests should include only those health care products likely to be used on a regular basis. A person rarely bothered by constipation, for instance, would have little need for a laxative.

Some drug products lose their potency on the shelf in time, especially after they are opened. Other drugs change in consistency. Milk of magnesia, for instance, dries out if it remains on the shelf for a while after opening. Buying the large "family size" of a product infrequently used may seem like a bargain, but it is poor economy if it has to be thrown out before the contents are used up. Ideally, supplies in the medicine chest should be bought to last over a period of no more than twelve months.

Obviously, selecting health care items for the family medicine chest is a matter of common sense. Here are some suggested items that will meet the needs of most families:

Nondrug Products

Adhesive bandages of assorted sizes
Sterile gauze in pads and a roll
Absorbent cotton
Adhesive tape
Elastic bandage
Small blunt-end scissors
Tweezers
Fever thermometer, including rectal type for young child
Hot water bottle
Heating pad
Ice bag
Dosage spoon (common household teaspoons are rarely the correct dosage size)
Vaporizer or humidifier

Drug Items

Analgesic (aspirin and/or acetaminophen. Both reduce fever and relieve pain, but only aspirin can reduce inflammation.)
Emetic (syrup of ipecac to induce vomiting and activated charcoal. Read the instructions on how to use these products.)
Antacid
Antiseptic solution—rubbing alcohol
Hydrocortisone creams for skin problems
Calamine for poison ivy and other skin irritations
Petroleum jelly as a lubricant
Antidiarrheic
Cough syrup (suppressant type)
Decongestant
Antibacterial topical ointment
Seasonal items (e.g., insect repellents and sunscreens)

When it comes to storing these health care items, the cardinal rule is to keep all medicines out of the reach of children. In addition, be sure all medications have child-resistant caps. Elderly people who have difficulty opening such caps can ask the pharmacist for caps with regular closure. However, they should be extra careful to see that young visitors cannot get to these drugs.

Both prescription and nonprescription drugs should be kept in a cool, dry place away from foods and other household products. Some drugs may require refrigeration. This should be indicated on the label. If in doubt, ask the pharmacist.

Many people keep medicines on a high shelf in a hall or bedroom closet. Some experts suggest using a locking box. A tackle box might do. A word of warning, however: Be sure all responsible adults in the family know where the key is kept.

To avoid confusion keep prescription and nonprescription drugs in separate boxes clearly labeled to distinguish one type of drug from another. A list of what is in each box, attached to the outside if possible, will make it easier to find specific items, particularly in an emergency.

The medicine chest should be checked periodically to be sure supplies are adequate and to get rid of drugs that may have gone bad or become outdated. Many drug labels have an expiration date beyond which the product should not be used. If there is no date, put a label on the container with the date of purchase and the date it was first opened. Then, if there are any questions in the future, a pharmacist can tell whether the product is safe to use.

Tablets that have become crumbly and medicines that have changed color, odor, or consistency, or are outdated should be destroyed. Empty the bottle of medicine into the toilet, flush it down, and rinse out the bottle. Do not put leftover drugs in the trash basket, where they can be dug out by inquisitive youngsters. Newly purchased drug products that do not look right should be returned to the pharmacy. Drug products that have lost their labels should also be destroyed.

Keep the telephone numbers of the local poison control center, physician, hospital, rescue squad, and fire and police departments near every phone in the house. Tape the emergency phone list inside the bathroom medicine cabinet door, and also keep it with the emergency supplies.

Each family's medicine chest is bound to contain some different items. For help in selecting appropriate health care products, check with a physician and a pharmacist.

First Aid Supplies

Activated charcoal
Adhesive strip bandages, assorted sizes
Adhesive tape, 1- and 2-inch rolls
Alcohol (70 percent)
Alcohol wipes
Antimicrobial skin ointment
Baking soda
Calamine lotion
Cotton balls
Elastic bandages, 2- and 3-inch widths
Face mask with one-way valve
Epsom salts
Flashlight and extra batteries
Gauze pads, 2 × 2 and 4 × 4 inches
Hot-water bottle
Ice bag (plastic)
Latex or vinyl gloves
Matches

Measuring cup and spoons
Needles
Paper and pencil
Paper drinking cups
Roller, self-adhering gauze, 2- to 4-inch widths
Safety pins, various sizes
Salt
Scissors
Sugar
Syrup of ipecac
Telfa pads, 3 × 4 inch
Thermometer—1 oral, 1 rectal
Triangular bandages, 2 or 3
Tweezers

These items can be placed in a fishing tackle box for storage and transporting.

Common Complaints

Abdomen Pain

Many disorders cause abdominal pain. It will be neither feasible nor useful to distinguish among the many causes of abdominal pain here because, in general, first aid will be similar regardless of the cause.

To assess abdominal pain determine the following:

- Location of the pain
- Quality of the pain (Constant abdominal pain suggests inflammation; intermittent cramping suggests obstruction of a hollow organ.)
- Duration of the pain
- Intensity of the pain
- Nature of onset (sudden or gradual onset of pain)
- Change in bowel habits

The victim can tell you where the pain is. First examine the other three quadrants, so that any pain you elicit from the trouble spot does not tighten the rest of the abdominal muscles. Except for examining the painful area last, the order in which the quadrants are examined is not important.

Help the victim relax by explaining what you are doing. If possible, have him or her urinate before the examination. Ask the victim to remove all clothing from the abdomen. Then place the victim comfortably on his or her back, knees bent and arms at the sides to keep the abdominal muscles from tensing. Your hands should be warm; keep the victim covered and warm except for the part you are examining.

Use light pressing or palpation. In light palpation, use the fingertips to depress the abdominal wall a little more than a half inch. Light palpation will reveal large masses and tender areas. This type of palpation will cause guarding of the abdominal wall when a sensitive area is reached. Most victims will guard (hold the abdominal muscle tight and/or cover the area with their hands) when a sensitive area is reached. First aiders should perform only light palpations.

Do *not* evaluate the abdomen extensively. Extensive palpation is of little value, will delay transportation, and may cause unnecessary pain.

First Aid

The acute abdomen may require surgery, although some acute abdomens may be treated medically. In either case, seek immediate medical attention.

- Do *not* give anything to eat or drink. Food or fluid can aggravate many of the symptoms. If emergency surgery is needed, food in the stomach will make the surgery more dangerous. In some cases, food will not have passed out of the stomach and will only increase the likelihood of vomiting.
- Do *not* give any pain medication. Pain medication will hide the symptoms and delay the diagnosis by a physician.
- Do *not* give an enema or a laxative; they may cause the appendix to rupture.
- Recognize the possibility of vomiting and be prepared for it by transporting the victim on his or her side so that any vomitus can quickly drain or be cleansed from the mouth.
- Keep the victim in a comfortable position, usually with knees bent.
- Do *not* waste time palpating the abdomen extensively.
- Save any stool, urine, or vomitus so it can be tested at the hospital for the presence of blood or poison.
- Do *not* attempt to diagnose the victim's condition.
- Seek medical attention if any of these occur:
  1. Severe abdominal pain that lasts more than 24 hours.
  2. Abdominal injury
  3. Vomiting
  4. Black or bloody stool

Constipation

Constipation is the passage of hard, dry stools or none at all. It is seldom a serious condition, although it may be very painful. Most cases respond well to diet changes or bowel movement habits.

First Aid

- Drink extra glasses of water, especially in the morning.
- Avoid laxatives; eat more fiber.
- Seek medical attention if any of these occur:
  1. Condition persists after treatment for three days (infants), seven days (adults).
  2. Dark blood is seen in stools.

Cough

There are two types of coughs. One is the dry, irritative, nonproductive cough (produces no mucus or phlegm to spit out). The other is the loose, productive cough (produces large amounts of secretions that can be spit out).

First Aid

- Nonmedical cough remedies include sucking on hard candy to increase the flow of saliva, drinking liquids to keep the throat moist, and breathing steam from a vaporizer or hot shower to loosen secretions.
- For an annoying, exhausting cough, consider using a nonprescription, medicine containing dextromethorphan, which acts on the cough center in the brain. Do *not* use it to control a productive cough; do *not* use for more than three consecutive days.
- Seek medical attention if coughing lasts for more than five days without improvement or is accompanied by high fever, rash, or persistent headache.

Diarrhea

Most diarrhea is caused by a stomach virus that overstimulates the intestines to empty themselves and push the stools through before water can be reabsorbed by the intestines. The body becomes dehydrated when a large amount of fluid is lost and not replaced. Adult diarrhea is often caused by stress or emotional problems.

First Aid

- Avoid solid foods for one day.
- Add mild foods the next day (e.g., banana, rice, applesauce).
- Replace lost fluids.
- Seek medical attention if any of these occur:
  1. Severe abdominal pain or cramps

2. No improvement after 24 hours
3. Mild diarrhea lasting more than one week
4. Black or bloody stools
5. No urine for more than eight hours

Earache

Earache, or inflammation of the middle ear, is common in children and youth, but it may happen in people of all ages.

First Aid

- Apply heat by placing a warm washcloth or a heating pad on the ear.
- Take oral nasal decongestant.
- Use nasal decongestant spray for no more than three days.
- Increase humidity by using a humidifier.
- Chew gum to relieve pain from pressure.
- Seek medical attention if any of these occur:
  1. Severe pain lasts more than one hour.
  2. Temperature rises above 102°F.
  3. Eardrum ruptures.

Fever

Unless it is very high, a fever is not to be feared. It is not a disease, simply a sign—a warning sign—that something is wrong with the body. A fever may even serve a useful purpose by fighting an infection.

First Aid

- Keep room at a moderate temperature and bed coverings to a minimum.
- Sponge with lukewarm water, which increases heat loss through evaporation.
- Increase fluid intake.
- Seek medical attention if any of these occur:
  1. Child with fever over 101°F
  2. Older children and adults with fever over 102°F
  3. Fever persists or recurs for more than three days.
  4. Seizures
  5. Vomiting
  6. Heat stroke

Headache

When the muscles of the head or neck become tense, blood vessels of the head go into spasm. These headaches can be very painful and last for hours or even days. Most headaches are minor and will go away in time.

First Aid

- Use aspirin or acetaminophen as needed.
- Massage scalp and neck muscles.
- Apply heat or take a hot shower.
- Lie down with cool cloth on forehead.
- Seek medical attention if any of these occur:
    1. Severe pain not relieved by pain depressant
    2. Fever
    3. Visual problems
    4. Pain related to bending head forward; stiff neck
    5. More than three to five headaches per week

Sore Throat

Most sore throats are minor. However, those caused by bacteria are known as strep throats and should be medically treated with an antibiotic. The only way to accurately determine a strep throat is by taking a throat culture. If a strep infection is not treated with antibiotics for 10 days, complications such as rheumatic fever or kidney inflammation may result.

First Aid

- Use a humidifier
- Gargle with hot saltwater (one teaspoonful in eight ounces of water) or with commercial mouthwash every two hours
- Suck cough drops, hard candy, or honey
- Drink more fluids
- Take a pain reliever (aspirin or acetaminophen) for severe discomfort.
- Seek medical attention if any of these occur:
    1. Exposure to someone with strep throat

2. Soreness that lasts more than three days or after treatment (four days in adults)
3. Throat that is bright red or has white spots or pus on it
4. Fever of 102°F
5. Skin rash

Vomiting

A forceful, active oral explusion of stomach contents, vomiting is usually a sign of a viral infection of the stomach and intestine, excessive drinking of alcohol, or emotional upsets.

Dehydration is a threat. Signs of dehydration include thirst, dark yellow urine, dry mouth, sunken eyes, and skin that has lost its elasticity (pinched skin should normally spring back immediately).

First Aid

- Do *not* eat or drink anything for four hours.
- Drink clear liquids (apple juice, ginger ale) during next 20 hours.
- When vomiting stops, take soups, mild foods, and liquids on second day.
- Rest in bed.
- Seek medical attention if any of these occur:
    1. Severe vomiting (ejected in large amounts)
    2. Vomiting that continues after 12 hours of treatment
    3. Signs of dehydration
    4. Blood or dark, coffee-groundlike material in vomit
    5. Severe or constant abdominal pain
    6. Vomiting that occurs after a recent head injury
    7. Vomit that is yellow or green on several occasions
    8. Fever and dizziness

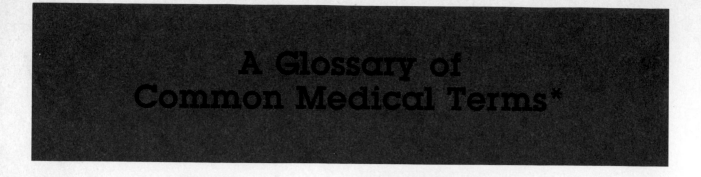

A Glossary of
Common Medical Terms*

A

abandonment: A termination of a helping relationship by a first aider without consent of the victim and without replacement care to the victim by qualified medical personnel.

ABC's: Airway, Breathing and Circulation; the first three steps in the examination of any victim; basic life support.

abdomen: The large body cavity below the diaphragm and above the pelvis.

abnormal: Not normal; malformed.

abrasion: An injury consisting of the loss of a partial thickness of skin from rubbing or scraping on a hard, rough surface; also called a brush burn, friction burn.

acetone: A chemical compound found normally in small amounts in the urine; diabetic victims are said to produce a fruity odor when larger amounts are produced in blood and urine.

activated charcoal: Powdered charcoal that has been treated to increase its powers of absorption; used in a slurry to absorb ingested poison.

acute: Having rapid onset, severe symptoms, and a relatively short duration.

acute abdomen: A serious intra-abdominal condition causing irration or inflammation of the peritoneum, attended by pain, tenderness, and muscular rigidity (boardlike abdomen).

acute myocardial infarction: The acute phase of a heart attack wherein a spasm or blockage of a coronary artery produces a spectrum of signs and symptoms, commonly including chest pain, nausea, diaphoresis, anxiety, pallor, and lassitude.

Adam's apple: The projection on the anterior surface of the neck, formed by the thyroid cartilage of the larynx.

addiction: The state of being strongly dependent upon some agent; drugs or tobacco, for example.

adjunct: An accessory or auxiliary agent or measure; an oropharyngeal airway is an airway management adjunct.

adrenalin: The proprietary name for epinephrine.

afterbirth: The placenta and membranes expelled after the birth of a child.

air: The gaseous mixture which composes the Earth's atmosphere; composed of approximately 21 percent oxygen, 79 percent nitrogen, plus trace gases.

air embolism: The presence of air bubbles in the heart or blood vessels, causing an obstruction.

air splint: A double-walled plastic tube that immobilizes a limb when sufficient air is blown into the space between the walls of the tube to cause it to become almost rigid.

airway: An air passage.

allergic reaction: A local or general reaction to an allergen, usually characterized by hives or tissue swelling or dyspnea.

allergy: Hypersensitivity to a substance, causing an abnormal reaction.

AMI: Abbreviation for acute myocardial infarction.

amnesia: Loss or impairment of memory.

amniotic fluid: The fluid surrounding the fetus in the uterus, contained in the amniotic sac.

amniotic sac: A thick, transparent sac that holds the fetus suspended in the amniotic fluid.

amputation: Complete removal of an appendage.

analgesic: A pain-relieving drug; a class of drugs used to reduce pain.

anaphylaxis: An exaggerated allergic reaction, usually caused by foreign proteins.

anatomic position: The presumed body position when referring to anatomical landmarks; upright, facing the observer, with hands and arms at sides, thumbs pointing away from the body, legs and feet pointing straight ahead.

anesthesia: A partial or complete loss of sensation with or without loss of consciousness; can result from drug administration or from injury or disease.

aneurysm: A permanent blood-filled dilation of a blood vessel resulting from disease or injury of the blood vessel wall.

angina pectoris: A spasmodic pain in the chest, characterized by a sensation of severe constriction or pressure on the anterior chest; associated with insufficient blood supply to the heart, aggravated by exercise or tension, and relieved by rest or medication.

Source: Adapted from National Highway Traffic Safety Administration, Emergency Medical Care (Washington, D.C., U.S. Government Printing Office).

angulation: The formation of an angle; an abnormal angle in an extremity or organ.

anoxia: Without oxygen; a reduction of oxygen in body tissues below required physiology levels.

ante-: A prefix meaning *before* in time or place.

anterior: Situated in front of, or in the forward part of; in anatomy, used in reference to the ventral, or belly, surface of the body.

anti-: A prefix that shows a negative or reversal of the word root placed after it.

antibody: A substance produced in the body in response to an antigen that destroys or inactivates the antigen.

antidote: A substance to counteract or combat the effect of poison.

antigen: A substance that causes the formation of antibodies.

antihistamine: A substance capable of counteracting the effects of histamine.

antipyretic: A class of drugs that reduces fever.

antiseptic: Any preparation that prevents the growth of bacteria.

antivenin: An antiserum containing antibodies against reptile or insect venom.

arm: The upper extremity, specifically that segment between the shoulder and hand.

arterial blood: Oxygenated blood.

artery: A blood vessel, consisting of three layers of tissue and smooth muscle, that carries blood away from the heart.

artificial ventilation: Movement of air into and out of the lungs by artifical means.

asphyxia: Suffocation.

aspirate: To inhale foreign material into the lungs; to remove fluid or foreign material from the lungs or elsewhere by mechanical suction.

aspirin: Salicylic acid acetate; a drug known for its analgesic, fever-reducing, and anti-inflammatory properties.

asthma: A condition marked by recurrent attacks of dyspnea with wheezing, due to spasmodic constriction of the bronchi, often as a response to allergens, or to mucous plugs in the bronchioles.

avulsion: An injury that leaves a piece of skin or other tissue either partially or completely torn away from the body.

axilla: The armpit.

axillary temperature: A body temperature measured by placing a thermometer in the axilla while holding the arm close to the body for a period of ten minutes.

B

Babinski reflex: A reflex response of movement of the big toe; positive reflex is determined when, as the sole is stroked, the toe turns upward; negative is determined by a downward movement, or no movement of the toe.

bag of waters: The amniotic sac and the fluid it contains.

ball-and-socket joint: A joint wherein the distal bone has a rounded head (ball) that fits into the proximal bone's cuplike socket; the hip and shoulder joints, for example.

bandage: A material used to hold a dressing in place.

basal skull fracture: A fracture involving the base of the cranium.

basic life support: Maintenance of the ABC's (airway, breathing, and circulation) without adjunctive equipment.

Battle's sign: A contusion on the mastoid area of either ear; sign of a basal skull fracture.

biological death: A condition present when irreversible brain damage has occurred, usually from three to ten minutes after cardiac arrest.

blanch: To become white or pale.

blister: A collection of fluid under or within the epidermis.

blood: The fluid that circulates through the heart, arteries, capillaries, and veins, carrying nutriment and oxygen to the body cells, and removing waste products such as carbon dioxide and various metabolic products for excretion.

blood clot: A soft, coherent, jellylike mass resulting from the conversion of fibrinogen to fibrin, thereby entrapping the red blood cells and other formed elements within the fibrinic web.

bone: The hard form of connective tissue that constitutes most of the skeleton in a majority of vertebrates.

bowel: See *intestine*.

brachial artery: The artery of the arm that is the continuation of the axillary artery, that in turn branches at the elbow into the radial and ulnar arteries. Used to determine an infant's pulse.

brain: A soft, large mass of nerve tissue that is contained within the cranium.

breech birth (breech delivery): The delivery during which the presenting part of the fetus is the buttocks or foot instead of the head.

bronchial asthma: The common form of asthma.

bruise: An injury that does not break the skin but causes rupture of small underlying blood vessels, with resulting tissue discoloration; a contusion.

burn: An injury caused by heat, electrical current, or a chemical of extreme acidity or alkalinity.

> **first-degree burn:** A burn causing only reddening of the outer layer of skin; sunburn is usually a first-degree burn.
>
> **second-degree burn :** A burn extending through the outer layer of skin, causing blisters and edema; a scald is usually a second-degree burn.
>
> **third-degree burn:** A burn extending through all layers of skin, at times through muscle or connective tissue, having a white, leathery look and lacking sensation; grafting is more often necessary with a third-degree burn; a flame burn is usually third-degree.

burn center: A medical facility especially designed, equipped, and staffed to treat severely burned patients.

C

capillary: Any one of the small blood vessels that connect arteriole and venule, and through whose walls various substances pass into and out of the interstitial tissues, and thence on to the cells.

carbon monoxide: CO_2; a colorless, odorless, and dangerous gas formed by incomplete combustion of carbon; it combines four times more quickly with hemoglobin than oxygen; when in the presence of heme, replaces oxygen and reduces oxygen uptake in the lungs.

cardiac arrest: The sudden cessation of cardiac function, with no pulse, no blood pressure, unresponsiveness.

cardiopulmonary arrest: The cessation of cardiac and respiratory activity.

cardiopulmonary resuscitation (CPR): The application of artificial ventilation and external cardiac compression in victims with cardiac arrest to provide an adequate circulation to support life.

carotid artery: The principal artery of the neck, palpated easily on either side of the thyroid cartilage.

carpals: The eight small bones of the wrist.

cartilage: A tough, elastic, connective tissue that covers opposite surfaces of movable joints and also forms parts of the skeleton, such as ear and nose.

caustic: Corrosive, destructive to living tissue.

centigrade scale: The temperature scale in which the freezing point of water is 0° and the boiling point at sea level is 100°; Celsius scale.

cerebral contusion: A bruise of the brain, causing a characteristic symptomatic response.

cerebral hemorrhage: Bleeding into the cerebrum; one form of stroke or cerebrovascular accident.

cerebrospinal fluid: The fluid contained in the four ventricles of the brain and the space around the brain and spinal cord.

cerebrovascular accident (CVA): The sudden cessation of circulation to a region of the brain due to thrombus, embolism, or hemorrhage; also, a stroke or apoplexy.

cervical: Pertaining to the neck.

cervical collar: A device used to immobilize and support the neck.

chief complaint: The problem for which a person seeks help, stated in a word or short phrase.

chills: A sensation of cold, with convulsive shaking of the body.

circulatory system: The body system consisting of the heart and blood vessels.

clammy: Damp and usually cool.

clavicle: The collarbone; attached to the uppermost part of the sternum at a right angle, and joined to the scapular spine to form the point of the shoulder.

clinical death: A term that refers to the lack of signs of life, when there is no pulse and no blood pressure; occurs immediately after the onset of cardiac arrest.

clot: A semisolid mass of fibrin and cells.

closed fracture: A fracture in which there is no laceration in the overlying skin.

closed wound: A wound in which there is no tear or cut in the epidermis.

coffee grounds vomitus: A vomitus having the appearance and consistency of coffee grounds; indicates slow bleeding in the stomach and represents the vomiting of partially digested blood.

coma: A state of unconsciousness from which the victim cannot be aroused even by powerful stimulation.

comminuted fracture: A fracture in which the bone ends are broken into many fragments.

communicable disease: A disease that is transmissible from one person to another.

compound fracture: An open fracture; a fracture in which there is an open wound of the skin and soft tissues leading down to the location of the fracture.

compress: A folded cloth or pad used for applying pressure to stop hemorrhage or as a wet dressing.

concussion: A violent jar or shock which injures the central nervous system.

conscious: Capable of responding to sensory stimuli and having subjective experiences.

consent: An agreement by patients to accept treatment offered as explained by medical personnel and/or first aiders.

> **implied consent:** An assumed consent given by an unconscious adult when emergency lifesaving treatment is required.
>
> **informed consent:** A consent given by a mentally competent adult who understands what the treatment will involve; it can also be given by the parent or guardian of a child, as defined by the state, or for a mentally incompetent adult.

constrict: To be made smaller by drawing together or squeezing.

constricting band: A band used to restrict the lymphatic flow of blood back to the heart.

contagious: A term that refers to a disease that is readily transmitted from one person to another.

contagious disease: An infectious disease transmissible by direct or indirect contact; now synonymous with *communicable disease*.

contaminated: A term used in reference to a wound or other surface that has been infected with bacteria; may also refer to polluted water, food, or drugs.

contusion: A bruise; an injury that causes a hemorrhage in or beneath the skin but does not break the skin.

convulsion: A violent involuntary contraction or series of contractions of the voluntary muscles; a fit or seizure.

core temperature: A body temperature measured centrally, from within the esophagus or rectum.

coronary: A term applied to the cardiac blood vessels that supply blood to the walls of the heart.

coronary artery: One of the two arteries arising from the aortic sinus to supply the heart muscle with blood.

CPR: Abbreviation for cardiopulmonary resuscitation.

cramp: A painful spasm, usually of a muscle; a gripping pain in the abdominal area; colic.

cravat: A type of bandage made from a large triangular piece of cloth and folded to form a band; used as a temporary dressing for a fracture or wound.

crepitus: A grating sound heard and the sensation felt when the fractured ends of a bone rub together.

crowning: The stage of birth when the presenting part of the baby is visible at the vaginal orifice.

CVA: Abbreviation for *cerebrovascular accident.*

cyanosis: A blueness of the skin due to insufficient oxygen in the blood.

D

defibrillation: Applying direct current electrical shock to stop fibrillation of the heart.

dehydration: Loss of water and electrolytes; excessive loss of body water.

depressed fracture: A skull fracture with impaction, depression, or a sinking in of the fragments.

diabetes: A general term referring to disorders characterized by excessive urine excretion, excessive thirst, and excessive hunger.

diabetes mellitus: A systemic disease marked by lack of production of insulin, which causes an inability to metabolize carbohydrates, resulting in an increase in blood sugar.

diabetic coma: Loss of consciousness due to severe diabetes mellitus that has not been treated or to treatment that has not been adequately regulated.

diarrhea: The passage of frequent watery or loose stools.

digestive tract: The passages of tubes leading from the mouth and pharynx to the anus; the alimentary tract; mouth, pharynx, esophagus, stomach, small intestine, large intestine, rectum, and anus.

dilated pupil: A pupil enlarged beyond its normal size.

dilation: The process of expanding or enlarging.

dispatcher: One who transmits calls to service units and vehicles and personnel on assignments.

distal: Farthest from any point on the center or median line; in extemities, farthest from the point of junction of the trunk of the body.

drag: A general term referring to methods of moving victims without a stretcher or litter, usually employed by a single rescuer.

    blanket drag: A method by which one rescuer encloses a victim in a blanket and then drags the victim to safety.

    clothes drag: A method by which one rescuer can drag a victim to safety by grasping the victim's clothes and pulling him away from danger.

    fireman's drag: A method by which one rescuer crawls with a victim, looping the victim's tied wrists over the rescuer's neck to support the victim's weight.

dressing: A protective covering for a wound; used to stop bleeding and to prevent contamination of the wound.

E

-ectomy: Suffix meaning surgical removal, as in *appendectomy.*

edema: A condition in which fluid escapes into the body tissues from the vascular or lymphatic spaces and causes local or generalized swelling.

electrocution: Death caused by passage of electrical current through the body.

embolism: The sudden blocking of an artery or vein by a clot or foreign material that has been brought to the site of lodgement by the blood current.

emesis: Vomiting.

EMS: Emergency Medical Services.

EMT: Emergency Medical Technician.

epidermis: The outermost and nonvascular layer of the skin.

epiglottis: The lidlike cartilaginous structure overhanging the superior entrance to the larynx and serving to prevent food from entering the larynx and trachea while swallowing.

epilepsy: A chronic brain disorder marked by paroxysmal attacks of brain dysfunction, usually associated with some alteration of consciousness, abnormal motor behavior, psychic or sensory disturbances; may be preceded by aura.

epinephrine: A hormone released by the adrenal medulla which stimulates the sympathetic nervous system, producing vasoconstriction, increased heart rate and bronchodilation.

epistaxis: Nosebleed.

esophagus: The portion of the digestive tract that lies between the pharynx and the stomach.

exhalation: The act of breathing out; expiration.

extremity: A limb, an arm, or a leg.

extrication: Disentanglement; freeing from entrapment.

F

Fahrenheit scale: The temperature scale in which the freezing point is 32° and the boiling point at sea level is 212°.

fainting: A momentary loss of consciousness caused by insufficient blood supply to the brain; syncope.

feces: The product expelled by the bowels; semisoft waste products of digestion.

femoral artery: The principal artery of the thigh, a continuation of the iliac artery; supplies blood to the lower abdomen wall, the external genitalia, and the lower body extremities; pulse may be palpated in the groin area.

femur: The bone that extends from the pelvis to the knee; the longest and largest bone of the body; the thigh bone.

fever: An elevation of body temperature beyond normal.

fibrillation: Ineffective contractions of the heart muscles.

fibula: The smaller of the two bones of the lower leg; the most lateral bone of the lower leg.

first-degree burn: A burn causing only reddening of the outer layer of skin; sunburn usually is a first-degree burn.

first responder: A person who has been trained to provide emergency care before the EMTs arrive; usually police or fire fighters.

flail chest: A condition in which several ribs are broken, each in at least two places, or a sternal fracture or separation of the ribs from the sternum producing a free floating segment of the chest wall that moves paradoxically on respiration.

forearm: The part of the upper extremity between the elbow and the wrist.

fracture: A break or rupture in a bone.

> **closed fracture:** A simple fracture, one that does not cause a break in the skin.
>
> **comminuted fracture:** A fracture in which the bone is shattered.
>
> **compound fracture:** An open fracture, one in which the bone ends pierce the skin.
>
> **greenstick fracture:** An incomplete fracture (the bone is not broken all the way through); seen most often in children
>
> **impacted fracture:** A fracture in which the ends of the bones are jammed together.
>
> **oblique fracture:** A fracture in which the break crosses the bone at an angle.
>
> **open fracture:** A compound fracture, one in which the skin is open.
>
> **simple fracture:** A closed fracture, one in which the skin is not broken.
>
> **spiral fracture:** A fracture in which the breakline twists around and through the bone.
>
> **transverse fracture:** A fracture in which the breakline extends across the bone at a right angle to the long axis.

fracture of the hip: A fracture that occurs at the upper end of the femur, most often at the neck of the femur.

frostnip: The superficial local tissue destruction caused by freezing; it is limited in scope and does not destroy the full thickness of skin

frostbite: The damage to tissues as a result of prolonged exposure to extreme cold.

G

gangrene: Local tissue death as the result of an injury or inadequate blood supply.

gastrointestinal tract: The digestive tract, including stomach, small intestine, large intestine, rectum, and anus.

grand mal: A type of epileptic attack; characterized by a short-term, generalized, convulsive seizure.

gullet: Esophagus; the passage from the pharynx to the stomach.

H

half-ring splint: A traction splint with a hinged half-ring at the upper end that allows the splint to be used on either the right or left leg.

heart: A hollow muscular organ that receives the blood from the veins, sends it through the lungs to be oxygenated, then pumps it to the arteries.

heart attack: A layman's term for a condition resulting from blockage of a coronary artery and subsequent death of part of the heart muscle; an acute myocardial infarction; a coronary.

heat cramps: A painful muscle cramp resulting from excessive loss of salt and water through sweating.

heat exhaustion: A prostration caused by excessive loss of water and salt through sweating; characterized by clammy skin and a weak, rapid pulse.

hematoma: A localized collection of blood in an organ, tissue, or space as a result of injury or a broken blood vessel.

heme: The deep red, iron-containing group of hemoglobin.

hemiplegia: Paralysis of one side of the body.

hemoglobin: The oxygen-carrying substance of the red blood cells; when it has absorbed oxygen in the lungs, it is bright red and called *oxyhemoglobin;* after it has given up its oxygen to the tissues, it is purple in color and is called *caroxyhemoglobin.*

hemophilia: An inherited blood disease occurring mostly in males, characterized by the inability of the blood to clot.

hemorrhage: Abnormally large amount of bleeding.

hemorrhagic shock: A state of inadequate tissue perfusion due to blood loss.

hemothorax: Bleeding into the thoracic cavity.

hives: Red or white raised patches on the skin, often attended by severe itching; a characteristic reaction in allergic responses.

humerus: The bone of the upper arm.

hyper-: Prefix meaning excessive, or increased.

hyperglycemia: An abnormally increased concentration of sugar in the blood.

hypertension: High blood pressure, usually in reference to a diastolic pressure greater than 90–95 mm Hg.

hyperthermia: An abnormally increased body temperature.

hyperventilation: An increased rate and depth of breathing resulting in an abnormal lowering of arterial carbon dioxide, causing alkalosis.

hyphema: Hemorrhage within the anterior chamber of the eye.

hypo-: A prefix meaning less than, lack of; a deficiency.

hypoglycemia: An abnormally diminished concentration of sugar in the blood; insulin shock.

hypothermia: Decreased body temperature.

hypovolemic shock: Shock caused by a reduction in blood volume, such as caused by hemorrage.

hypoxia: A low oxygen content in the blood; lack of oxygen in inspired air.

I

immobilization: To hold a part firmly in place, as with a splint.

impaled object: An object that has caused a puncture wound and remains embedded in the wound.

incision: A wound usually made deliberately in connection with surgery; a clean cut as opposed to a laceration.

infarction: The death (*necrosis*) of a localized area of tissue by cutting off its blood supply.

infection: An invasion of a body by disease-producing organisms.

inferior: Anatomically, situated below, or the lower surface or part of a structure.

inflammation: A tissue reaction to disease, irritation, or infection; characterized by pain, heat, redness, and swelling.

ingestion: Intake of food or other substances through the mouth.

inhalation: The drawing of air or other substances into the lungs.

insulin: A hormone secreted in the pancreas; essential for the proper metabolism of blood sugar.

insulin shock: Not a true form of shock; hypoglycemia caused by excessive insulin dosage, characterized by sweating, tremor, anxiety, unusual behavior, and vertigo; may cause death of brain cells.

intestine: The portion of the alimentary canal extending from the stomach to the anus.

intoxicate: To poison; commonly, to cause diminished control by means of drugs or alcohol.

ipecac syrup: A medication used to induce vomiting.

-itis: A suffix meaning inflammation

J

jaw-thrust maneuver: A procedure for opening the airway, wherein the jaw is lifted and pulled forward to keep the tongue from falling back into the airway.

joint: The point at which two or more bones articulate; commonly, marijuana cigarette.

jugular: Pertaining to the neck; large vein on either side of the neck, draining the head via its portion named *external jugular,* or draining the brain via the internal jugular.

K

kidneys: The paired organs that filter blood and produce urine; they also act as adjuncts to keep a proper acid-base balance.

knee: A hinge joint between the femur and the tibia.

L

labor: The process or period of childbirth; especially, the muscular contractions of the uterus designed to expel the fetus from the mother.

laceration: A wound made by tearing or cutting of body tissues.

ladder splint: A flexible splint consisting of two stout parallel wires and finer crosswires; resembles a ladder.

laryngospasm: A severe constriction of the vocal cords, often in response to allergy or noxious stimuli.

larynx: The organ of voice production.

lateral: Of or toward the side; away from the midline of the body.

leg: The lower limb generally, specifically, that part of the lower limb extending from the knee to the ankle.

lesion: A distinct area of pathologically altered tissue; an injury or wound.

lethal: Fatal.

lethargy: A lack of activity; drowsiness; indifference.

ligament: A tough band of fibrous tissue that connects bone to bone or that supports any organ.

limb presentation: A delivery in which the presenting part of a fetus is an arm or a leg.

linear fracture: A fracture running parallel to the long axis of the bone.

linear skull fracture: A skull fracture that runs in a straight line.

litter: Stretcher.

liver: The large organ in the right upper quadrant of the abdomen that secretes bile, produces many essential proteins, detoxifies many substances, and stores glycogen..

log roll: A method for placing a person on a carrying device, usually a long spineboard or a flat litter; the person is rolled on his or her side, then back on the litter.

lungs: The paired organs in the thorax that effect ventilation and oxygenation.

lymph: A straw-colored fluid that circulates in the lymphatic vessels and interstitial space.

M

mastoid: A portion of the temporal bone that lies behind the ear and contains spongy bone tissue.

medial: Toward the midline of the body.

metacarpal bones: The five cylindrical bones of the hand extending from the wrist to the fingers.

metatarsal bones: The five cylindrical bones of the foot extending from the ankles to the toes.

morbidity: A synonym for illness; generally used to refer to an untoward effect of an illness or injury.

mortality: Refers to death from a given disease or injury; generally thought of as a statistic to state the ratio of death to recovery.

motion sickness: A sensation induced by repetitive motion, characterized by nausea and lightheadedness.

mottled: Characterized by a patchy, discolored appearance.

mouth-to-mouth ventilation: The preferred emergency method of artificial ventilation when adjuncts are not available.

mouth-to-nose ventilation: An emergency method of artificial ventilation when mouth-to-mouth cannot be used.

mucus: A viscid, slippery secretion that lubricates and protects various body structures.

muscle: A tissue composed of elongated cells that have the ability to contract when stimulated, thus causing bone and joints to move, or other anatomical structures to be drawn together.

myocardial infarction: The damaging or death of an area of the heart muscle resulting from a lack of blood supplying the area; a heart attack.

N

nausea: An unpleasant sensation, vaguely referred to the epigastrium and abdomen, often culminating in vomiting.

necrosis: A death of an area of tissue, usually caused by the cessation of blood supply.

nerve: A cordlike structure composed of a collection of fibers that convey impulses between a part of the central nervous system and some other region.

nervous system: The brain, spinal cord, and nerve branches from the central, peripheral, and autonomic systems.

nitroglycerin: A drug used in the treatment of angina pectoris.

noxious: Injurious.

O

oblique fracture: A fracture that runs diagonally to the long axis of the bone.

occipital: Pertaining to the back of the head.

ointment: A semisolid preparation for external application to the body, usually containing a medicinal substance.

open fracture or dislocation: A fracture or dislocation exposed to the exterior; an open wound lies over the fracture or dislocation.

open wound: A wound in which the affected tissues are exposed by an external opening.

oral: Pertaining to the mouth.

-otomy: A suffix meaning surgical incision into an organ, as in *tracheotomy*.

oxygen: A colorless, odorless, tasteless gas that is essential to life and comprises 21 percent of the atmosphere; chemical formula: O_2.

P

pallor: A paleness of the skin.

palpation: The act of palpating; the act of feeling with the hands for the purpose of determining the consistency of the part beneath.

palpitation: A sensation felt under the left breast when the heart "skips a beat" because of premature ventricular contractions.

paralysis: Loss or impairment of motor function of a part due to a lesion of the neural or muscular mechanism.

paraplegia: The loss of both sensation and motion in the lower extremities; most commonly due to damage to the spinal cord.

patella: A small, flat bone that protects the knee joint; the kneecap.

pediatrics: The medical specialty devoted to the diagnosis and treatment of diseases of children.

penetrate: To pierce; to pass into the deeper tissues or into a cavity.

perfusion: The act of pouring through or into; the blood suffusing the cells in order to exchange gases, nutrients, etc., with the cells.

petit mal seizure: A type of epileptic attack, characterized by a momentary loss of awareness but not accompanied by loss of motor tone.

pharynx: The portion of the airway between the nasal cavity and the larynx.

placenta: A vascular organ attached to the uterine wall that supplies oxygen and nutrients to the fetus; also called *afterbirth*.

pneumothorax: An accumulation of air in the pleural cavity, usually entering after a wound or injury that causes a penetration of the chest wall or laceration of the lung.

point tenderness: An area of tenderness limited to two or three centimeters in diameter; point tenderness can be located in any area of the body; usually associated with acute inflammation, as in peritonitis (abdominal point tenderness).

posterior: Situated in the back of or behind a surface.

presenting part: The part of the baby that emerges first during delivery.

pressure dressing: A dressing with which enough pressure is applied over a wound site to stop bleeding.

pressure point: One of several places on the body where the blood flow of a given artery can be restricted by pressing the artery against an underlying bone.

pressure splints: An inflatable plastic circumferential splint that can be applied to an extremity and inflated to achieve stability after a fracture.

prognosis: A probable outcome of a disease based on assumptive knowledge.

prolapsed cord delivery: A delivery in which the umbilical cord appears at the vaginal opening before the head of the infant.

prone: A position of lying face down.

psychogenic shock: A fainting spell resulting from transient generalized cerebral ischemia; not a true shock condition.

psychosomatic: An indication of an illness in which some part of the cause is related to emotional factors.

pulse rate: The heart rate determined by counting the number of pulsations occurring in any superficial artery.

pump failure: A partial or total failure of the heart to pump blood effectively.

pupil: The small opening in the center of the iris.

Q

quadrant: One of the four quarters of the abdomen.

quadriplegia: A paralysis of both arms and legs.

R

radial artery: One of the major arteries of the forearm; the pulse is palpable at the base of the thumb.

radiation sickness: The condition that follows excessive irradiation from any source.

radius: The bone on the thumb side of the forearm.

rape: Sexual intercourse by force.

rash: An eruption of the skin, either localized or generalized.

rectal temperature: The core body temperature obtained by inserting a thermometer into the rectum and retaining it for a minute; normally 1°F higher than oral temperature.

regurgitation: A backward flowing, as the casting up of undigested food from the stomach to the mouth.

respiration: The act of breathing; the exchange of oxygen and carbon dioxide in the tissues and lungs.

respiratory arrest: The cessation of breathing.

respiratory system: A system of organs that controls the inspiration of oxygen and the expiration of carbon dioxide.

resuscitation: The act of reviving an unconscious victim.

rib: One of the 24 bones forming the thoracic cavity wall.

rigid splint: A splint made of a firm material that can be applied to an injured extremity to prevent motion at the site of a fracture or dislocation.

roller dressing: A strip of rolled-up material used for dressings.

S

saliva: The clear, alkaline fluid secreted by the salivary glands.

scab: A crust formed by the coagulation of blood, pus, serum, or any combination of these on the surface of an ulcer, erosion, abrasion, or any other type of wound.

scapula: The shoulder blade.

sclera: The white, opaque, outer layer of the eyeball.

second-degree burn: A burn penetrating beneath the superficial skin layers, producing edema and blisters.

seizure: A sudden attack or recurrence of a disease; a convulsion; an attack of epilepsy.

semiconscious: Stuporous; partially conscious.

shell temperature: The temperature of the extremities and surface of the body.

shivering: A trembling from cold or fear; it produces heat by muscular contractions.

shock: A state of inadequate tissue perfusion that may be a result of pump failure (cariogenic shock), volume loss or sequestration (hypovolemic shock), vasodilation (neurogenic shock), or any combination of these.

>   **anaphylactic shock:** A rapidly occurring state of collapse caused by hypersensitivity to drugs or other foreign materials (insect venom, certain foods, inhaled allergens); symptoms may include hives, wheezing, tissue edema, bronchospasm, and vascular collapse.

>   **septic shock:** A shock developing in the presence of, and as a result of, severe infection.

sign: Any objective evidence of physical manifestation of a disease.

simple fracture: A fracture that is not compound; the skin is not broken over the break in the bone.

skeleton: The hard, bony structure that forms the main support of the body.

skin: the outer integument or covering of the body, consisting of the dermis and the epidermis; the largest organ of the body; it contains various sensory and regulatory mechanisms.

skull: The bony structure surrounding the brain; it consists of the cranial bones, the facial bones, and the teeth.

sling: A triangular bandage applied around the neck to support an injured upper extremity; any material long enough to suspend an upper extremity by passing the material around the neck; used to support and protect an injury or the arm, shoulder, or clavicle.

sling and swathe: A bandage in which the arm is placed in a sling and is bound to the body by another bandage placed around the chest and arm to hold the arm close to the body.

small intestine: The portion of the intestine between the stomach and colon.

snowblindness: Obscured vision caused by sunlight reflected off snow.

spasm: A sudden, violent, involuntary contraction of a muscle, or group of muscles, attended by pain and interference with function; a sudden but transitory constriction of a passage, canal, or orifice.

spineboard: A wooden or metal device primarily used for extrication and transportation of victims with actual or suspected spinal injuries.

spiral fracture: A fracture in which the line of break runs diagonally around the long axis of the bone.

spleen: The largest lymphatic organ of the body; located in the left upper quadrant of the abdomen.

splint: Any support used to immobilize a fracture or to restrict movement of a part.

sprain: A trauma to a joint that injures the ligaments.

sputum: Expectorated matter, especially mucus or matter resulting from diseases of the air passages.

status asthmaticus: A severe, prolonged asthmatic attack that cannot be broken with epinephrine.

status epilepticus: The occurrence of two or more seizures with a period of complete consciousness between them.

sterile: Free from living organisms, such as bacteria.

sterilize: to render sterile or free from bacterial contamination; to make an organism unable to reproduce.

sternum: The long, flat bone located in the midline in the anterior part of the thoracic cage; articulates above with the clavicles and along the sides with the cartilages of the first seven ribs.

stomach: A hollow digestive organ in the epigastrium that receives food from the esophagus.

stool: Feces; the matter discharged at defecation.

stove-in chest: See *flail chest.*

strain: An injury to a muscle caused by a violent contraction or an excessive, forcible stretching.

stretcher: A carrying device that enables two or more persons to lift and carry a patient who is lying down.

stroke: A cerebrovascular accident of sudden onset.

sublingual: Under the tongue.

sucking chest wound: An open pneumothorax.

suffocate: to impede breathing, to asphyxiate.

suicide: The act of deliberately taking one's own life.

sunstroke: A form of heatstroke due to prolonged sun exposure.

superior: In anatomy, used to refer to an organ or part that is located above another organ or part.

supine: Lying in a face-upward position.

suture: The material used to close a surgical wound or to repair a gaping wound.

swathe: A cravat tied around the body to decrease movement of a part.

symptom: A subjective sensation or awareness of disturbance of bodily function.

syncope: Fainting; a brief period of unconsciousness.

syndrome: A complex of symptoms and signs characteristic of condition.

synovial fluid: A clear fluid that lubricates joints; it is secreted by the synovial membrane.

T

tachycardia: Abnormally rapid heart rate, over 100 beats per minute.

tarsal: Pertaining to the tarsus, the ankle.

temperature: The degree of heat of a living body; varies in cold-blooded animals with environmental temperature and is constant, within a narrow range, for warm-blooded animals; 98.6°F oral temperature and 99.6°F rectal are considered normal for humans.

tendon: a tough band of dense, fibrous, connective tissue that attaches muscles to bone and other parts.

tetanus: An infectious disease caused by bacteria, *Clostridium tetani,* that is usually introduced through a wound, characterized by extreme body rigidity and spasms of voluntary body muscles.

thermal: Pertaining to heat.

thigh: The portion of the lower extremity between the hip and knee.

third-degree burn: A full-thickness burn destroying all skin layers and underlying tissue; has a charred or white, leathery appearance; insensitive.

thoracic: Pertaining to the chest.

thrombosis: Formation of a blood clot, or *thrombus.*

tibia: The larger of the two bones in the leg; the shin bone.

tissue: An aggregation of similarly specialized cells and their intercellular substance, united in the performance of a particular function.

tourniquet: A constrictive device used on the extremities to impede venous blood return to the heart or obstruct arterial blood flow to the extremities.

toxin: Any poison manufactured by plant or animal life.

trachea: The cartilaginous tube extending from the larynx to its division into the primary bronchi; windpipe.

traction: The act of exerting a pulling force.

triage: A system used for sorting victims to determine the order in which they will receive medical attention.

triangular bandage: A piece of cloth cut in the shape of a right-angled triangle; used as a sling or folded for a cravat bandage.

trunk: The body, excluding the head and limbs; torso.

U

ulcer: An open lesion of the skin or mucous membrane.

ulna: The larger bone of the forearm, on the side opposite that of the thumb.

umbilical cord: A flexible structure connecting the fetus to the placenta.

umbilicus: The navel.

unconscious: Without awareness; the state of being comatose.

universal access number: A telephone number that can be called in emergency situations of all kinds, which ties in with the police, fire, and emergency medical services; in most areas the number is 9-1-1.

universal dressing: A large (9 × 36″) dressing of multilayered material that can be used open, folded, or rolled to cover most wounds, to pad splints, or to form a cervical collar.

uterus: The muscular organ that holds and nourishes the fetus, opening into the vagina through the cervix; the womb.

V

vagina: The canal in the female extending from the uterus to the vulva; the birth canal.

vasoconstriction: The narrowing of the diameter of a blood vessel.

vein: Any blood vessel that carries blood from the tissues to the heart.

venom: A poison, usually derived from reptiles or insects.

venous blood: Unoxygenated blood, containing hemoglobin in the carboxyhemoglobin state.

ventilation: Breathing; supplying fresh air to the lungs.

ventricular fibrillation: A rapid, tremulous, and ineffectual contraction of the cardia myofibrils, producing no cardiac output; cardiac arrest.

vertebra: Any one of the 33 bones of the spinal column.

vertigo: A dizziness; a hallucination of movement; a sensation that the external world is spinning; it may be right or left, upward or downward.

vital signs: The indication of life through values that reflect mental status, blood pressure, pulse rate, and respiration rate.

vitreous fluid: A jellylike, transparent substance filling the inside of the eyeball.

voice box: The larynx.

vomiting: A forceful, active expulsion of stomach contents through the mouth, as opposed to regurgitation, which is passive.

vomitus: The matter ejected from the stomach by vomiting.

W

wheal: A swelling on the skin, produced by a sting, an injection, external force, or internal reaction.

wheeze: A high-pitched, whistling sound characterizing an obstruction or spasm of the lower airways.

wind-chill factor: The relationship of wind velocity and temperature in determining the effect of the factor on a living organism.

windpipe: The trachea.

womb: The uterus.

wrist: The joint or the region of the joint between the forearm and the hand.

X

xiphoid process: A sword-shaped cartilaginous process at the lowest portion of the sternum that ossifies in the aged and has no ribs attached to it.

Quick Emergency Index